Spine Surgery and Peripheral Nerve Surgery

Khaled Fares AlAli • Hashim Talib Hashim

Spine Surgery and Peripheral Nerve Surgery

Springer

Khaled Fares AlAli
Department of Neurosurgery
Zayed Military Hospital
Abu Dhabi, Abu Dhabi
United Arab Emirates

Hashim Talib Hashim
Vascular Surgery Department
Oregon Health and Science University
Portland, OR, USA

Research Department
University of Warith Al-Anbiyaa, College of Medicine
Karbala, Iraq

Emergency Department
Qal'at Sukkar General Hospital
Qal'at Sukkar, Thi Qar, Iraq

ISBN 978-3-031-98542-3 ISBN 978-3-031-98543-0 (eBook)
https://doi.org/10.1007/978-3-031-98543-0

This Springer imprint is published by the registered company Springer Nature Switzerland AG
The registered company address is: Gewerbestrasse 11, 6330 Cham, Switzerland

May this book carry the warmth of my heart,
As every word is a reflection of you.
Holding your light in every chapter,
Always and forever, everything I do is
for you.

Khaled Fares AlAli

Introduction

Having practiced spine and peripheral nerve surgery in both peaceful settings and conflict zones for over ten years, we have seen the changing difficulties neurosurgeons and spine experts deal with on a daily basis. From treating complex spinal deformities to doing delicate peripheral nerve repairs, our path has molded our approach to both surgical methods and clinical judgment.

Designed as a thorough study of multiple-choice questions (MCQs), this book provides a disciplined yet interesting approach to reinforce important surgical ideas. What makes this book unique?

- Uniquely Illustrated: The author provides detailed medical illustrations to enhance understanding.
- Highly Referenced: Reliable sources support answers, therefore guaranteeing correctness and depth.
- Complete Coverage: From principles to advanced techniques, the material covers all facets of spine and peripheral nerve surgery.
- Balanced Question Difficulty: Readers are ready for both tests and clinical practice by means of questions ranging from fundamental ideas to demanding real-world situations.
- Detailed Explanations: Each answer is carefully explained, reinforcing key surgical and anatomical insights.

This book is a great tool for learning and revision regardless of your level of experience, resident, fellow, or senior surgeon. In the always-changing disciplines of spine and peripheral nerve surgery, our aim is to provide a useful, high-yield resource bridging the gap between theory and real surgical experience.

Contents

Part I

Spine Surgery

Spine Anatomy

1

1. Identify the structures (1–10) in the following image (Fig. 1.1):
   Correct Answer: 1. Anterior tuberculum. 2. Anterior arch. 3. Odontoid process of C2. 4. Transverse foramen. 5. Spinal canal. 6. Posterior tuberculum. 7. Lateral mass. 8. Superior articular surface. 9. Transverse ligament. 10. Posterior arch
2. Identify the structures (1–13) in the following image (Fig. 1.2):
   Correct Answer: C2 vertebra: 1. Odontoid process. 2. Body. 3. Superior articular surface. 4. Superior articular facet. 5. Pars articularis. 6. Pedicle. 7. Inferior articualr surface. 8. inferior articular facet. 9. Spinous process. 10. Lamina. 11. Transverse foramen. 12. Transverse process. 13. Spinal canal

Fig. 1.1 C1 superior view

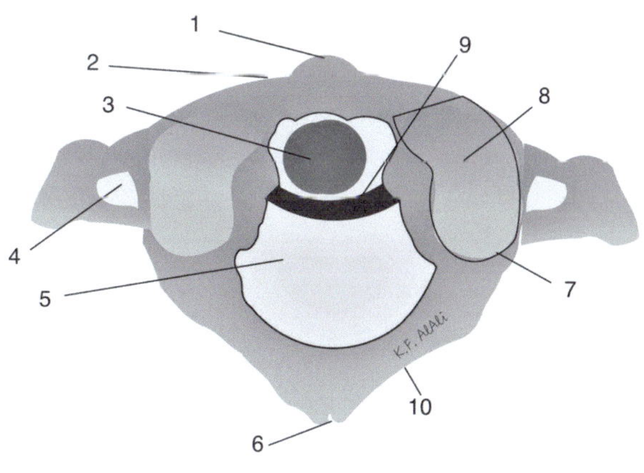

K. F. AlAli, H. T. Hashim, *Spine Surgery and Peripheral Nerve Surgery*,
https://doi.org/10.1007/978-3-031-98543-0_1

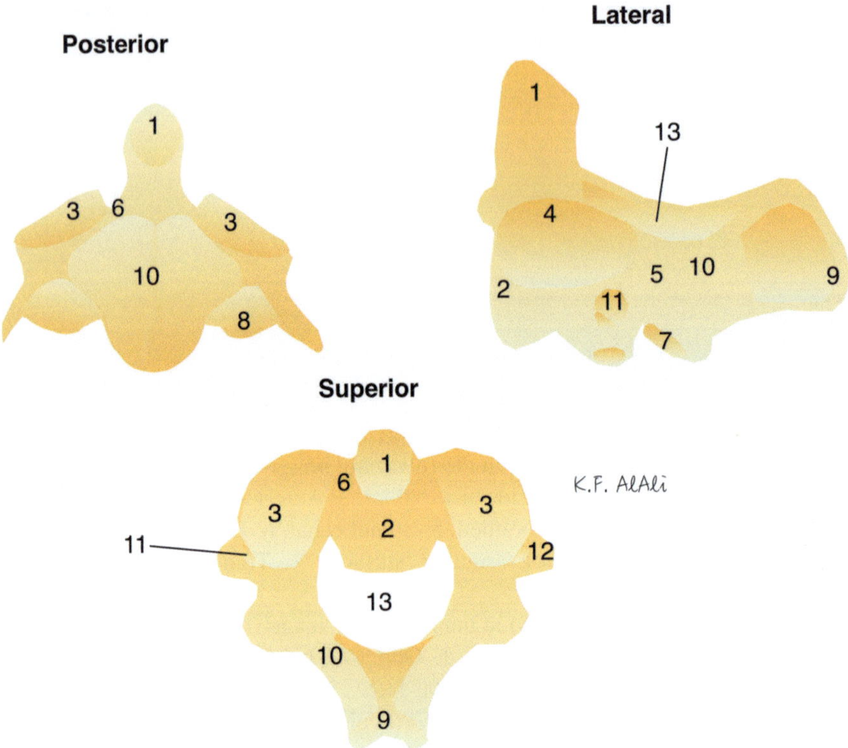

Fig. 1.2 C2 vertebra views

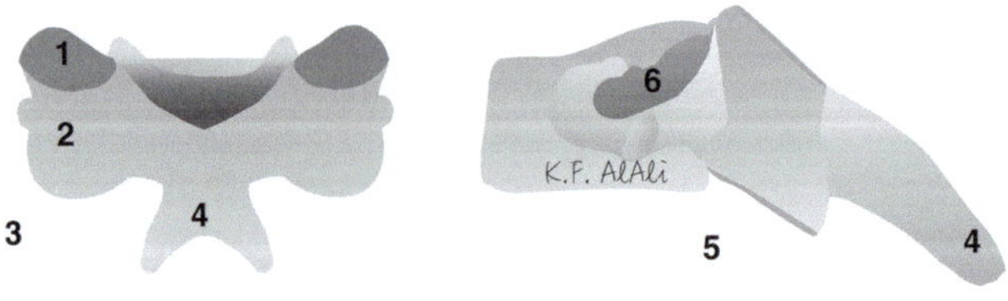

Fig. 1.3 Subaxial cervical vertebra

3. Which vertebral level is this, and identify the structures (1–6) in the following image (Fig. 1.3):

   Correct Answers: These are illustrations of the subaxial cervical spine, posterior, and lateral views. 1. Superior articular surface. 2. Lateral mass. 3. Lamina. 4. Spinous process. 5. Inferior articular surface. 6. Transverse foramen

4. Which vertebral level is this, and identify the structures (1–7) in the following image (Fig. 1.4):

   Correct Answers: This is a lateral view of a typical thoracic vertebra. 1. Vertebral body. 2. Superior costal surface. 3. Inferior costal surface. 4. Superior articular surface. 5. Transverse costal surface. 6. Spinous process. 7. Inferior articular surface
5. Which vertebral level is this, and identify the structures (1–5) in the following image (Fig. 1.5):

   Correct Answers: This is a lumbar vertebra (posterior and axial views). 1. Superior articular surface. 2. Pars articularis. 3. Spinous process. 4. Transverse process. 5. Spinal canal
6. Identify the structures (1–6) in the following image (Fig. 1.6):

   Correct Answers: 1. Anterior longitudinal ligament. 2. Posterior longitudinal ligament. 3. Intervertebral disc.4. Flavum ligament. 5. Interspinal ligament. 6. Nuchal ligament. 6. Facet capsule.

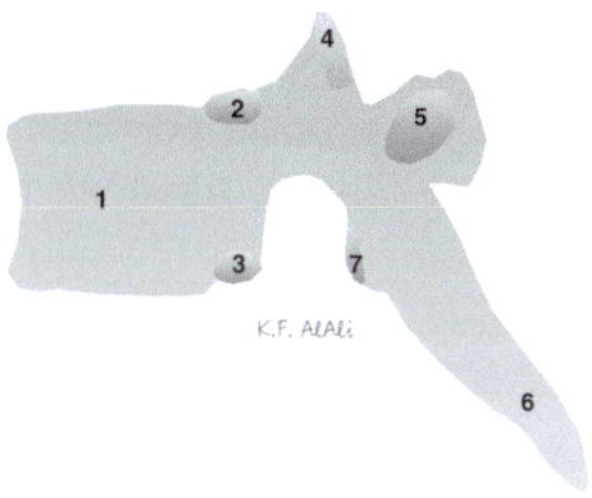

Fig. 1.4 Thoracic spine - lateral view

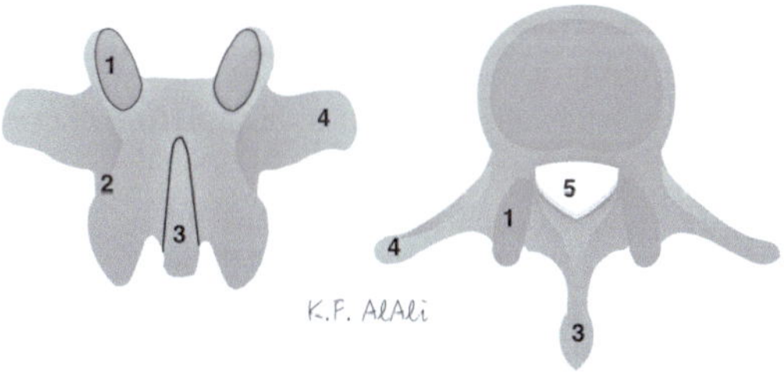

Fig. 1.5 Lumbar spine

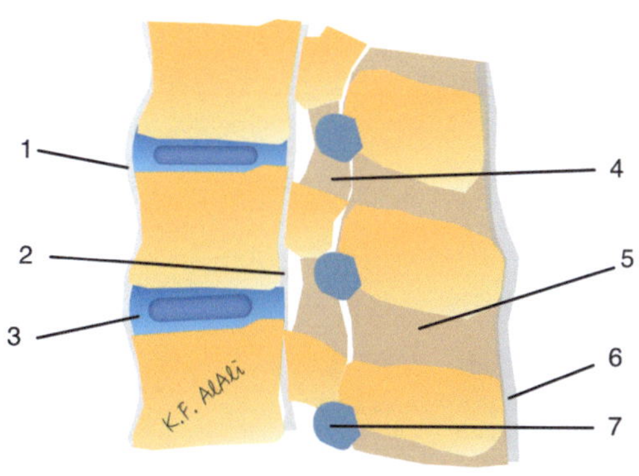

Fig. 1.6 Cervical spinal ligaments - lateral view

7. Identify the structures (1–5) and (A–G) in the following image (Fig. 1.7):

   Correct Answers:

   This shows cross cross-section of a spinal cord. Ascending tracts: 1. Fasciculus gracilis (medial) and cuneatus (lateral). 2. Dorsal spinocerebellar tract. 3. Ventral spinocerebellar tract. 4. Lateral spinothalamic tract. 5. Ventral spinothalamic tract.

   Descending tracts: A. Lateral corticospinal tract. B. Lateral reticuospinal tract. C. Rubrospinal tract. D. Vestibulospinal tract. E. Medial reticuospinal tract. F. Ventral corticospinal tract. G. Tectospinal tract.

8. All of the following are features of the C7 vertebra, EXCEPT:
   A. Non-bifid spinous process
   B. Small transverse foramen
   C. Large lateral recess
   D. Bigger pedicle

   Correct Answer: C.

   Explanation:

   Cervical vertebra 7 is an atypical vertebra with C1 and C2. It has distinctive features: non-bifid spinous process, small transverse foramen, **small lateral recess,** and bigger pedicle (Fig. 1.8).

9. A surgeon is performing a spinal fusion procedure and is concerned about maintaining adequate blood supply to the mid-thoracic spinal cord (T3–T9). Which of the following arteries is primarily responsible for supplying this region, and why is it important to avoid compromising it?
   A. The artery of Adamkiewicz, as it directly supplies the anterior spinal artery in the mid-thoracic spine
   B. Segmental spinal arteries branching from the posterior intercostal arteries, as they feed the segmental medullary arteries that support the mid-thoracic ASA
   C. Vertebral arteries branching from the subclavian arteries, providing direct support to the ASA at T3–T9
   D. Radiculomedullary arteries from the cervicothoracic trunk, as they supply the ASA along the entire thoracic region

   Correct Answer: B

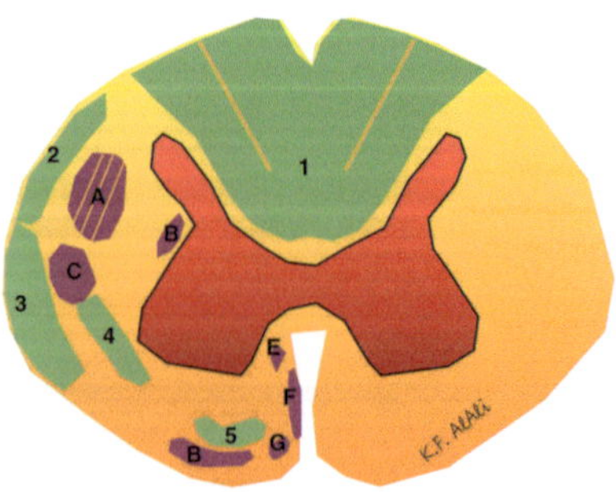

Fig. 1.7 Cervical spinal cord - cross section

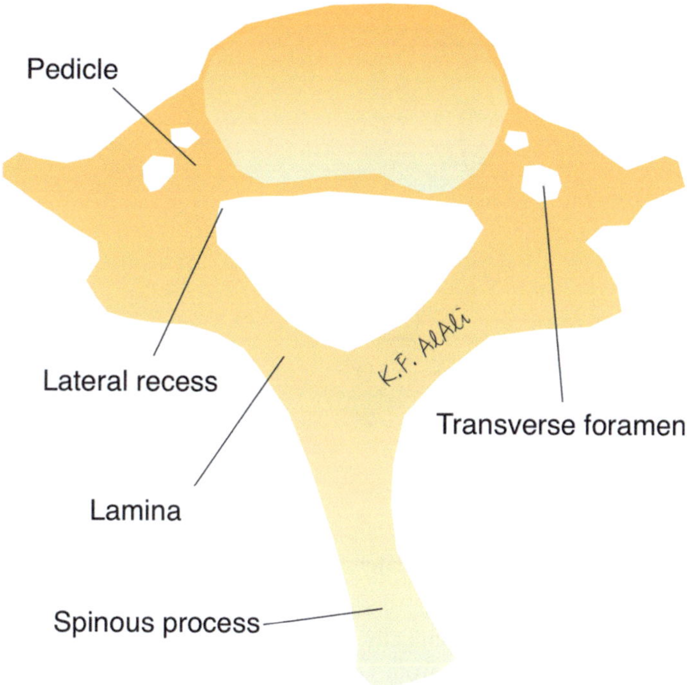

Fig. 1.8 C7 vertebra

Explanation:

The mid-thoracic spinal cord (T3–T9) is supplied by segmental spinal arteries branching from the posterior intercostal arteries, which in turn feed into the anterior spinal artery (ASA) via segmental medullary arteries. This area is particularly vulnerable due to its reliance on segmental blood supply, making preservation of these arteries critical for preventing ischemia and maintaining function (Fig. 1.9).

(RS, p. 44)

10. A 45-year-old patient undergoing thoracoabdominal surgery suffers an intraoperative injury that disrupts the artery of Adamkiewicz. Which of the following consequences is most likely if the injury is not immediately addressed?
    A. Ischemia of the lower cervical spinal cord
    B. Ischemia of the anterior thoracolumbar spinal cord, potentially leading to paraplegia
    C. Decreased blood flow to the posterior two-thirds of the thoracic spinal cord
    D. Reduced venous drainage in the lumbosacral region, causing swelling in the Batson plexus

    Correct Answer: B

    Explanation:

    The artery of Adamkiewicz, also known as the great radicular artery, is the primary vessel supplying blood to the lower two-thirds of the spinal cord via the

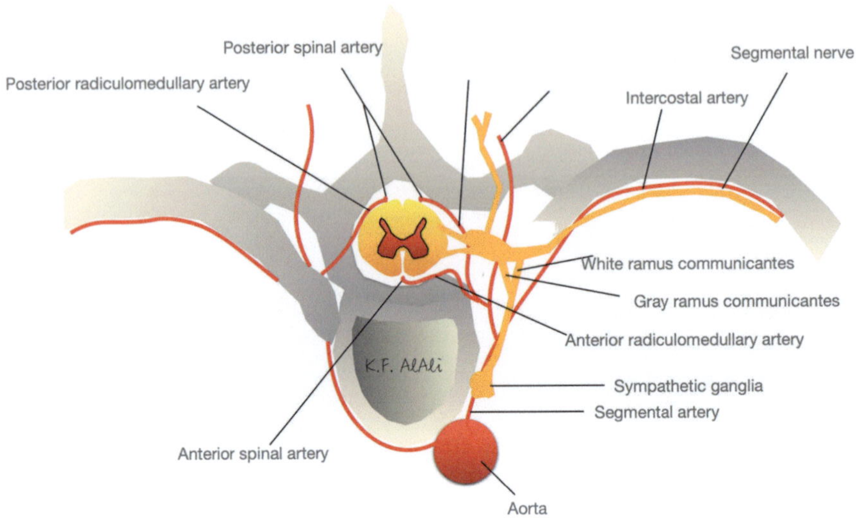

Fig. 1.9 Cross-section of thoracic spinal level showing vascular anatomy of the spinal cord

anterior spinal artery. Anatomically, it typically originates between T9 and T12, although its origin can vary from T8 to L3, and it most often arises from a left-sided intercostal or lumbar artery. Functionally, this artery plays a crucial role in maintaining spinal cord viability, particularly in the thoracolumbar region, where it supplies the anterior two-thirds of the thoracolumbar spinal cord, including the ventral horns that house motor neurons essential for lower limb movement.

Clinically, the artery of Adamkiewicz is of significant importance in spinal and aortic surgeries. Damage or interruption to this artery during procedures, such as thoracoabdominal aortic surgeries, can lead to spinal cord ischemia and result in irreversible outcomes like paraplegia. For this reason, it is often mapped preoperatively using MRI or angiography to avoid inadvertent injury.

(RS, p. 44)

11. The origin of the segmental arteries supplying the L5 vertebra is variable. Which of the following is NOT a potential source?
    A. Iliolumbar artery
    B. Middle sacral artery
    C. Middle sacral artery
    D. Renal artery
    Correct Answer: D
    (SS, p. 42)
12. What is the primary function of Batson's plexus in the lumbar spine?
    A. It provides a pathway for arterial blood to the spinal canal.
    B. It acts as an alternate venous drainage route to the inferior vena cava.
    C. It supplies blood to the paraspinous muscles.
    D. It controls blood flow to the lumbar vertebrae during increased abdominal pressure.

Correct Answer: B

Explanation:

Batson's plexus is a network of valveless veins situated within the spinal canal and around the vertebral body, serving as an alternative venous drainage route to the inferior vena cava. Due to the absence of valves, increases in abdominal pressure, such as those occurring during spine surgery positioning, can redirect blood flow toward the spinal canal and adjacent bony structures. Additionally, Batson's plexus acts as a pathway for the spread of metastatic tumors and infections to the lumbar spine.

(SS, p. 42)

13. What is the clinical significance of the iliolumbar vein during anterior lumbar spine surgery?
   A. It supplies the abdominal wall with blood.
   B. It limits the mobilization of the iliac vessels, requiring careful isolation and ligation.
   C. It supplies blood to the spinal canal and its contents.
   D. It connects directly with Batson's plexus to prevent venous congestion.

   Correct Answer: B

   Explanation:

   The iliolumbar vein, a branch of the iliac vein, restricts the mobilization of the iliac vessels from the anterior spine. To access the anterior aspect of the spine at the L4–L5 disc level, this vein must be carefully isolated and securely ligated before moving the vascular structures.

   (SS, p. 42)

14. The least rotation in the spine is seen at:
   A. Atlanto-occipital joint
   B. C1–C2
   C. C3–C6
   D. C6–C7

   Correct Answer: A

   Explanation:

   The principal movement at the atlantooccipital joint is flexion-extension. There is limited lateral flexion (abduction/adduction) and almost no rotation of the head.

   (SS. p16)

15. An axial CT scan of the C1 vertebra of a 6-month-old baby will usually show:
   A. One primary ossification center
   B. Two primary ossification centers
   C. Three primary ossification centers
   D. Four primary ossification centers

   Correct Answer: C

   Explanation:

   Atlas (C1) has 2–5 primary ossification centers (commonly 3): Anterior arch (1), posterior arch (1) + lateral masses (2). It has no secondary ossification center. (BSA, p. 2498)

16. What are the boundaries of the lateral recess in the spine?
    A. Anterior: Intervertebral disc and posterior longitudinal ligament; Posterior: Ligamentum flavum; Lateral: Pedicle
    B. Anterior: Posterior vertebral body and intervertebral disc; Posterior: Superior articular facet; Lateral: Pedicle
    C. Anterior: Intervertebral disc; Posterior: Inferior articular facet; Lateral: Transverse process
    D. Anterior: Vertebral body; Posterior: Lamina; Lateral: Intervertebral foramen

    Correct Answer: B

    Explanation:

    The lateral recess is an anatomical corridor located between the spinal canal and the neural foramina. It allows the traversing nerve root to pass before exiting the spine. Its boundaries are (Fig. 1.10):

    - Anteriorly: Formed by the posterior aspect of the vertebral body and intervertebral disc
    - Posteriorly: Bordered by the superior articular facet of the inferior vertebra
    - Laterally: Limited by the pedicle of the vertebra

    (RP)

17. The origin of the segmental arteries for L5 is variable, and it could originate from all of the following, EXCEPT:
    A. Iliolumbar artery
    B. Fourth lumbar segmental artery

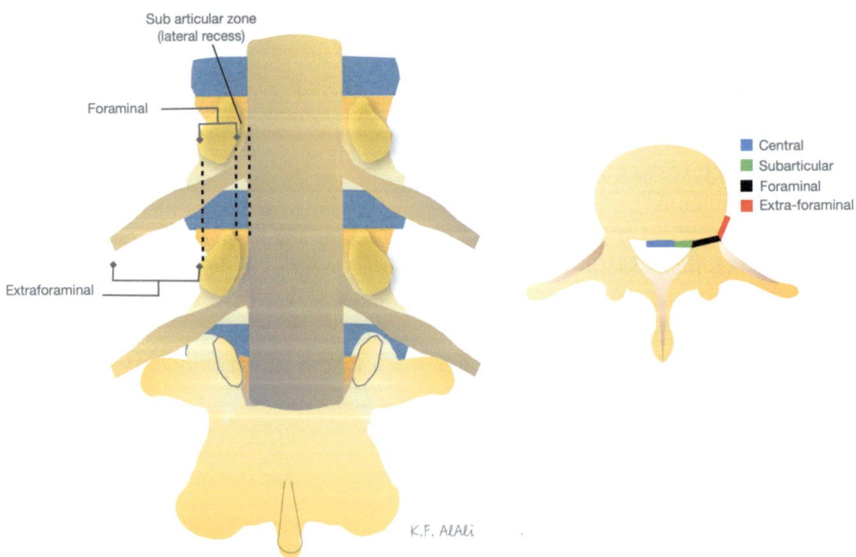

Fig. 1.10 Illustration of the posterior view of the lumbar spine showing the boundaries of the lateral recess and nerve root foramen. It also shows the common locations of lumbar disc herniations

C. Middle sacral artery
D. First and second sacral artery

Correct Answer: D

Explanation:

Each lumbar vertebra receives blood supply from paired lumbar segmental arteries. The segmental arteries for L1 through L4 originate from the aorta, while the source of the L5 segmental arteries is variable. They may arise from the iliolumbar artery, the fourth lumbar segmental artery, the middle sacral artery, or directly from the aorta.

(SS, p. 42)

18. Which of the following statements about interspinous ligaments is correct?
A. They connect the transverse processes of adjacent vertebrae.
B. They are situated lateral to the interspinal muscles.
C. They connect the base of one spinous process to the apex of the next inferior spinous process.
D. They are single, continuous ligaments with no cleft.

Correct Answer: C

Explanation:

The interspinous ligaments are thin, membranous fibers that connect adjacent spinous processes. They lie medial to the interspinal muscles, which span the tips of the spinous processes. The fibers of these ligaments are obliquely oriented, **attaching the base of one spinous process to the superior ridge and apex of the next inferior spinous process**. These ligaments are paired, with a distinct cleft separating the two halves.

(RS, p. 25)

19. The arterial supply to the anterior two-thirds of the spinal cord is predominantly provided by the:
A. Posterior spinal arteries
B. Radicular arteries
C. Anterior spinal artery
D. Artery of Adamkiewicz

Correct Answer: C

Explanation:

The anterior spinal artery is the primary blood supply to the anterior two-thirds of the spinal cord, including the motor tracts and anterior horns. It runs along the anterior median fissure of the spinal cord, receiving reinforcement from radicular arteries at various levels. The posterior spinal arteries mainly supply the posterior one-third of the spinal cord. The artery of Adamkiewicz is a large radicular artery that provides significant reinforcement to the anterior spinal artery in the thoracolumbar region.

(RS, pp. 44–45)

20. The vertebral artery passes through the transverse foramina of which cervical vertebrae?
A. C1–C6
B. C1–C7

C. C3–C7
D. C1–C5

Correct Answer: A

Explanation:

The vertebral arteries (VA) are paired vessels originating from the subclavian arteries. They ascend through the neck to supply blood to the posterior fossa, occipital lobes, and provide segmental blood flow to the vertebrae and spinal column. The V2 segment travels upward through the transverse foramina of the cervical vertebrae, typically from C6 to C3, alongside the vertebral veins and sympathetic nerves. At C2, the artery takes a superolateral turn through the inverted L-shaped transverse foramen.

(DI, p. 5)

21. In cases of atlantoaxial instability, the most commonly affected ligament is the:
A. Alar ligament
B. Tectorial membrane
C. Apical ligament
D. Transverse ligament of the atlas

Correct Answer: D

Explanation:

The transverse ligament is a robust horizontal part of the cruciate ligament, spanning from behind the C2 dens to the medial surfaces of the lateral masses of C1. It is the main ligament for **atlantoaxial (C1–C2) stability**. The vertical component consists of a fibrous band extending superiorly from the transverse ligament to the foramen magnum and inferiorly to C2.

(DI, p. 5)

22. The posterior longitudinal ligament is most intimately associated with which structure?
A. Vertebral bodies
B. Vertebral pedicles
C. Spinal cord
D. Annulus fibrosus of the intervertebral discs

Correct Answer: D

Explanation:

The posterior longitudinal ligament (PLL) extends along the dorsal surface of the vertebral bodies from the skull to the sacrum. It has a segmental denticulate pattern, being wider at the intervertebral disc spaces and narrowing while becoming thicker at the level of the vertebral bodies. It is immediately posterior to the annulus fibrosus of the intervertebral discs.

(DI, p. 5)

23. Which type of collagen predominates in the inner portion of the annulus fibrosus?
A. Type I collagen
B. Type II collagen
C. Type III collagen
D. Type IV collagen

Correct Answer: B

Explanation:

The annulus fibrosus comprises concentrically arranged collagen fibers that encase the nucleus pulposus. These fibers anchor to the vertebral cortex through Sharpey fibers and connect to the anterior and posterior longitudinal ligaments. The outer annulus primarily consists of type I collagen, while **type II collagen** predominates in the inner annulus. The posterior anular contour reflects the adjacent endplate's shape, which is typically slightly concave in the axial plane. At L4–L5 and L5–S1 levels, this contour may be flat or convex. Importantly, a convex contour on axial imaging alone does not necessarily indicate degenerative bulging.

(DI, p. 4)

24. Which of the following is a distinctive feature of C1 (atlas)?
   A. Presence of a vertebral body
   B. Superior facets shaped as large ovals
   C. Small transverse processes without tubercles
   D. Inferior facets facing upward

   Correct Answer: B

   Explanation:

   C1, also known as the atlas, lacks a vertebral body and forms a ring-shaped bony structure. Its **superior articular facets are large ovals that face upward**, while the inferior articular facets are circular. The transverse processes of C1 are prominent and feature fused anterior and posterior tubercles.

   (DI, p. 4)

25. Which spinal tract is most responsible for transmitting pain and temperature sensations?
   A. Dorsal column-medial lemniscus
   B. Corticospinal tract
   C. Spinothalamic tract
   D. Rubrospinal tract

   Correct Answer: C

   Explanation:

   Spinothalamic tracts are ascending tracts located in the anterior and lateral portions of the spinal cord and are responsible for transmitting sensations of pain, temperature, and light touch. The anterior spinothalamic tract primarily carries light touch, while the lateral spinothalamic tract predominantly transmits **pain and temperature.** These tracts cross to the opposite side of the spinal cord shortly after entering, resulting in the transmission of sensations from the contralateral side of the body.

   (SS, p. 21)

26. One of the following is CORRECT about the uncinate process of the cervical spine:
   A. It is also found between T1–T4
   B. It joins the inferolateral portion of the vertebral body to form the Luschka joint.

C. It limits cervical spine extension
D. It can be found unilaterally between C6 and C7

Correct Answer: B

Explanation:

The uncinate process is a hook-shaped structure located bilaterally on the superolateral margins of the cervical vertebral bodies from C3 to C7. These processes are positioned more anteriorly in the upper cervical spine and shift posteriorly in the lower cervical spine. They form **uncovertebral (Luschka) joints through their articulation with the inferolateral portion of the vertebral body above**. The uncinate processes play critical roles in limiting lateral flexion to preserve the integrity of the ipsilateral intervertebral foramen and maintaining the position of intervertebral discs during axial rotation.

(RP)

27. Which of the following best describes the course of the recurrent laryngeal nerve on the right side?
A. Passes under the aortic arch
B. Loops around the subclavian artery
C. Runs alongside the carotid sheath
D. Courses between the trachea and the esophagus

Correct Answer: B

Explanation:

The recurrent laryngeal nerve, which originates from the vagus nerve, enters the tracheoesophageal groove with distinct courses on the left and right sides. On the right side, it **loops around the subclavian artery**, while on the left, it passes under the aortic arch. During anterior surgical exposure of the lower cervical spine, meticulous dissection in the interval between the tracheoesophageal sheath and the carotid sheath is essential to prevent injury to this nerve.

(SS, p. 22)

28. The denticulate ligaments attach the spinal cord laterally to the:
A. Anterior longitudinal ligament
B. Vertebral bodies
C. Dura mater
D. Posterior longitudinal ligament

Correct Answer: C

Explanation:

Denticulate ligaments are bands of pia mater composed of longitudinally oriented fibers that extend from the surface of the spinal cord to the **dura mater**, helping to centralize the spinal cord within the subarachnoid space. It is used surgically to slightly retract the spinal cord.

(SS, p. 20)

29. At which vertebral level does the thoracic duct typically cross from right to left behind the esophagus?
    A. T2
    B. T4
    C. T8
    D. T10

    Correct Answer: B

    Explanation:

    The thoracic duct begins as a continuation of the cisterna chyli at approximately the L1 vertebral level (range T10–L3) and enters the thoracic cavity through the aortic hiatus. It ascends in the posterior mediastinum to the right of the midline, between the aorta and the azygos vein, and behind the esophagus. At the T4–T6 vertebral level, it crosses to the left of the midline and continues through the thoracic inlet. In the neck, it arches behind the left carotid sheath, crosses over the dome of the left pleura and subclavian artery, and drains into the venous angle formed by the left subclavian and internal jugular veins.

    (RP)
30. The ligamentum flavum is attached to the facet capsule in:
    A. Cervical spine
    B. Thoracic
    C. Lumbar
    D. All of the above

    Correct Answer: D

    Explanation:

    The ligamentum flavum is a segmental ligament that connects adjacent laminae. It attaches to the ventral surface of the superior lamina and the dorsal surface of the inferior lamina. Laterally, it is attached to the facet joint capsules at all spinal levels.

    (SS. p. 17)
31. The posterior spinal arteries typically originate from which vessels?
    A. Vertebral arteries
    B. Posterior inferior cerebellar
    C. Subclavian artery
    D. A and B

    Answer: D.

    Explanation:

    The posterior spinal arteries, originating from the **posterior inferior cerebellar or vertebral arteries**, run along the posterolateral aspect of the spinal cord. They descend on the spinal cord's surface and are reinforced by branches entering through the intervertebral foramina. The spinal cord's blood supply is divided into three main sections, with predictable feeders:

    C1–T3: Supplied by anterior segmental medullary arteries (~C3) and ascending cervical artery (~C6–C7).

T3–T7: Supplied by posterior intercostal arteries (~T7).

T8–Conus: Includes the artery of Adamkiewicz (T9–T12) and cone artery (artery of Desproges-Gotteron from iliolumbar arteries).

The posterior spinal arteries often anastomose with their contralateral counterparts and the anterior spinal artery via a surrounding pial plexus.

32. The filum terminale is an extension of which meningeal layer?
    A. Dura mater
    B. Arachnoid mater
    C. Pia mater
    D. Ligamentum flavum

    Correct Answer: C

    Explanation:

    The filum terminale, a unique structure of the **pia mater**, is a slender, bluish-white filament composed of glial cells and ependymal cells and is encased in pia mater. The initial 5–6 mm of the filum terminale contains the central canal. It spans approximately 20 cm, extending from the tip of the conus medullaris within the lumbar cistern to the dorsum of the coccyx, where it merges with the connective tissue covering the coccyx.

    (CA, p. 117)
33. The intervertebral disc is classified as what type of joint?
    A. Synovial
    B. Fibrocartilaginous
    C. Amphiarthrosis
    D. Synarthrosis

    Correct Answer: B

    Explanation:

    Intervertebral discs are resilient, cushion-like structures composed primarily of connective tissue, specifically specialized **fibrocartilage**.

    (CA, p. 740)
34. A 52-year-old man presents with weakness predominantly affecting the proximal muscles of his right lower extremity. On examination, he exhibits spasticity and hyperreflexia in the right leg. His distal muscle strength is relatively preserved, and there is no sensory deficit. An MRI of the thoracic spinal cord reveals a small, focal lesion in the anterior funiculus on the right side at the T10 level. Which of the following best explains the patient's neurological findings?
    A. Damage to the right lateral corticospinal tract causes ipsilateral distal muscle weakness.
    B. Damage to the left lateral corticospinal tract causes contralateral proximal muscle weakness.
    C. Damage to the right anterior corticospinal tract, causing bilateral proximal muscle weakness, more pronounced on the right
    D. Damage to the right dorsal columns affects proprioception and vibration sense.

Correct Answer: C

Explanation:

The **anterior corticospinal tract** primarily mediates control of **proximal muscles**, including those involved in postural adjustments and gross motor movements. These tracts do not decussate completely, meaning they affect both sides of the body but predominantly the ipsilateral muscles. In this case, the lesion at **T10 in the anterior funiculus** would damage the right anterior corticospinal tract, resulting in **proximal muscle weakness** that is more pronounced on the right side.

Other incorrect options:

A. **Damage to the right lateral corticospinal tract causing ipsilateral distal muscle weakness**: The lateral corticospinal tract primarily controls distal musculature. Damage to this tract would result in **distal weakness**, not proximal, and does not match the clinical findings.
B. **Damage to the left lateral corticospinal tract causing contralateral proximal muscle weakness**: The lateral corticospinal tract predominantly affects **distal muscle groups** and crosses at the medulla. Proximal weakness is more associated with anterior corticospinal tract damage.
C. **Damage to the right dorsal columns affecting proprioception and vibration sense**: The dorsal columns transmit **sensory information** (e.g., proprioception and vibration). This option does not explain the motor findings, spasticity, or hyperreflexia observed in the patient.

(SS, p. 20–21)

35. The posterior longitudinal ligament extends superiorly and attaches to the skull base as:
    A. Tectal ligament
    B. Tectorial membrane
    C. Tented membrane
    D. Tectonium ligament

    Correct Answer: B

    Explanation:

    The posterior longitudinal ligament (PLL) is a significant ligament situated directly behind the vertebral bodies, to which it is loosely attached, and intervertebral discs, to which it is firmly secured.

    This ligament extends from the posterior surface of the sacrum and widens progressively as it ascends. At the level of C2, it expands to form the **tectorial membrane**, which ultimately attaches to the base of the skull.

36. The epidural venous plexus (Batson's plexus) is notable for which characteristic?
    A. It is valveless
    B. It drains directly into the internal jugular veins
    C. It only drains the posterior spinal elements
    D. It has valves to prevent backflow

Correct Answer: A

Explanation:

Batson's plexus is a network of **valveless** veins situated within the spinal canal and around the vertebral body, serving as an alternative venous drainage route to the inferior vena cava. Due to the absence of valves, increases in abdominal pressure, such as those occurring during spine surgery positioning, can redirect blood flow toward the spinal canal and adjacent bony structures. Additionally, Batson's plexus acts as a pathway for the spread of metastatic tumors and infections to the lumbar spine.

(SS, p. 42)

37. The sacral promontory is part of which structure?
    A. Sacral ala
    B. S1 vertebral body
    C. Lumbosacral joint
    D. Sacroiliac joint

    Correct Answer: B

    Explanation:

    The **sacral promontory** is the anterior-superior part of the S1 body.

    (SS, p. 36)

38. The vertebral levels at which the cauda equina begins are:
    A. T12–L1
    B. L1–L2
    C. L3–L4
    D. S1–S2

    Correct Answer: B

    Explanation:

    The spinal cord typically ends at the **L1–L2** level in adults, forming the conus medullaris. Below this level, the thecal sac contains the cauda equina.

    (SS, p. 1)

39. The motor innervation to the diaphragm is primarily through which spinal nerve roots?
    A. C3, C4, C5
    B. C5, C6, C7
    C. T1, T2, T3
    D. T4, T5, T6

    Correct Answer: A

    Explanation:

    The diaphragm is innervated by the phrenic nerve, which arises from the C3, C4, and C5 spinal segments (Mnemonic: C3, C4, C5 makes the diaphragm alive). Due to its central innervation and blood supply, the diaphragm can be incised and retracted from its thoracic wall insertion during surgical procedures involving the thoracolumbar vertebral bodies without disrupting its neurovascular integrity.

    (SS, p. 30)

40. A 35-year-old male presents with loss of proprioception and vibratory sensation below the T8 level on the right side, along with left-sided loss of pain and temperature sensation below T8. Motor function is weakened on the right side below T8. Which of the following spinal cord lesions best explains his symptoms?
   A. Central cord syndrome at T8
   B. Anterior cord syndrome at T8
   C. Right-sided hemisection of the spinal cord at T8
   D. Posterior cord syndrome at T8

   Correct Answer: C

   Explanation:

   Brown-Séquard syndrome results from **hemisection** of the spinal cord and is characterized by **ipsilateral loss of motor function and proprioception, along with contralateral loss of pain and temperature sensation below the level of injury.** The prognosis for recovery is generally favorable, with many patients regaining some level of ambulation and bowel and bladder function. Common causes include penetrating trauma, missile injuries, unilateral laminar or pedicle fractures, and rotational injuries with subluxation.

   (SS, p. 520)

41. During a posterior cervical spine surgery, a neurosurgeon needs to identify the dorsal root entry zone to avoid damaging the sensory fibers. Which of the following structures marks the separation between the dorsal and ventral roots in the spinal cord?
   A. Anterior median fissure
   B. Posterior median sulcus
   C. Posterolateral sulcus
   D. Anterolateral sulcus

   Correct Answer: C

   Explanation:

   The **posterolateral sulcus** is the anatomical landmark where the dorsal rootlets of the spinal nerves enter the spinal cord. It separates the dorsal sensory roots from the ventral motor roots, making it critical for surgeons to identify this structure during procedures to avoid damaging sensory fibers.

   Anterior median fissure marks the midline on the anterior surface of the spinal cord, housing the anterior spinal artery.

   The posterior median sulcus is a shallow groove along the midline on the dorsal side of the spinal cord and does not separate sensory and motor roots.

   The anterolateral sulcus is where the ventral motor rootlets exit the spinal cord.

   (CA, p. 104)

42. In the thoracic spine, the orientation of the facet joints primarily limits which of the following movements?
   A. Flexion
   B. Extension

C. Rotation
D. Lateral flexion

Correct Answer: C

Explanation:

The thoracic facets are oriented 60° in the sagittal plane and slightly medially inclined (20°). Motion in the thoracic spine is limited by anatomical constraints, including the rib cage, ligamentous attachments, narrow intervertebral discs, and overlapping laminae and spinous processes. **Rotation is limited by the coronal orientation of the thoracic facets.** Flexion-extension increases from T1–T2 to T12–L1, while axial rotation is greatest at T1–T2 and minimal at the thoracolumbar junction. Lateral bending is more evenly distributed across the thoracic region.

(SS, p. 27–28)

43. A patient presents with difficulty in neck extension and rotation to the same side. Which muscle, innervated by the dorsal rami of spinal nerves, is most likely affected?
A. Sternocleidomastoid
B. Anterior scalene
C. Levator scapulae
D. Splenius capitis

Correct Answer: D

Explanation:

The splenius capitis is a strap-like muscle in the superficial layer of intrinsic back muscles, working alongside the splenius cervicis. It originates from the ligamentum nuchae and the spinous processes of C7 and the upper thoracic vertebrae, inserting onto the mastoid process and the occipital bone below the lateral third of the superior nuchal line. Located deep to the trapezius and superficial to the semispinalis capitis and longissimus capitis, it forms part of the floor of the posterior neck triangle. The muscle receives blood supply from the occipital and deep cervical arteries and is innervated by lateral branches of the second and third cervical dorsal rami. Its actions include **rotating the head to the same side** when acting unilaterally (synergistically with the sternocleidomastoid) and **extending the head** when acting bilaterally.

(RP)

44. Compression of the anterior horn cells at the spinal cord level would most likely result in which of the following deficits?
A. Loss of fine touch and proprioception
B. Loss of pain and temperature sensation
C. Flaccid paralysis of the muscles innervated at that level
D. Spastic paralysis below the level of the lesion

Correct Answer: C

Explanation:

Each spinal nerve consists of both motor and sensory fibers, which contribute to the formation of peripheral nerves. The cell bodies of motor axons, forming the ventrally exiting motor roots, are located in the **anterior horn** of the spinal cord (**primary motor neurons**). Compression of the anterior horn at a spinal level will result in **paralysis of the muscles innervated at that level**. The cell bodies of sensory axons (primary sensory neurons) reside outside the spinal cord in the dorsal root ganglion.

(SS, p. 170)

45. Which of the following spinal cord tracts is responsible for transmitting unconscious proprioceptive information from the lower limbs to the cerebellum?
    A. Fasciculus cuneatus
    B. Dorsal (posterior) spinocerebellar tract
    C. Ventral (anterior) spinocerebellar tract
    D. Lateral corticospinal tract

    Correct Answer: B

    Explanation:

    The dorsal spinocerebellar tract (DSCT) is located in the lateral funiculus, ventral to the dorsolateral tract of Lissauer and lateral to the lateral corticospinal tract. Originating at the L2–L3 spinal segments, it ascends to relay proprioceptive and tactile information from the trunk and lower extremities. The cell bodies of DSCT fibers reside in Clarke's nucleus (nucleus dorsalis), found in lamina VII of spinal segments C8/T1 to L2/L3, with prominent development in the upper lumbar and lower thoracic regions. Additional contributions to the DSCT come from axons in the intermediate and dorsal laminae of nearby segments. The tract processes **proprioceptive** input and may include mechanisms for different types of sensory information integration.

    (CA, p. 473)

46. A lesion affecting the dorsal columns on the right side at the T6 level would result in which of the following deficits?
    A. Loss of pain and temperature sensation on the left side below T6
    B. Loss of motor function on the right side below T6
    C. Loss of proprioception and vibratory sense on the right side below T6
    D. Loss of pain and temperature sensation on the right side below T6

    Correct Answer: C

    Explanation:

    The dorsal columns, also known as the posterior columns, are ascending sensory pathways that transmit **vibration**, conscious **proprioception**, and fine (discriminative) touch. These columns are divided into two tracts: the medial fasciculus gracilis and the lateral fasciculus cuneatus. Fasciculus gracilis is responsible for carrying sensory information from the lower half of the body, including the trunk and lower extremities, while fasciculus cuneatus carries sensory signals from the upper trunk, arms, and neck.

    (CA, p. 456)

47. Which of the following best explains the link between Horner's syndrome and the carotid artery?
    A. Damage to sympathetic fibers in the carotid sheath alongside the vagus nerve
    B. Injury to preganglionic fibers ascending with the internal carotid artery

C. Disruption of postganglionic fibers in the adventitia of the internal carotid artery
D. Compression of the sympathetic trunk by the carotid artery

Correct Answer: C.

Explanation:

Horner's syndrome is a condition in which the oculosympathetic pathway is disrupted. It is manifested clinically by ipsilateral miosis, ptosis, and anhidrosis. This 3-neuron pathway originates from the hypothalamus and goes through the brainstem, spinal cord (C8–T2), cervicothoracic ganglia, and along the carotid artery to the eye.

The first-order neuron originates from the hypothalamus and synapses at the levels of C8–T2.

The second-order neuron: At T1, preganglionic pupillomotor fibers leave the spinal cord and ascend to the superior cervical ganglion, situated close to the angle of the jaw and the bifurcation of the common carotid artery. They then pass through the brachial plexus and over the lung apex.

The third-order neuron, Postganglionic pupillomotor fibers, ascends along the internal carotid artery to enter the cavernous sinus and joins the trigeminal nerve's ophthalmic division to reach the eye.

(BS, p. 326; GB, p. 594)

48. In spinal cord anatomy, Clarke's nucleus plays a crucial role in which of the following pathways?

A. Anterolateral (spinothalamic) pathway
B. Dorsal spinocerebellar tract
C. Lateral corticospinal tract
D. Medial lemniscus pathway

Correct Answer: B

Explanation:

Fibers of the posterior spinocerebellar tract, also known as the Flechsig tract, originate in the posterior root ganglion and enter the spinal cord. These fibers synapse with neurons in the thoracic nucleus, or **Clarke's column**, located in the posterior horn of all 12 thoracic segments and the first two lumbar segments. From there, the tract ascends along the dorsal lateral funiculus, adjacent to the lateral corticospinal tract, and continues to the medulla. It ultimately reaches the cerebellum through the ipsilateral inferior cerebellar peduncle. Importantly, the fibers of the posterior spinocerebellar tract remain ipsilateral to their origin and do not cross (decussate).

(RP)

49. A neurosurgeon performing a lumbar puncture needs to know the correct anatomical layers to traverse. Which of the following lists the correct order of structures pierced, from superficial to deep?

A. Skin → Supraspinous ligament → Interspinous ligament → Ligamentum flavum → Dura mater → Arachnoid mater
B. Skin → Ligamentum flavum → Supraspinous ligament → Interspinous ligament → Dura mater → Arachnoid mater

C. Skin → Supraspinous ligament → Interspinous ligament → Ligamentum flavum → Epidural space → Dura mater → Arachnoid mater
D. Skin → Interspinous ligament → Supraspinous ligament → Ligamentum flavum → Dura mater → Pia mater

Correct Answer: C

Explanation:

Option (C) represents the structures the needle passes through from superficial to deep.

50. Which of the following best describes the anatomical location of the nucleus pulposus within an intervertebral disc?
A. Peripheral fibrous ring
B. Central gelatinous core
C. Posteriorly located fibrous tissue
D. Superior cartilaginous endplate

Correct Answer: B

Explanation:

Each intervertebral disc consists of **a central gelatinous core**

Known as the nucleus pulposus, surrounded by a fibrous annulus fibrosus. The disc is bound to the vertebral bodies via hyaline cartilage endplates. The annulus (mainly type 1 collagen) connects to the endplates through obliquely arranged collagen fibers, while the nucleus (rich in glycosaminoglycans and type 2 collagen) retains water to generate intradiscal pressure, distributing loads to the annulus. Aging leads to dehydration of the nucleus pulposus, reducing its water-binding capacity and increasing stress on the annulus.

(SS, p. 18)

51. Which of the following ligaments connects the tips of the spinous processes from C7 to the sacrum?
A. Interspinous ligament
B. Ligamentum flavum
C. Anterior longitudinal ligament
D. Supraspinous ligament

Correct Answer: D

Explanation:

The supraspinous ligament runs from the sacrum to C7, where it transitions into the ligamentum nuchae. The ligamentum nuchae extends from C7 to the occiput, forming a sheet-like structure that provides muscle attachment and functions as a posterior tension band, supporting an upright neck posture.

(SS, p. 17)

Spine Radiology

2

1. Identify the following structures (A, B, C, D, E) in the following cervical lateral X-ray (Fig. 2.1).

   Correct Answer: A. Occipital bone. B. C1 anterior arch. C. C1 posterior arch. D. C2 body. E. C3 lamina. F. C4–C5 facet joint. G. C7 spinous process
2. Identify the following structures (A, B, C, D, E) in the following cervical MRI (Fig. 2.2).

   Correct Answer: A. Clivus of the occipital bone. B. Cerebellar tonsils. C. Odontoid process of C2. D. C1 posterior arch. E. C2 spinous process
3. Identify the following structures (A, B, C, D, E, F) in the following cervical MRI at the level of C4–C5 disc (Fig. 2.3).

   Correct Answers: A. Trachea. B. Carotid artery. C. C4–C5 disc. D. Right C5 nerve root. E. Spinal cord. F. left C4–C5 facet joint
4. Identify the following structures (A, B, C, D, E, F, G) in the following lumbar lateral X-ray (Fig. 2.4).

   Correct Answer: A. L1 vertebral body. B. Twelfth rib. C. L2 spinous process. D. L3 pedicle. E. L3-L4 facet joint. F. L3–L4 intervertebral disc. G. S1 vertebral body
5. Identify the following structures (A, B, C, D, E) in the following lumbar lateral X-ray (Fig. 2.5).

   Correct Answers: A. Twelfth rib. B. left L2 transverse process. C. Left L3 pedicle. D. L4 spinous process. E. L4-L5 intervertebral space
6. Identify the following structures (A, B, C, D, E) in the following lumbar oblique X-ray (Fig. 2.6).

   Correct Answer: The X-ray shows the "scotty dog appearance." A. Superior articular facet (ear of the scotty dog). B. Pedicle (eye). C. Pars interarticularis (neck). D. Inferior articular facet (leg). E. Transverse process (nose)

K. F. AlAli, H. T. Hashim, *Spine Surgery and Peripheral Nerve Surgery*,
https://doi.org/10.1007/978-3-031-98543-0_2

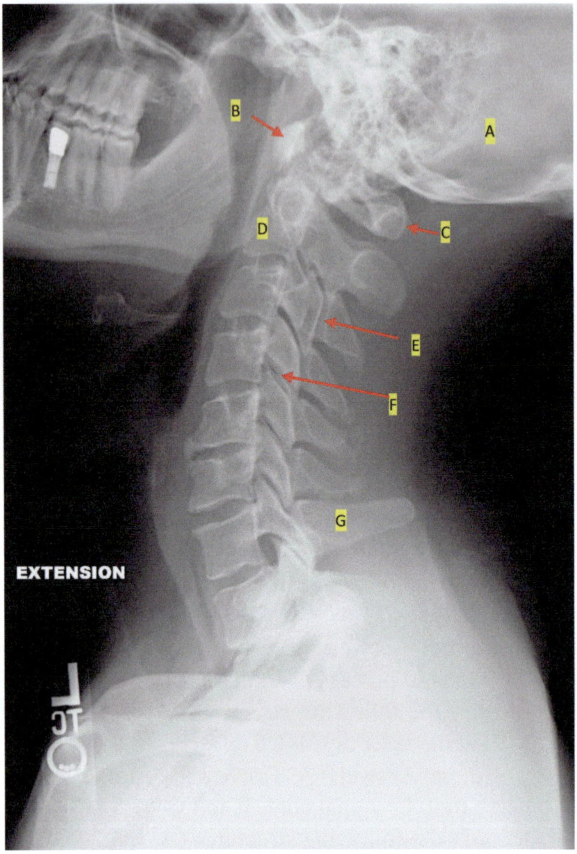

Fig. 2.1 Case 1 x-ray

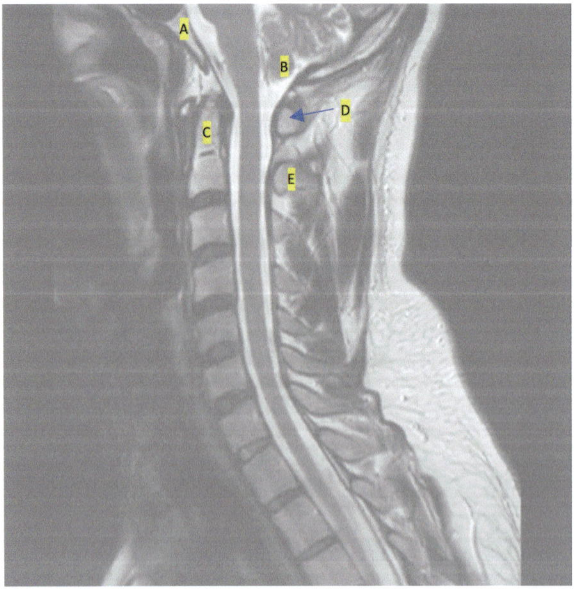

Fig. 2.2 Case 2 MRI

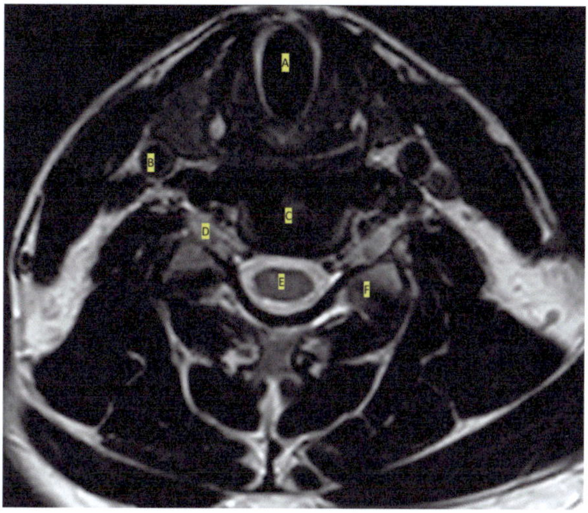

Fig. 2.3 Case 3 cervical MRI

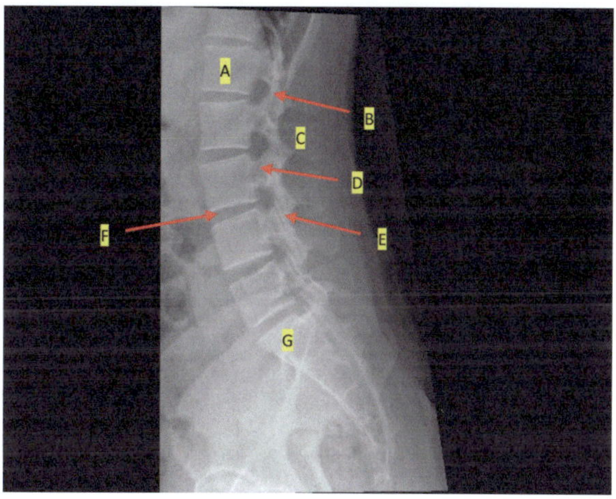

Fig. 2.4 Case 4 X-ray

7. Identify the following structures (A, B, C, D, E) in the following axial MRI at the L4–L5 level (Fig. 2.7).

   Correct Answers: A. Psoas muscle. B. L4–L5 intervertebral disc. C. Right L4 nerve root (exciting nerve). D. Right L5 nerve root (traversing nerve). E. flavum ligament. F. L4 lamina. G. L4 spinous process. H. Multifidus muscle. I. Longismus muscle. J. Iliocostalis muscle
8. All of the following can be MRI features of spinal ependymoma are EXCEPT:
   A. Enhanced with gadolinium contrast
   B. Cap sign
   C. Target sign
   D. Cervical spine predominance

   Correct Answer: C

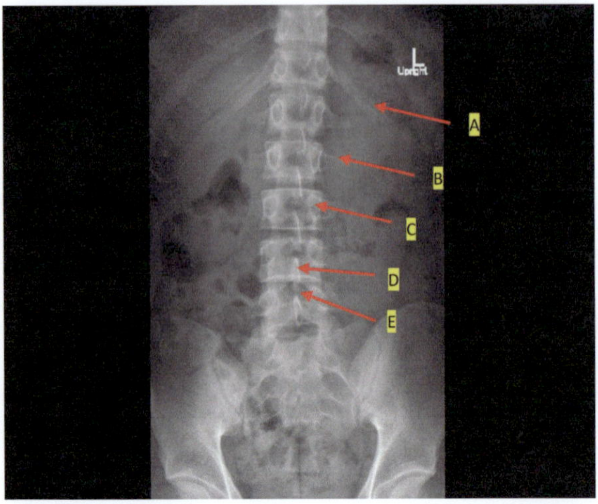

Fig. 2.5 Case 5 X-ray

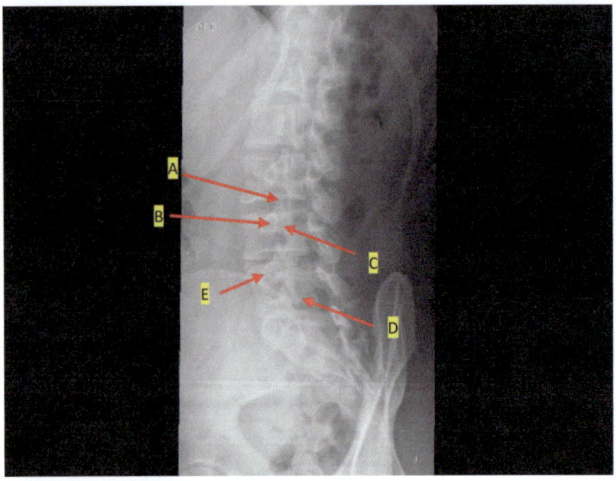

Fig. 2.6 Case 6 X-ray

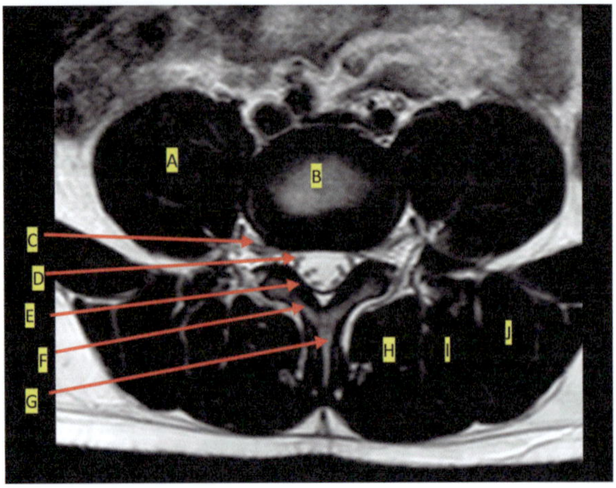

Fig. 2.7 Case 7 axial MRI

Explanation:

Target sign is not a typical MRI feature of spinal ependymoma. Spinal ependymomas typically appear as an intramedullary mass. That strongly enhances with gadolinium contrast, has a **haemosiderin cap sign,** where a cap of T2 hypointense haemosiderin is seen because of previous haemorrhage. It is commonly found in the cervical spine, followed by the thoracic spine.

Target sign is not a typical feature of spinal ependymomas. Instead, the target sign is more commonly associated with peripheral nerve sheath tumors, such as schwannomas or neurofibromas.

(DI, p. 806)

9. The "Corduroy sign" on axial T2-weighted MRI images is characteristic of which spinal pathology?
   A. Ependymoma
   B. Hemangioma
   C. Metastatic lesion
   D. Cavernous malformation

   Correct Answer: B

   Explanation:

   Corduroy sign is a radiological feature typically associated with **vertebral hemangiomas** on T2-weighted MRI sequences, characterized by a pattern of alternating low and high signal intensities due to the presence of fat and vascular components within the lesion.

   (RP)

10. A 55-year-old patient presents with chronic low back pain. His MRI is attached (Fig. 2.8). Which is the best describing describes the findings at L5–S1 level?
    A. Modic type 1
    B. Modic type 2
    C. Modic type 3
    D. None of the above

    Correct Answer: A

    Explanation:

    Modic has categorized three types of changes in vertebral endplates on a lumbar MRI, which are closely associated with disc degeneration and low back pain. Acute disruption and inflammation are linked to **Type I** changes, which appear as low signals on T1 and high signals in T2 images due to bone marrow edema. **Type II** changes are a result of bone marrow degeneration that is marked by high T1 signals and either strong or low T2 signals, suggesting that the condition is more chronic and stable. Bone sclerosis is the focus of **Type III** changes, which are demonstrated as dark on T1 and T2 sequences. The prevalence of Modic changes in patients with low back pain is much higher than that of the general population, with 46% of them experiencing these changes. Type I changes are strongly linked to both symptoms and spinal hypermobility.

    (SS, p. 460)

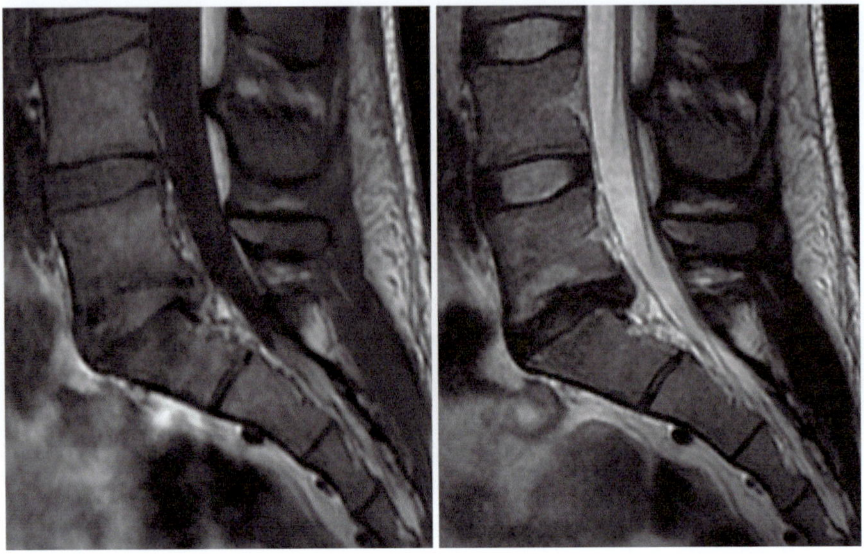

Fig. 2.8 Case 10 MRI

11. An 18-year-old presented with abdominal pain. A bone window of the abdominal CT scan is shown (Fig. 2.9). What is the abnormality seen in the CT scan?
   A. Diastematomyelia
   B. Spina bifida occulta
   C. Unsegmented S1 vertebra
   D. Butterfly S1 vertebrae
   Correct Answer: B
   Explanation:
   Spina bifida occulta, the most common form of spina bifida, affects 10–20% of the population. It is characterized by a congenital defect where the posterior element of the spine fails to completely form, resulting in a spinous or paraspinal cleft, typically in the lower lumbosacral region. Covered by intact skin with no developmental abnormalities of the spinal cord or nerve roots, it is usually asymptomatic and lacks neurological symptoms. On plain radiographs and CT scans, it appears as a midline or para-midline bony defect in the posterior vertebral arch.
   (RP)
12. In the context of lumbar degenerative disc disease, which statement best describes the significance of a vacuum phenomenon observed on imaging studies?
   A. Indicates infection within the disc space
   B. Sign of advanced disc degeneration with gas formation
   C. Suggests recent disc herniation
   D. Represents a normal variant without clinical significance
   Correct Answer: B

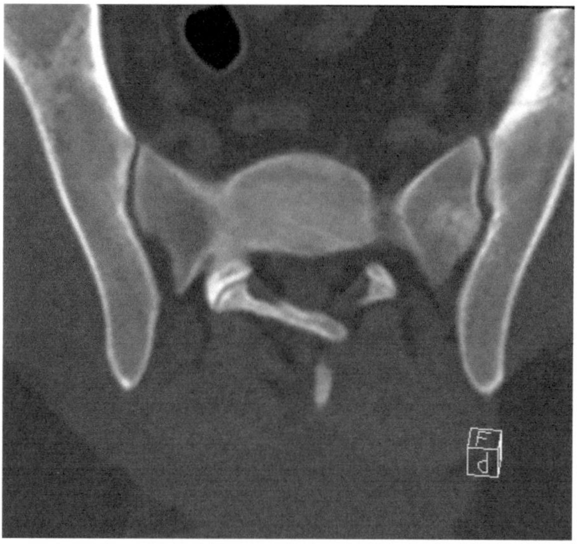

Fig. 2.9 Case 11 CT scan

Explanation:

Vacuum phenomena refer to aseptic gas collections, primarily nitrogen with traces of oxygen and carbon dioxide, found within intervertebral discs, bones, joints, or adjacent tissues due to migration. These phenomena can be physiological, commonly associated with aging or joint movement, or pathological, and in the intervertebral disc, **degeneration**. Intradiscal vacuum phenomena are prevalent in the elderly, affecting up to 20% of cases. They are typically asymptomatic but may rarely cause complications, such as pneumatic nerve root compression.

(RP)

13. What radiographic feature is commonly associated with a teardrop fracture on an AP cervical spine X-ray?
    A. Prevertebral soft-tissue swelling
    B. Separation of facet joints
    C. A sagittal split fracture of the vertebral body
    D. Hyperextension deformity

    Correct Answer: C

    Explanation:

    Teardrop fractures, originally described by Schneider and Kahn, occur due to hyperflexion or axial loading of the cervical spine, often eliminating normal cervical lordosis. These injuries result from two forces: anterior column compression and tension on the dorsal longitudinal complex. In severe cases, the injury disrupts all ligaments, facet joints, and intervertebral discs, with ≥3 mm posterior displacement of the vertebral body into the spinal canal. Radiographic features include a small chip of bone, known as the "teardrop," located just beyond the anterior-inferior edge of the involved vertebral body on lateral cervical spine X-rays. Other features are a sagittal split through the vertebral body, visible on AP views and better delineated on thin-cut CT scans, which may appear midline or off-center. Additionally, a large triangular fragment of the anterior-inferior vertebral body is a hallmark finding, emphasizing the severity of the injury.

Typically unstable, teardrop fractures are seen in ~5% of cervical spine trauma cases and may cause quadriplegia or anterior cervical cord syndrome.

(GB, p. 1185)

14. In the context of degenerative disc disease, Modic type 2 changes on MRI most likely represent:
    A. Edema in the vertebral body
    B. Fibrosis and fatty replacement in bone marrow
    C. Osteonecrosis
    D. Chronic inflammation

    Correct Answer: B

    Explanation:

    Type II Modic changes represent fibrosis and fatty degeneration of marrow with high T1 and isointense or slightly high T2 signals, indicating a chronic and more stable degenerative state.

    (RP)

15. Which of the following is NOT a feature of a Jefferson fracture on radiographic examination?
    A. Lateral displacement of C1 lateral masses
    B. Fracture of the anterior and posterior arches of C1
    C. Spinous process avulsion
    D. Absence of displacement on the lateral cervical radiograph

    Correct Answer: C

    Explanation:

    A Jefferson fracture typically involves lateral displacement of the C1 lateral masses and fractures of the anterior and/or posterior arches of C1. Displacement of the lateral masses is often visible on radiographic examination, particularly in the open-mouth odontoid view. Displacement of lateral masses of C1 relative to the lateral margins of C2 of ≥7 mm, suggesting transverse ligament disruption. An avulsion fragment from the inner C1 pillar at the transverse ligament insertion further indicates instability. Widening of the atlantoaxial interval is concerning, with ≥4 mm suggesting transverse ligament involvement and ≥ 7 mm strongly indicative of its disruption. Associated fractures of C2, such as hangman's or odontoid fractures, are frequently observed, along with potential fractures at lower levels.

    Spinous process avulsion is not characteristic of a Jefferson fracture, making it the incorrect feature in this context.

    (DI, p. 244)

16. On MRI, the "owl's eye" appearance in the cervical spinal cord is typically associated with:
    A. Syringomyelia
    B. Amyotrophic lateral sclerosis
    C. Central cord syndrome
    D. Spinal cord infarction

    Correct Answer: D

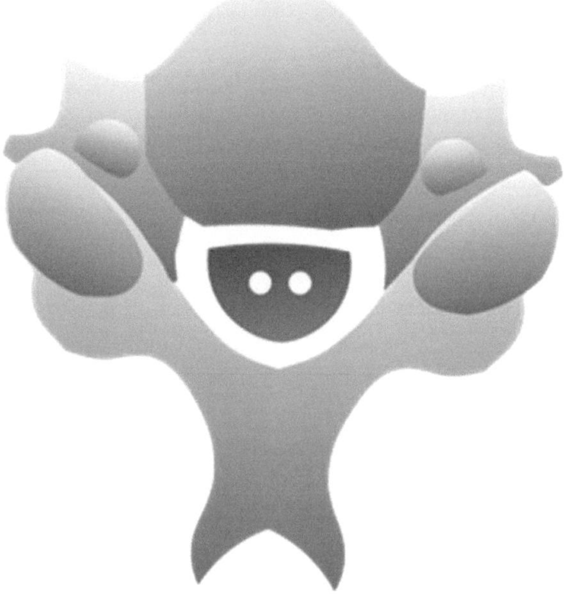

Fig. 2.10 An illustration of axial T2 MRI of a cervical spine showing Owl eyes sign in spinal cord infarction

Explanation:

The owl-eyes sign, also referred to as the snake-eyes sign or fried-eggs sign, is characterized by bilaterally symmetrical, circular to ovoid areas of high T2-weighted signal intensity located in the anterior horn cells of the spinal cord, visible on axial MRI. On sagittal imaging, this finding corresponds to a "pencil-like" vertical linear high T2-weighted signal, typically extending across multiple segments (Fig. 2.10).

(RP)

17. A 50-year-old patient undergoes T11–T12 fixation, and a follow-up CT scan is performed to assess fusion (see Fig. 2.11). Which of the following findings seen on CT is most indicative of successful bony fusion?
    A. Presence of bridging trabecular bone across the facet joint
    B. Sclerosis surrounding the pedicle screws
    C. Persistent lucency around the hardware
    D. Loss of disc height at adjacent levels

    Correct Answer: A

    Explanation:

    The presence of bridging trabecular bone across the facet joint is the most reliable indicator of successful bony fusion on this follow-up CT scan. This finding demonstrates the formation of continuous, solid bone, confirming a stable and fused segment. Assessing bony fusion is an essential part of post-surgical follow-up to ensure the spine's stability and the absence of motion at the fused segment.

    Successful bony fusion after spine fixation is typically assessed 6 to 12 months postoperatively, as this timeframe allows sufficient bone healing. The gold standard for evaluating fusion is a high-resolution CT scan, which

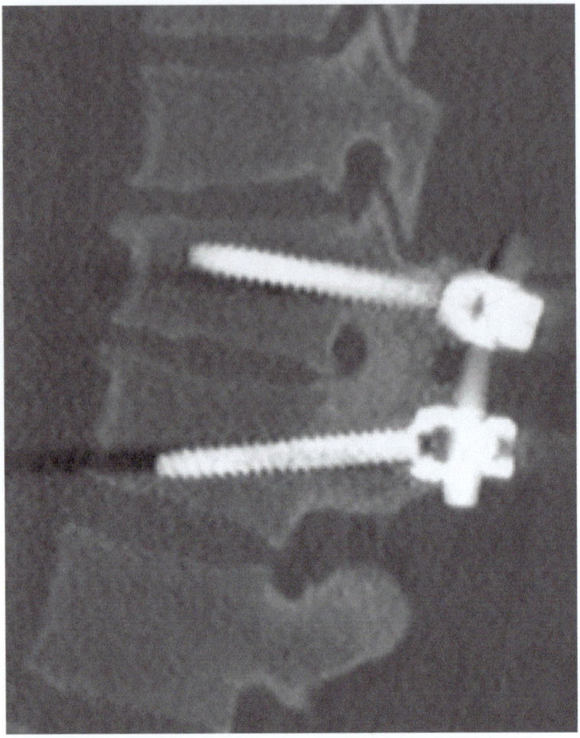

Fig. 2.11 Case 17 CT scan

provides detailed visualization of bridging trabecular bone across the facet joint or interbody space, a key indicator of successful fusion. Radiographs, including flexion-extension X-rays, can assess segmental motion, with a lack of movement suggesting a stable fusion. Persistent lucency around hardware or gaps in the fusion mass, as well as signs of hardware loosening or breakage, may indicate nonunion. The presence of continuous bone formation and the absence of radiolucent gaps are the most reliable indicators of a successful fusion.

(SS, p. 328)

18. In the context of spondylolisthesis, a "scotty dog" sign is seen on:
    A. Lateral cervical radiographs
    B. umbar radiographs
    C. Oblique lumbar radiographs
    D. Axial CT images

    Correct Answer: C

    Explanation:

    On an oblique lumbar radiograph, the vertebral structures can be visualized as resembling the shape of a "Scotty dog": the superior articular process forms the ear, the pedicle represents the head, the pars interarticularis corresponds to the neck or collar, the inferior articular process makes up the front leg/foot, the lamina represents the body, the contralateral inferior articular process forms the hind leg/foot, and the spinous process represents the tail. A defect in the pars interarticularis, seen as a radiolucent line at the Scotty dog's neck or collar, indicates spondylolysis (Fig. 2.12).

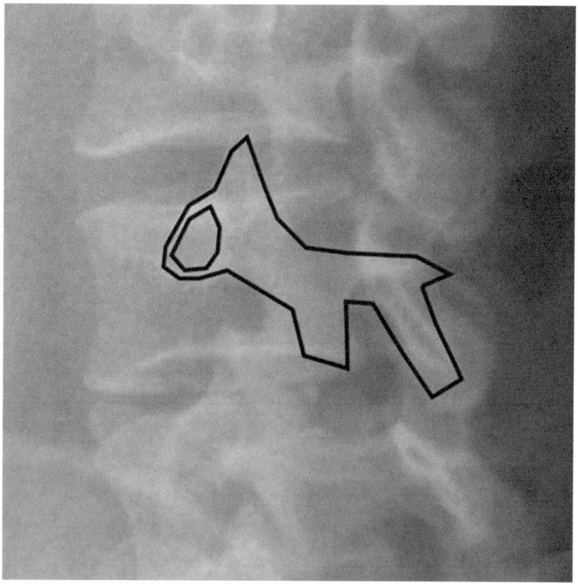

Fig. 2.12 Oblique lumbar X-ray showing the "Scotty dog" and outlined

19. Regarding ankylosing spondylitis:
    19a. Which of the following is an early radiographic finding of it in the sacroiliac joints?
    A. Bilateral joint fusion
    B. Sclerosis with end-stage ankylosis
    C. Loss of definition of the subchondral bone plate
    D. Syndesmophyte formation
    19b. Which of the following is a late radiographic finding of ankylosing spondylitis?
    A. Romanus lesions
    B. Andersson lesions
    C. Bamboo spine
    D. Widened intervertebral joint spaces
    Correct Answer: 19a: C, 19b: C
    Explanation:
    Radiographic features of ankylosing spondylitis include characteristic findings in the sacroiliac joints (SIJs), vertebral bodies, facet joints, and sites of enthesopathy. Sacroiliitis presents as a bilaterally symmetric erosive arthropathy, initially seen on the iliac side of the joint. Early changes **include loss of subchondral bone plate** definition, followed by erosions, joint space widening, and eventual sclerosis with end-stage fusion. In the vertebral bodies, early findings include vertebral body squaring and corner erosions (Romanus lesions), progressing to "shiny corner" sclerosis and discovertebral inflammation (Andersson lesion). Later stages show thin, vertically oriented syndesmophytes bridging vertebrae, culminating in widespread ankylosis (**bamboo spine**). Facet and uncovertebral joints may exhibit erosions progressing to

fusion. Enthesopathy involves erosions and periosteal new bone formation at tendon and ligament attachment sites.

(DI, p. 515)

20. The "curtain sign" in postoperative spinal infections refers to:
    A. Bilateral abscesses in the paraspinal muscles extending into the epidural space
    B. Bilobed posterior bulging of an abscess on both sides of the meningovertebral ligament
    C. Curtain-like clumping of nerve roots adhering to the thecal sac
    D. Enhancement patterns of inflammatory tissue extending across multiple vertebral levels

    Correct Answer: B

    Explanation:

    A curtain sign is seen in MRI, usually T1 or T1 with contrast. It is typically seen in post-spine surgery infections, plasmacytoma, and spinal metastasis.

    (DI, p. 693, 749, 1097)

21. Which MRI sequence is most sensitive in detecting multiple sclerosis plaques in the cervical spine?
    A. T1-weighted
    B. T2-weighted
    C. Proton density
    D. FLAIR

    Correct Answer: D

    Explanation:

    FLAIR (Fluid-Attenuated Inversion Recovery) is highly sensitive for detecting periventricular MS lesions in the brain and in the cervical spine. T2-weighted imaging is also sensitive in detecting MS. FLAIR is more sensitive than T2-weighted imaging for detecting juxtacortical, periventricular, and cervical plaques, whereas T2-weighted imaging is better at identifying infratentorial lesions.

    T1-weighted imaging is less sensitive for detecting MS plaques but can show hypointense lesions ("black holes") in advanced disease.

    Proton density sequences can help identify plaques but are generally less commonly used for MS compared to T2-weighted imaging.

    (DI, p. 643, RP)

22. Based on Lee's classification, the degree of central lumbar spinal stenosis in this axial T2 MRI is (Fig. 2.13).
    A. Grade 0
    B. Grade 1
    C. Grade 2
    D. Grade 3

    Correct Answer: C

    Explanation:

    Lee classification is a 4-grade classification system for lumbar central canal stenosis based on the degree of obliteration of the anterior CSF space in the dural sac, as observed on axial T2-weighted MRI:

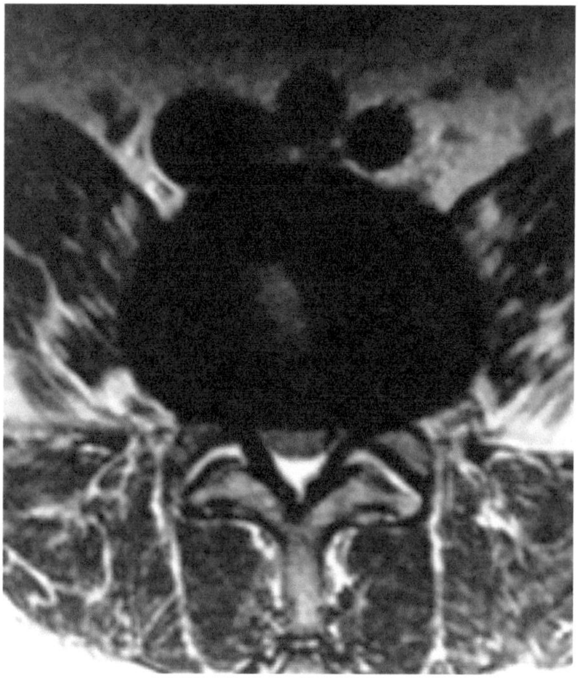

Fig. 2.13 Case 22 axial T2 MRI

Grade 0 (No stenosis): The anterior CSF space is intact, with no obliteration.

Grade 1 (Mild stenosis): The anterior CSF space is mildly obliterated, but all cauda equina nerve roots remain clearly separable.

Grade 2 (Moderate stenosis): The anterior CSF space is moderately obliterated, and some cauda equina nerve roots are aggregated, making visual separation impossible.

Grade 3 (Severe stenosis): The anterior CSF space is severely obliterated, with significant compression of the dural sac, causing the cauda equina to appear as a single, inseparable bundle.

(RP)

23. Based on Lee's classification, the degree of foraminal lumbar spinal stenosis in this axial T2 MRI is (Fig. 2.14).
    A. Grade 0
    B. Grade 1
    C. Grade 2
    D. Grade 3

    Correct Answer: D

    Explanation:

    Lee classification is a 4-grade classification system for lumbar foraminal c stenosis based on the degree of obliteration of fat around the exiting nerve root, as observed on sagittal T2-weighted MRI:

Grade 0 (Normal): The nerve root is surrounded circumferentially by perineural fat.

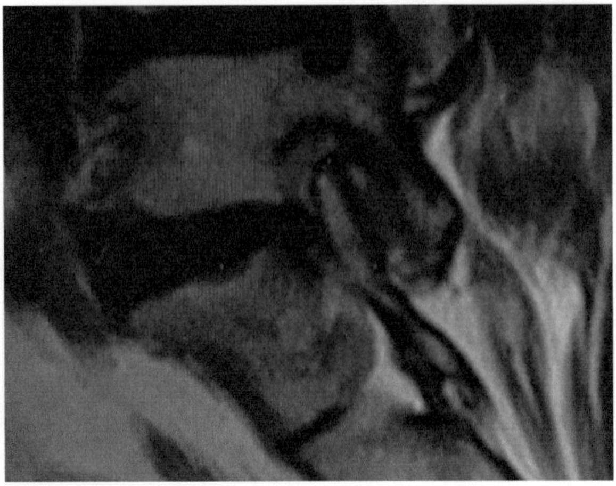

Fig. 2.14 Case 23 axial T2 MRI

Grade 1 (Mild): Partial loss of perineural fat visualization in one dimension, either vertical or horizontal. Anteroposterior narrowing caused by thickening or buckling of the ligamentum flavum.

Grade 2 (Moderate): Complete loss of perineural fat visualization circumferentially, but no visible compression of the nerve root.

Grade 3 (Severe): Complete absence of perineural fat visualization accompanied by visible compression and morphologic changes of the nerve root.

(RP)

24. Which of the following spinal conditions is typically associated with the presence of the "flow voids" on MRI?
    A. Disc herniation
    B. Arteriovenous malformations (AVMs)
    C. Spinal stenosis
    D. Vertebral hemangioma

    Correct Answer: B

    Explanation:

    Flow voids on MRI are hypointense areas seen on T1- and T2-weighted images, caused by rapid blood flow within vessels. These are characteristic findings of vascular lesions, such as arteriovenous malformations (AVMs), where abnormal connections between arteries and veins result in turbulent and high-velocity blood flow.

    (DI, p. 896)

25. 13. The "clay-shoveler's fracture" is typically an avulsion fracture of which spinal process?
    A. C7 spinous process
    B. C3 vertebral body
    C. T2 spinous process
    D. L1 transverse process

    Correct Answer: A

Explanation:

Clay-shoveler fractures are fractures of the spinous process of the lower cervical spine (C7) or T1. It results from hyperflexion.

(DI, p. 226)

26. A 46-year-old patient presents with low back pain radiating into the right leg. MRI reveals a herniation of the L4–5 disc, as seen in Fig. 2.15. Which nerve root is most likely compressed?
    A. L3 nerve root
    B. L4 nerve root
    C. L5 nerve root
    D. B and C

    Correct Answer: D

    Explanation:

    This herniated disc has with upward herniation, which can compress the traversing and the exiting nerve root. In this case, it is L4 (exciting) and it is compressed at the lateral recess of L4 as seen in the axial MRI and the L5 (traversing nerve root), as any paracentral disc herniation.

    [43]

27. The characteristic finding of a "burst fracture" on CT imaging is:
    A. Multiple comminuted fragments
    B. Compression of the vertebral endplates
    C. Retropulsion of posterior vertebral body fragments
    D. Pars interarticularis defect

    Correct Answer: C

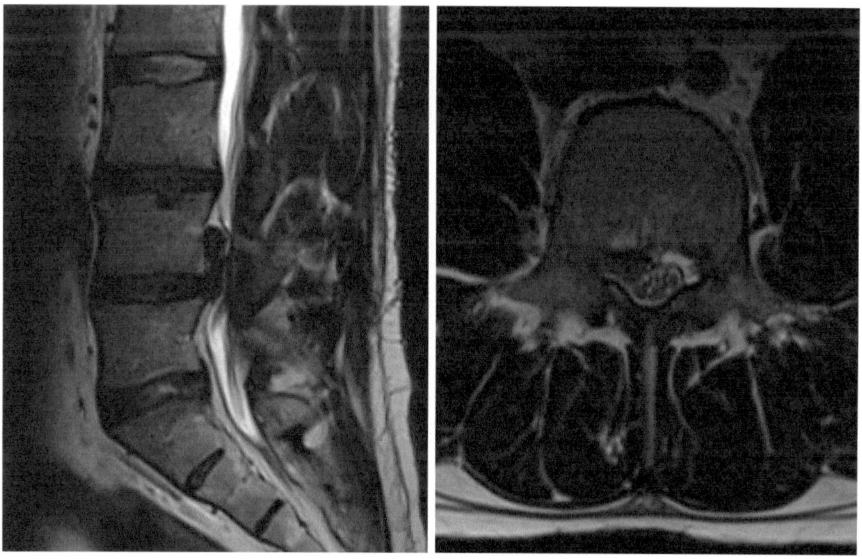

Fig. 2.15 Case 26 MRI reveals a herniation of the L4–5 disc

Explanation:

Burst fracture is defined as a fracture that results in a fracture line that extends to the posterior vertebral cortex and fragments projecting posteriorly into the spinal canal, narrowing the canal and potentially compressing neural elements.

(DI, p. 294)

28. Which of the following is true regarding the appearance of spinal meningiomas on MRI?
    A. Isointense on T1, hyperintense on T2, with enhancement post-contrast
    B. Hypointense on both T1 and T2
    C. Always associated with vertebral destruction
    D. Show restricted diffusion

    Correct Answer: A

    Explanation:

    Spinal meningiomas typically appear isointense to the spinal cord on T1-weighted MRI. On T2-weighted imaging, they are generally isointense but may be hypointense if calcified or hyperintense in cases with cystic degeneration, which occurs in 2–4% of cases. Highly vascular meningiomas may exhibit prominent flow voids on T2-weighted imaging. After contrast administration on T1-weighted imaging, spinal meningiomas show prominent, diffuse enhancement, often accompanied by a characteristic dural tail sign.

    (DI, p. 777)

29. The primary distinguishing feature of vertebral hemangioma on MRI is:
    A. Hypointensity on T1 and T2
    B. Hyperintensity on T1 and T2
    C. Irregular signal on T1 and hypo on T2
    D. Associated cord compression

    Correct Answer: B

    Explanation:

    Spinal hemangiomas on MRI are typically hyperintense on T1-weighted and T2-weighted imaging due to the high fat content within vascular channels. They often show a classic "polka-dot" appearance on CT and X-ray due to thickened trabeculae. On T1-weighted images with contrast shows variable enhancement. (DI, p. 697)

30. How do you know that the following image is a T1 post post-contrast MRI (Fig. 2.16):
    A. Hyperintensity between the spinous processes
    B. Hyperintensity intervertebral disc
    C. Hyperintensity basivertebral veins
    D. Hyperintensity of subcutaneous veins

    Answer: C.

    Explanation:

    Basivertebral veins are large venous structures located within the vertebral bodies. They are part of the internal vertebral venous plexus and function as a key component of the venous drainage system of the spine. These veins originate within the spongy bone of the vertebral body and exit **posteriorly** through the basivertebral foramen to communicate with the anterior and posterior internal

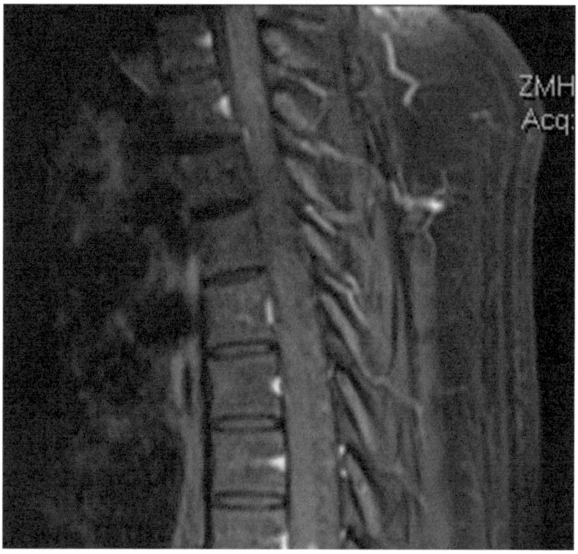

Fig. 2.16 Case 30 T1 post-contrast MRI

venous plexuses. Basivertebral veins enhance vividly in spine MRI with contrast as a hyperintense line in the middle of the posterior vertebral cortex.

(RP)

31. The presence of a "winking owl" sign on plain radiographs is indicative of:
    A. Osteoporotic compression fracture
    B. Pedicle destruction by metastasis
    C. Hemangioma
    D. Osteoid osteoma

    Correct Answer: B

    Explanation:

    The "winking owl" sign on plain radiographs is a classic radiological finding that indicates **pedicle destruction**, often caused by metastatic disease. The sign appears as the loss of one pedicle, resembling a "wink," with the intact pedicle representing the remaining "eye" of the owl. Metastatic lesions commonly involve the vertebral pedicles due to their rich vascular supply.

    - **Osteoporotic compression fracture** typically spares the pedicles and involve the vertebral body.
    - **Hemangioma** presents as vertical striations in the vertebral body, described as a "corduroy" pattern.
    - **Osteoid osteoma** is a small, benign tumor often seen in the posterior elements of the spine and does not cause pedicle destruction.

    (RS, p. 1516)

32. A 45-year-old patient presents with mild lower back pain. A CT scan reveals the lesion shown in the L1 vertebral body (Fig. 2.17). Which of the following best describes the typical radiographic feature of this lesion?
    A. Osteoblastic metastasis
    B. "honeycomb" appearance

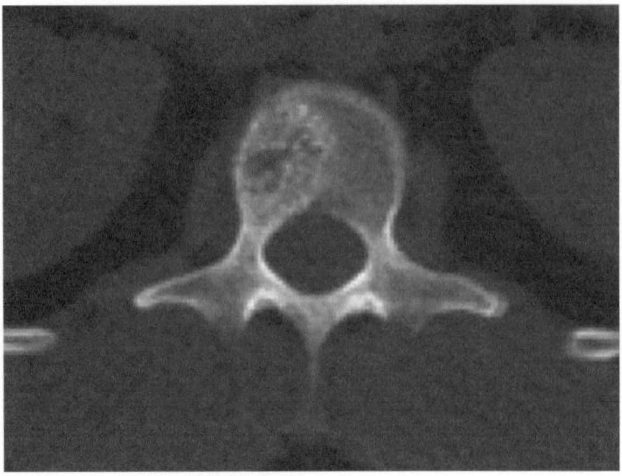

Fig. 2.17 Case 32
CT scan

C. Diffuse osteopenia
D. Ground-glass appearance
Correct Answer: B
Explanation:
This CT scan shows a spinal hemangioma. They are identified on X-ray or CT as vertebral body lesions with coarse vertical trabeculae, resembling a "corduroy" or "honeycomb" pattern. The hallmark of axial CT images is the "polka-dot" appearance, resulting from cross-sections of these trabeculae.
(DI, p. 670)

33. A Hangman's fracture classically involves which vertebral structure?
A. Pars interarticularis of C2
B. Anterior arch of C1
C. Odontoid process of C2
D. Body of C3
Correct Answer: A
Explanation:
Hangman's fracture is defined as a fracture through the bilateral C2 pars interarticularis. It results from hyperextension with axial loading or, less commonly, hyperflexion with axial loading.
(DI, p. 262)

34. Tethered cord syndrome on MRI is usually characterized by:
A. Low conus medullaris position
B. Thinned filum terminale
C. Enhancing intradural mass
D. Multiple nerve root clumping
Correct Answer: A
Explanation:
Tethered cord is characterized by a **low-lying conus medullaris**, often below the inferior border of L2 vertebra in postnatal cases, which lacks normal anterior motion in prone positioning. It may be associated with a thickened

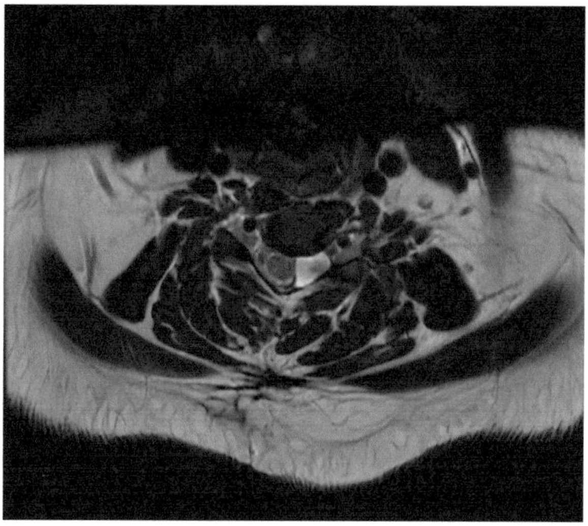

Fig. 2.18 Case 35 MRI

filum terminale (≥2 mm at L5–S1) or fatty infiltration and, in some cases, a lipomatous mass. The conus is abnormally positioned dorsally within the thecal sac, persisting even in the prone position. Normal spinal cords typically fall into the anterior two-thirds of the thecal sac in this posture. These findings are often accompanied by clinical signs and symptoms of tethering, such as lower extremity pain, weakness, spasticity, gait abnormalities, altered reflexes, and bladder dysfunction.

(DI, p. 103)

35. A 23-year-old who had a motorcycle crash and presented with left upper limb weakness. The MRI cervical is shown in Fig. 2.18. What is the diagnosis?
    A. Traumatic dural injury
    B. Ruptured cervical arachnoid cyst
    C. Cervical nerve root avulsion
    D. Traumatic spinal epidural hematoma

    Correct Answer: C

    Explanation:

    Nerve root avulsion on MRI or myelogram will show pseudomeningoceles at the avulsed levels. They are cerebrospinal fluid collections within dural sac outpouchings caused by dural or perineural tears. Retracted distal nerve roots or a nerve retraction ball may also be observed in MRI (Fig. 2.19).
36. Which of the following is the most characteristic imaging feature of Baastrup disease on MRI?
    A. Contact of adjacent spinous processes with sclerosis
    B. Diminished disc height
    C. Spondylolisthesis
    D. Hypertrophy of the ligamentum flavum

    Correct Answer: A

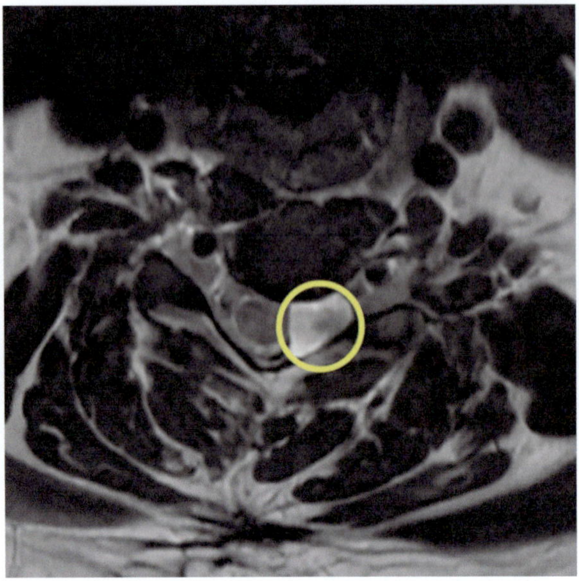

Fig. 2.19 T1 axial MRI cervical showing left pseudomeningoceles, which a cerebrospinal fluid collections within the dural sac seen in cervical root avulsion (yellow circle)

Explanation:

Baastrup disease, also known as “kissing spinous process disease,” is characterized by the contact and sclerosis of adjacent spinous processes. This is best visualized on MRI, where the apposing surfaces of spinous processes may show low signal intensity on T1-weighted images due to bony sclerosis and possible marrow edema. Flexion and extension radiographs can also show contact of spinous processes with sclerosis.

(DI, p. 431)

37. What is the percentage of spinal meningiomas that have dural tail signs?
    A. 10%
    B. 25%
    C. 50%
    D. 95%

    Answer: C.

    Explanation:

    The dural tail in spinal meningioma refers to a characteristic imaging feature where there is thickened, linear enhancement of the dura mater adjacent to the tumor on contrast-enhanced MRI. It represents reactive changes in the dura rather than direct tumor infiltration. It is found in approximately half of the patients.

    (DI, p. 777)

38. A “positive sagittal balance” on imaging is defined as:
    A. Anterior translation of the C7 plumb line
    B. Posterior displacement of the spinal cord
    C. Increased kyphotic angle
    D. Loss of lumbar lordosis

    Correct Answer: A

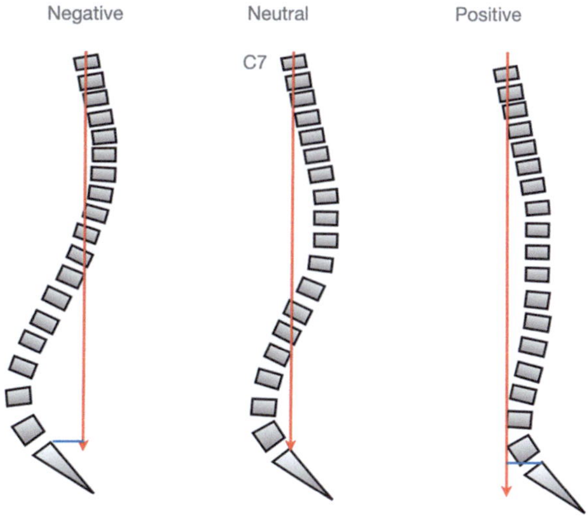

Fig. 2.20 The C7 plumb line is drawn vertically from the middle of the C7 vertebral body

Explanation:

Sagittal Balanc is a sagittal alignment which is assessed on a lateral view using the C7 plumb line, with the posterior superior aspect of the sacrum serving as the distal reference point. If the C7 plumb line falls anterior to this reference point, the value is considered positive; if it falls posterior, the value is negative.

Sagittal Balance Categories (Fig. 2.20):

Positive Balance: The C7 plumb line is positioned more than 2 cm anterior to the posterosuperior corner of the S1 vertebral body.

Neutral Balance: The C7 plumb line intersects the posterosuperior corner of the S1 vertebral body, with a mean sagittal vertical axis (SVA) of 0.5 cm ± 2.5 cm in asymptomatic adults.

Negative Balance: The C7 plumb line is located more than 2 cm posterior to the posterosuperior corner of the S1 vertebral body.

39. A 43-year-old who had C5-C6 ACDF 2 years ago. He presented with mechanical neck pain. A cervical CT scan is shown (Fig. 2.21). What is the most likely cause of the neck pain?
    A. Facet arthritis
    B. Adjacent degenerative disc disease
    C. Pseudoarthrosis
    D. All are possible causes

    Correct Answer: C

    Explanation:

    The coronal CT scan showed loss of the bony bridge in the interbody space between C5 and C6, which represents pseudoarthrosis (nonunion). Other signs of pseudoarthrosis seen in the CT scan is hollowing around the screws.

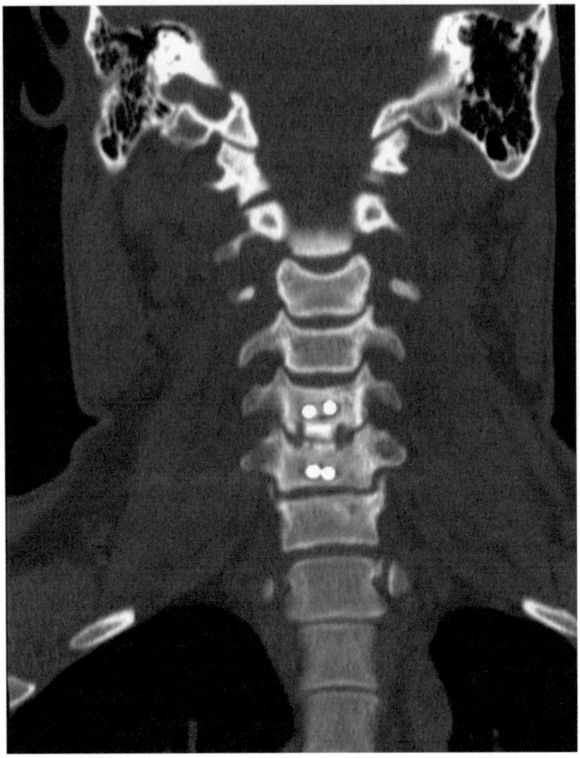

Fig. 2.21 Case 39
CT scan

40. On MRI, a "target sign" is typically associated with which of the following spinal tumors?
    A. Schwannoma
    B. Neurofibroma
    C. Meningioma
    D. Metastasis
    Correct Answer: B
    Explanation:
    Target sign is seen in nerve sheath tumors, schwannoma, and neurofibroma. It is more typical of neurofibroma. It is characterized as a high signal rim and low intensity center by MRI.
    (DI, p. 769)
41. Which of the following is a hallmark imaging feature of diffuse idiopathic skeletal hyperostosis (DISH)?
    A. Ossification of the anterior longitudinal ligament
    B. Ligamentous instability
    C. Syndesmophyte formation
    D. Erosive vertebral endplates
    Correct Answer: A
    Explanation:
    DISH, also known as Forestier disease or senile ankylosing hyperostosis, is characterized by **ossification of the anterior longitudinal ligament,** typically

affecting the thoracic (100%), cervical (65–80%), and lumbar (68–90%) spine, often more pronounced on the right. Imaging reveals anterior ossification over at least four contiguous vertebral bodies with minimal disc degeneration, no facet ankylosis, and absent sacroiliac joint involvement. Lateral radiographs are reliable for diagnosis, while MRI is reserved for evaluating coexistent ossification of the posterior longitudinal ligament (OPLL) or spinal cord compression. Pathologically, the condition is linked to exaggerated enthesial reactions, though the exact cause is unclear. Clinically, most cases are incidental, but symptoms like dysphagia may occur due to osteophytes, and treatment may involve osteophyte resection. Patients with DISH are at higher risk for extension-type fractures, which carry significant morbidity. Differential diagnoses include spondylosis, ankylosing spondylitis, and psoriatic or reactive arthritis.

(DI, p. 460)

42. A 38-year-old patient presents with low back pain. CT of the lumbar spine reveals a lesion at the L3 vertebra without soft tissue involvement (Fig. 2.22). What is the most likely diagnosis?
    A. Giant cell tumor
    B. Osteosarcoma
    C. Ostoid osteoma
    D. Paget disease

Answer: A.

Explanation:

A vertebral spine lytic lesion has an extensive differential diagnosis. It can be approached as follows:

Age Consideration

- **Child:** Likely diagnoses include Ewing's sarcoma and eosinophilic granuloma (Langerhans cell histiocytosis)
- **Middle-Aged to Elderly:** Commonly due to metastasis or multiple myeloma

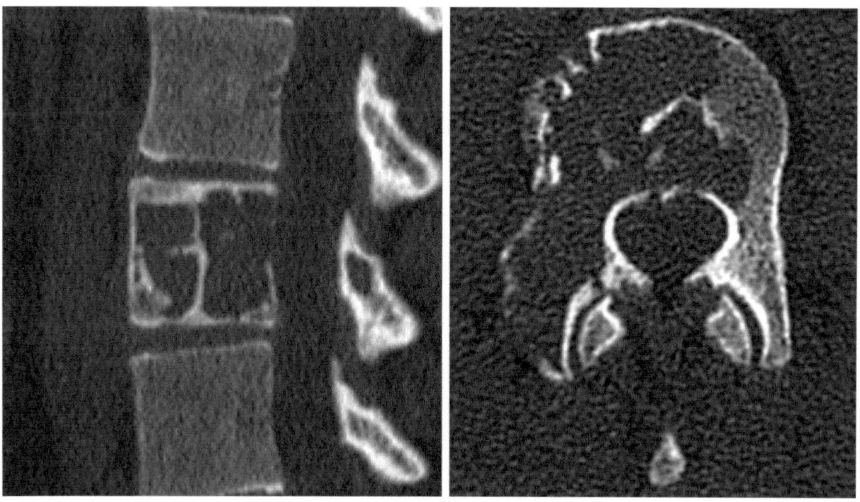

Fig. 2.22 Case 42 CT scan

- **Young to Middle-Aged Adults:** Possible causes are giant cell tumor, osteosarcoma, chondrosarcoma, hemangioma, and eosinophilic granuloma

Characteristics of the Lesion

- **Hemangioma:** Corduroy-patterned vertebral body
- **Paget's Disease:** Enlarged bone with coarsened trabeculae and thickened cortex
- **Langerhans Cell Histiocytosis:** Commonly affects the cervical spine and is the most frequent cause of vertebral plana (collapsed vertebral body with preserved disc)
  - Differential diagnosis for vertebral plana includes metastasis, lymphoma, myeloma, Ewing's sarcoma, osteoporosis, and eosinophilic granuloma.
- **Osteosarcoma:** Aggressive-appearing lesion with formation of immature bone. It is associated with soft tissue swelling.
- **Giant Cell Tumor:** Typically a lytic and expansile lesion, often found in the sacrum

  Given that it is a young adult patient with an expansile lytic lesion without soft tissue involvement, the likely diagnosis is giant cell tumor.

  (DI, p. 713)

43. The most common spinal level for cervical disc herniation is:
    A. C1–C2
    B. C3–C4
    C. C4–C5
    D. C5–C6

    Correct Answer: D

44. Which of the following best describes the "naked facet sign" on axial CT in the context of locked facet injury?
    A. The superior articular facet of the vertebra below is uncovered and displaced posteriorly.
    B. The inferior articular facet of the vertebra above is anteriorly displaced and covered by the intervertebral disc.
    C. The facet joint space appears widened but retains its "hamburger-like" configuration.
    D. The vertebral endplates exhibit a characteristic "step-off" deformity.

    Correct Answer:A

    Explanation:

    The naked facet sign (or hamburger sign/reverse hamburger bun sign) describes the CT appearance of an uncovered vertebral articular facet in cases of facet joint dislocation (Fig. 2.23), often associated with locked facets. This finding, seen in flexion-distraction injuries, signifies severe ligamentous disruption and spinal instability. Normally, on axial CT, the facet joint resembles a hamburger: the superior articular process of the vertebra below forms the top "bun," the inferior articular process of the vertebra above forms the bottom "bun," and the joint space resembles the "patty." In dislocation, the "top bun" (**superior articular facet) shifts posteriorly**, leaving the **facet joint uncovered**. This sign may be unilateral or bilateral, depending on the extent of dislocation.

    (RP)

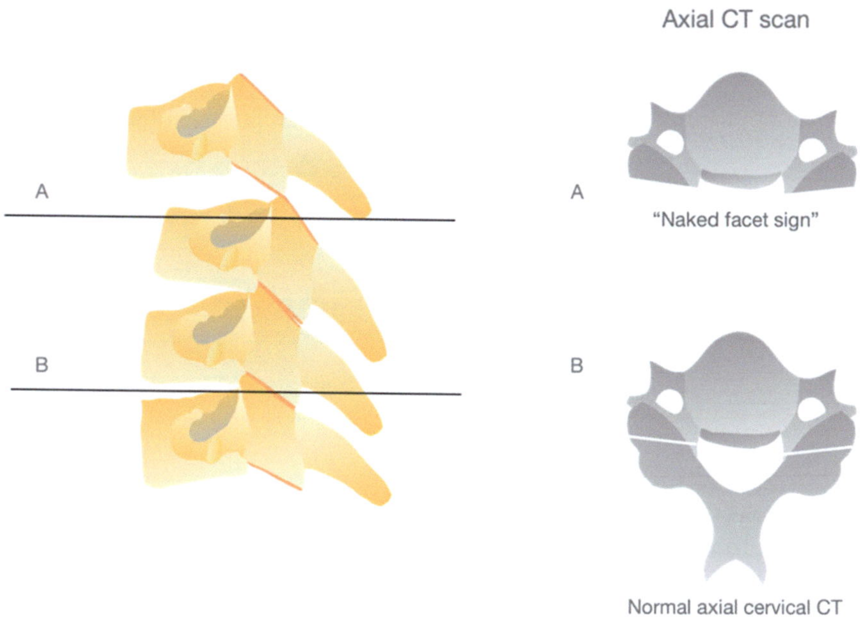

Fig. 2.23 The naked facet sign (or hamburger sign/reverse hamburger bun sign) describes the CT appearance

45. In a case of atlanto-axial instability in an adult patient, the predental space on the lateral cervical radiograph is increased. What is the normal upper limit for this space in adults?
    A. 3 mm
    B. 5 mm
    C. 7 mm
    D. 10 mm

    Correct Answer: A

    Explanation:

    The anterior atlantodental interval (ADI), also known as the predental space or interval, is the distance between the anterior margin of the dens and the closest point of the anterior arch of C1 on a lateral cervical spine X-ray.

    The normal upper limit of the anterior ADI is 3 mm in adults, with commonly accepted values outlined in guidelines. An increased ADI is indicative of a potential disruption of the transverse atlantal ligament, causing atlanto-axial instability (Fig. 2.24).

    (GB, p. 223)
46. A patient presents with a history of lumbar spine surgery and new radicular pain. MRI shows enhancement around the surgical site. What is the most likely diagnosis?
    A. Recurrent disc herniation
    B. Epidural fibrosis

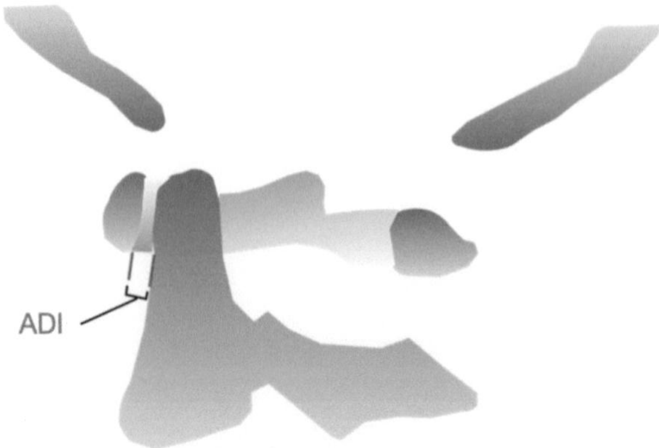

Fig. 2.24 The anterior atlantodental interval (ADI) on lateral X-ray

C. Discitis
D. Epidural hematoma

Correct Answer: B

Explanation:

Epidural fibrosis usually occurs after lumbar surgery that surrounds thecal sac and nerve root. It usually shows early enhancement in MRI. It can cause radicular pain. The main differential diagnosis of epidural fibrosis is recurrent disc herniation.

(DI, p. 407)

47. On a follow-up MRI after spinal decompression surgery, what finding would most strongly suggest recurrent disc herniation rather than postoperative scar formation?
A. Isointensity on T1-weighted images
B. Hypointensity on T2-weighted images
C. Lack of enhancement after contrast
D. High enhancement after contrast

Correct Answer: C

Explanation:

Recurrent disc herniation and epidural fibrosis (scar formation) present with distinct features on imaging and clinical evaluation. Because of its vascularity, epidural fibrosis shows immediate and substantial enhancement on MRI, whereas recurrent disc herniation shows modest, progressive enhancement, usually less than scar tissue. While epidural fibrosis exhibits fluctuating signal strength and an uneven appearance, recurrent disc herniation is isointense with the primary intervertebral disc. Although it is usually absent in epidural fibrosis, the mass effect is frequently seen with recurrent disc herniation and may result in the compression of the thecal sac. In contrast to epidural fibrosis, which does not preserve continuity with the parent intervertebral disc, recurrent disc herniation does.

Recurrent disc herniation may eventually become vascularized, but as epidural fibrosis ages, it usually becomes less pronounced. Contrast-enhanced MRI is the most effective imaging technique for both disorders. Non-contrast MRI can successfully assist in the initial diagnosis of epidural fibrosis, although it is restricted in its ability to distinguish recurrent disc herniation.

(DI, p. 407)

48. What is the best imaging modality for diagnosing a CSF leak after spinal surgery?
    A. Dynamic CT myelogram
    B. T2-weighted MRI
    C. Gadolinium-enhanced MRI
    D. X-ray with contrast injection

    Correct Answer: A

    Explanation:

    Dynamic CT myelography is the most sensitive imaging modality for diagnosing a CSF leak after spinal surgery. It allows real-time observation of the contrast flow and identification of the exact site of leakage. T2-weighted MRI can show CSF collections but may not identify active leaks or their source. Gadolinium-enhanced MRI is helpful in other contexts but is less specific for detecting CSF leaks. X-ray with contrast injection is outdated and less commonly used due to limited sensitivity and specificity.

    (DI, p. 857)

49. In a patient with ankylosing spondylitis and a history of trauma, which radiologic finding is most characteristic of a spinal fracture?
    A. Vertical fracture through multiple vertebral bodies
    B. Vertical fracture at the disc space
    C. Fracture involving the posterior elements
    D. A fracture through both anterior and posterior columns

    Correct Answer: D

    Explanation:

    Imaging of trauma in ankylosing spondylitis frequently reveals fractures at the C2 level, the cervicothoracic junction, and the thoracolumbar junction, often resulting from hyperextension injuries. These fractures, commonly called "chalk stick fractures," typically span **all three columns**, making them highly unstable and prone to complications. The fracture can involve the fused disc space.

    (DI, p. 515)

50. A patient presents with back pain and neurological deficits after spinal fusion surgery. CT shows a broken rod at the fusion site. What is the most likely explanation?
    A. Infection at the fusion site
    B. Stress shielding of the bone graft
    C. Hardware failure due to nonunion
    D. Over-tensioning of the hardware

    Correct Answer: C

    Explanation:

    Hardware breakage in the postoperative CT scan in a symptomatic patient likely indicates nonunion (pseudoarthrosis) at the operated spinal level. Other signs of nonunion are persistent lucency around hardware or gaps in the fusion mass and hardware loosening.

    (SS, p. 328)

51. A 34-year-old patient presents with the sudden onset of severe neck pain and posterior circulation ischemic symptoms, including dizziness and ataxia, following minor trauma. An MRI with T1 fat-saturation (FS) imaging is performed. What is the most likely radiologic finding to confirm vertebral artery dissection?
    A. Loss of normal flow void on T2-weighted imaging
    B. Crescentic hyperintense mural hematoma on T1 FS MRI
    C. Suboccipital rind sign on axial CT angiogram images
    D. Aneurysmal dilatation with intimal flap on MRA

    Correct Answer: B

    Explanation:

    Crescentic hyperintensity on T1 FS MRI, representing methemoglobin in the mural hematoma, is pathognomonic for vertebral artery dissection.

    (DI, p. 955)
52. A 45-year-old patient presents with neck pain and headache. CT angiogram reveals a tapered stenosis of the vertebral artery extending over a long segment ("string sign"). What type of vertebral artery dissection is most consistent with these findings?
    A. Steno-occlusive dissection
    B. Dissecting aneurysm
    C. Traumatic pseudoaneurysm
    D. Non-dissecting vasculopathy

    Correct Answer: A

    Explanation:

    A long segment of tapered stenosis, often called the "string sign," is characteristic of steno-occlusive dissection.

    Vertebral artery dissection commonly occurs at the atlantoaxial region (C1–C2). The srtery at that region is mobile and vulnerable to mechanical injury. The condition is classified into two types: **steno-occlusive dissection**, characterized by tapered long-segment stenosis ("string sign"), and dissecting aneurysm, presenting as focal or fusiform dilatation with or without stenosis, potentially causing subarachnoid hemorrhage. On axial T1-weighted fat-saturated (FS) MRI, a crescentic hyperintense mural hematoma is a key diagnostic clue. CT angiogram (CTA) reveals lumen contour changes and the "suboccipital rind sign," indicating a thickened wall from an intramural hematoma. T1. FS MRI and MP-RAGE sequences are the most effective in detecting intramural hematomas. Angiography can reveal aneurysmal dilatation, stenosis, and intimal flaps and is considered the gold standard. Non-contrast CT is used to exclude subarachnoid hemorrhage, brain imaging for infarction, and CTA/MRA are done to assess vertebral artery involvement. If the other investigations are inconclusive, then conventional angiography is used only when there is high suspicion. (DI, p. 955)
53. A postoperative MRI of a patient with spinal hardware shows abnormal signal intensity around the pedicle screws on T2-weighted images. What is the most likely explanation?
    A. Infection
    B. Pseudarthrosis

C. Metal artifact
D. Bone resorption

Correct Answer: C

Explanation:

In patients with spine fixation artifacts, MRI reveals a focal central signal loss with a peripheral "halo" of increased signal intensity on both T1- and T2-weighted images. These findings are attributed to spatial mismapping caused by metal hardware (artifact).

(DI, p. 1112)

A 52-year-old man underwent lumbar spine surgery three months ago. He now presents with persistent lower back pain, fever, and malaise. Lumbar X-ray shows loss of disc height. MRI shows T2 increased signal intensity, fluid collection at the surgical site, increased T2 signal intensity in paraspinal muscles, and persistent nerve root clumping on STIR sequences. CT scan shows bone destruction at the operated disc level.

- What is the best diagnostic clue for the patient's condition?
  A. Persistent nerve root clumping on STIR sequences
  B. Unexpected postoperative fluid collection with bone destruction
  C. Loss of disc height on radiographs
  D. Increased T2 signal intensity in paraspinal muscles

Correct Answer: B

Explanation:

The presence of an unexpected postoperative fluid collection and associated bone destruction is the most specific diagnostic clue for a postoperative spine infection. This finding, often observed on MRI or CT, should prompt further investigation and management to address the infection.

The best imaging tool for postoperative spine infection is contrast-enhanced MRI (C+ MRI), as it provides detailed visualization of infection-related changes. However, when hardware susceptibility affects MRI quality, FDG-PET can be considered as an alternative. For protocol optimization, STIR sequences are highly effective in detecting marrow edema, and fat-suppressed techniques enhance the conspicuity of infection, improving diagnostic accuracy.

(DI, p. 1097)

54. A 45-year-old man presents with persistent back pain and a palpable soft tissue mass over the lumbar region six months after lumbar laminectomy. MRI reveals a lobulated CSF signal collection dorsal to the thecal sac.
   (a) Which of the following findings on imaging best supports the diagnosis of pseudomeningocele?
      A. Hyperintense signal on T1-weighted images with enhancement
      B. CSF-like signal on T2-weighted images with communication to the thecal sac
      C. Hypointense signal on T2-weighted images with restricted diffusion
      D. Fluid collection with irregular soft tissue enhancement
   (b) What additional imaging feature would confirm pseudomeningocele?
      A. Thickened dural enhancement on T1-weighted MRI with contrast
      B. Peripheral fluid restriction on diffusion-weighted imaging

C. Identification of thecal sac communication on T2-weighted MRI
D. Presence of a lobulated fluid collection with gadolinium enhancement

Correct Answers: 45a: B, 45b: C

Explanation:

Pseudomeningocele, also known as dural dehiscence, is a collection of spinal fluid communicated with the thecal sac but not lined with meninges. It commonly occurs after trauma or surgery, such as laminectomy. The most common location is at the dorsal lumbar operative site, with rare intraosseous locations

Imaging Features:

Radiography: Generally nonspecific, showing postoperative changes like laminectomy defects.

CT: Reveals CSF-density cysts adjacent to the thecal sac, often aligned with the surgical approach. Intrathecal contrast may help demonstrate dural communication.

MRI: The gold-standard imaging modality. T1- and T2-weighted images show **CSF-intensity collections, with axial and sagittal T2 sequences identifying thecal sac communication.** Fat-saturated T2 sequences are particularly effective. Pseudomeningoceles lack restricted diffusion and enhancement unless infected or inflamed.

Ultrasound: May show a hypoechoic cyst.

Myelography: Useful for confirming the communication between the thecal sac and pseudomeningocele.

(DI, p. 1101)

55. A 68-year-old male presents with chronic low back pain that worsens with standing upright and extension, but improves with flexion. Radiographs reveal close apposition of adjacent spinous processes with sclerosis of their margins. MRI demonstrates T2 hyperintensity in the interspinous ligament and mild enhancement of adjacent soft tissues after contrast administration. No significant neural foraminal narrowing or disc herniation is noted.

Which of the following findings is least likely to be associated with this patient's condition?

A. Sclerosis of adjacent spinous processes on CT or radiographs
B. T2 hyperintensity of the interspinous ligament with cystic degeneration
C. Severe compression of the thecal sac causing spinal canal stenosis
D. Mild enhancement of the interspinous ligament on contrast-enhanced MRI

Correct Answer: C

Explanation:

Baastrup disease typically involves the interspinous ligament and adjacent spinous processes without direct involvement of the thecal sac or significant canal stenosis. Findings such as sclerosis on radiographs (A), T2 hyperintensity with cystic degeneration (B), and mild enhancement of the ligament (D) are characteristic. Severe thecal sac compression (C) is more indicative of other pathologies, such as disc herniation or ligamentum flavum hypertrophy.

(DI, p. 431)

56. A 35-year-old male is brought to the emergency department after a high-speed motor vehicle accident. He complains of severe back pain. Radiographs show a wedge-shaped vertebral body deformity at L2 with a loss of more than 50% anterior vertebral body height. AP view reveals an "empty body sign." No significant vertebral body subluxation is noted. A CT scan confirms a transverse fracture of the posterior elements and increased interspinous distance.
 Which of the following findings is LEAST likely associated with this patient's injury?
 A. Focal kyphosis at the level of the injury
 B. Discontinuous anterior longitudinal ligament (ALL)
 C. Separation of facet joints on axial imaging
 D. Buckling or mild retropulsion of the posterior cortex
 Correct Answer: B
 Explanation:
 Chance fractures are typically flexion-distraction, where the middle and posterior columns fail under tension and the anterior column is compressed.
 Radiographic findings of a chance fracture include anterior vertebral body wedging with trabecular impaction, >40–50% height loss, focal kyphosis, posterior column injuries like facet joint separation, and no vertebral body subluxation. The "empty body sign" on AP radiographs may be seen due to spinous process displacement. CT shows comminuted vertebral body fractures, posterior ligamentous injuries (e.g., naked facet sign), and retropulsed posterior cortex. MRI highlights fracture lines with low signal on all sequences, surrounding edema on T1 and T2/STIR, and potential ligament discontinuities mainly in the posterior element.
 (DI, p. 300)
57. What is the most typical imaging feature of an intradural extramedullary tumor, such as a schwannoma, on MRI?
 A. Isointense on T1 and T2 with no post-contrast enhancement
 B. Hypointense on T1, hyperintense on T2, with homogeneous contrast enhancement
 C. Hyperintense on T1 and hypo on T2, with homogeneous contrast enhancement
 D. Isointense on T1, isointense on T2, with homogeneous contrast enhancement
 Correct Answer: B
 Explanation:
 On MRI, schwannomas typically appear **iso- or hypointense** relative to the spinal cord or nerve roots on T1-weighted imaging, with melanotic schwannomas exhibiting hyperintensity. **On T2-weighted** imaging, 75% of schwannomas are **hyperintense**, with cystic changes seen in 40% of cases and occasional hemorrhage in 10%. Some may display a "target sign," characterized by a high-signal rim and a low-intensity center, though this is more common in neurofibromas. Spinal cord compression may result in associated myelomalacia or edema. On post-contrast T1-weighted imaging, schwannomas usually show

homogeneous enhancement but sometimes variable enhancement patterns, including uniform or peripheral enhancement.

(DI, p. 769)

58. In the evaluation of discitis-osteomyelitis, what imaging characteristic is most specific on MRI?
    A. High T2 signal intensity within the vertebral body
    B. Vivid gadolinium enhancement of the disc space
    C. Hypointensity on T1-weighted images with enhancement of endplates
    D. Loss of vertebral body height with paraspinal muscle enhancement

    Correct Answer: C

    Explanation:

    In discitis and vertebral osteomyelitis, the most characteristic imaging characteristic on MRI is T1 hypointensity of the vertebral endplates with contrast enhancement following. This finding indicates inflammation and infection of the endplates, a characteristic in discitis and vertebral osteomyelitis.

    High T2 signal intensity within the vertebral body (A): This is suggestive but nonspecific, as it may also be seen in other inflammatory or neoplastic conditions.

    Vivid gadolinium enhancement of the disc space (B): The Disc space usually has a variable enhancement pattern, either diffuse or rim enhancement. Not a vivid enhancement

    Loss of vertebral body height with paraspinal muscle enhancement (D): Loss of height may occur in severe cases, but paraspinal enhancement is not exclusive to discitis-osteomyelitis.

    T1 hypointensity with endplate enhancement best correlates with the pathophysiological process of the infection spreading from the disc to the adjacent vertebrae.

    (DI, p. 563)

59. What is the most reliable radiologic finding of atlanto-occipital dissociation (AOD) in trauma patients?
    A. Atlanto-dens interval (ADI) > 3 mm
    B. Disruption of the alar ligaments on MRI
    C. Basion-dens interval (BDI) > 12 mm
    D. Lateral displacement of C1 lateral masses

    Correct Answer: C

    Explanation:

    Various methods have been developed to diagnose atlanto-occipital dissociation (AOD) radiographically. None are entirely reliable. Measurements on CT scans are more precise than those on plain radiographs. Some of the commonly used measurements (Fig. 2.25):

    - **Basion-Axial Interval (BAI)**: This measurement represents the distance from the basion to the upper margin of the posterior axial line (PAL) on C2. It is effective for detecting both anterior and posterior AOD. Normal BAI values on plain X-ray are ≤12 mm in adults and up to 12 mm in pediatric cases. On CT, it may be used, but reliability is limited.

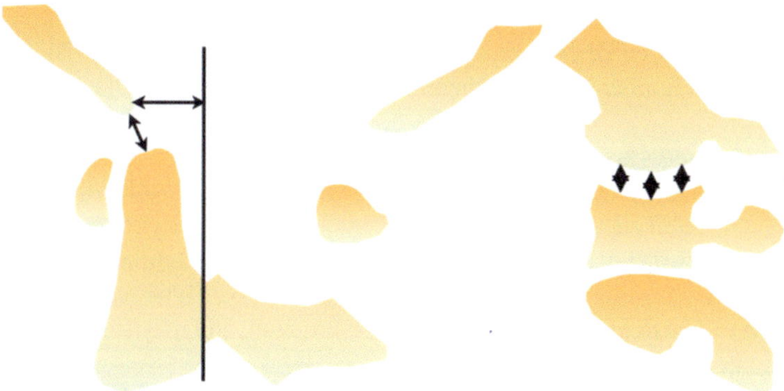

Fig. 2.25 Atlanto-occipital dissociation measurements (AOD)

- **Basion-Dental Interval (BDI)**: This interval is the distance from the basion to the tip of the odontoid and is useful for identifying distracted AOD. **It is one of the most specific findings with the condylar gap**. Normal BDI values on X-ray for adults are ≤12 mm. In children under 13, BDI is unreliable due to varying ossification ages and fusion stages of the odontoid. For adults on CT, the normal BDI should be <8.5 mm, while for pediatric patients, it should be <10.5 mm.
- **The condylar-C1 Interval (CCI)** or **condylar gap**, measures the distance between the occipital condyle and the superior articular surface of C1. On plain X-ray, the interval should be ≤2 mm in adults and ≤ 5 mm in pediatric patients. On CT, the normal value for adults is <1.4 mm. For pediatric patients, it should be <2.5 mm

Power's ratio: The power's ratio is calculated as ratio is measured as the ratio of the distance in the midsagittal plane between (AB/CD):

- Basion (A) and the posterior spinolaminar line of the atlas (B) and
- Opisthion (C) and the anterior arch of the atlas (D).

Normal values are <1 on CT or X-ray.

(RP)

60. On spinal imaging, what radiological feature distinguishes a benign hemangioma from a malignant lesion?

A. Diffuse T1 and T2 hyperintensity
B. Heterogeneous signal intensity with involvement of the posterior elements
C. Retropulsion of bony fragments into the spinal canal
D. Presence of a fat signal on T1-weighted imaging

Correct Answer: D

Explanation:

The radiological features of **spinal hemangioma** and **metastasis can,** in most cases, differ. **Spinal hemangiomas** typically demonstrate hyperintensity on **T1 MRI due to fatty marrow** and T2 hyperintensity, because of vascular content and edema. On CT, they exhibit a classic "corduroy" or "honeycomb" pattern on sagittal images and a "polka-dot" appearance on axial scans due to thickened vertical trabeculae. Post-gadolinium, hemangiomas demonstrate mild, homogeneous enhancement. They usually remain confined to a single vertebra without significant involvement of posterior elements or adjacent soft tissues.

In contrast, **metastases** appear hypointense on T1-weighted MRI as they replace normal marrow and show variable T2-weighted signal, often hyperintense with associated edema. MRI with contrast typically shows heterogeneous enhancement, and metastases frequently involve multiple vertebrae with possible soft tissues or epidural space extension. CT scan shows lytic, sclerotic, or mixed lesions with irregular margins, cortical destruction, and may show pathological fractures.

These imaging differences, combined with clinical history, provide critical insights for diagnosis. Sometimes it is difficult to distinguish both them specifically in the case of aggressive hemangioma.

(DI, p. 670)

61. A 35-year-old patient presents with progressive sensory deficits and intermittent sharp pain in the upper extremities. MRI of the cervical spine shows a fluid-filled cavity within the spinal cord, extending from C4 to C7. The cavity is eccentric, with septations visible on T2-weighted imaging, and there is evidence of spinal cord edema. Which of the following imaging findings would most likely help distinguish this lesion from a benign central canal dilatation?
    A. Smooth, regular margins of the cavity following CSF intensity
    B. Septations within the cavity with associated cord edema
    C. Lack of spinal cord atrophy or structural distortion
    D. Hypointensity on T1 and hyperintensity on T2 without inflammation

    Correct Answer: B

    Explanation:

    Central canal dilatations and syrinx in most cases differ in their radiographic features. Central canal dilatation is an enlargement of the normal central canal of the spinal cord. They are congenital and asymptomatic. On MRI, they appear smooth with regular margins. They resemble cerebrospinal fluid in signal intensity, showing T1 hypointensity and T2 hyperintensity. They do not have associated spinal cord changes like edema or atrophy. Contrarily, a syrinx is a fluid-filled cavity within the spinal cord, often associated with underlying conditions such as Chiari malformations, trauma, tumors, or arachnoiditis. Syrinxes are usually eccentric and have irregular shapes, with possible septations or debris. They usually expand asymmetrically. On MRI, they also demonstrate T1 hypointensity and T2 hyperintensity. They may show contrast enhancement if there is inflammation or tumor involvement. In extreme cases, syrinxes can be associated with spinal cord edema, atrophy, or tethering.

    (DI, pp. 330–334)

62. A 17-year-old male presents with chronic, localized back pain that worsens at night and is relieved by NSAIDs. Imaging shows focal scoliosis concave on the

symptomatic side. Radiography reveals an area of sclerosis in the posterior elements of a lumbar vertebra. A CT scan is performed.
What is the most likely CT finding confirming the diagnosis?
A. Sclerotic vertebral body with loss of height
B. Central radiolucent nidus surrounded by reactive sclerosis
C. Diffuse vertebral marrow edema with cortical thickening
D. Enhancing soft tissue mass extending into adjacent structures
Correct Answer: B
Explanation:
Osteoid osteoma is a small, benign bone tumor that affects young patients. They usually cause back pain that responds to NSAIDs. Radiographically, they usually have a radiolucent nidus surrounded by reactive sclerosis. They are seen in the spine in 10% of cases, predominantly in the posterior element of the lumbar region (59%), followed by cervical (27%) and thoracic (12%) regions. The nidus is usually less than 1.5 cm, if larger lesions are considered as osteoblastomas.

X-ray often reveals a central lucent nidus, though it may be obscured by surrounding sclerosis. Focal scoliosis concave to the tumor side is a typical finding. CT is the gold standard, showing details of the central nidus that may show variable ossification. IT might show reactive changes like dense sclerosis, periosteal reaction, and occasionally soft tissue masses or ossification of adjacent structures like the ligamentum flavum.

MRI usually shows nidus as low-intensity on T1 and variable signal intensity on T2 and STIR. It can also show surrounding edema, which appears low T1 and high T2 signal with gadolinium enhancement. The nidus can be missed on MRI because of its small size, oblique orientation, or partial volume effects, leading to potential misdiagnosis as infection or malignancy.

Bone scans with Tc-99 m MDP show positive uptake in all three phases, making them highly sensitive.
(DI, p. 701)

63. A 28-year-old patient with a history of sickle cell disease presents with chronic lower back pain. Physical examination is unremarkable. What is the best diagnostic clue for identifying spine involvement in sickle cell disease on imaging?
A. Generalized osteopenia with biconcave vertebrae
B. Presence of patchy sclerosis in long bones
C. H-shaped vertebral bodies due to central endplate compression deformities
D. Increased signal intensity on MRI in the vertebral body marrow spaces
Correct Answer: C.
Explanation:
Sickle cell disease has characteristic findings on spinal imaging. The key finding is **H-shaped vertebral bodies caused by central endplate compression deformities**, best seen on sagittal views of X-ray or CT. Sickle cell disease affects the spine in 40–70% of patients, although bone infarcts more commonly

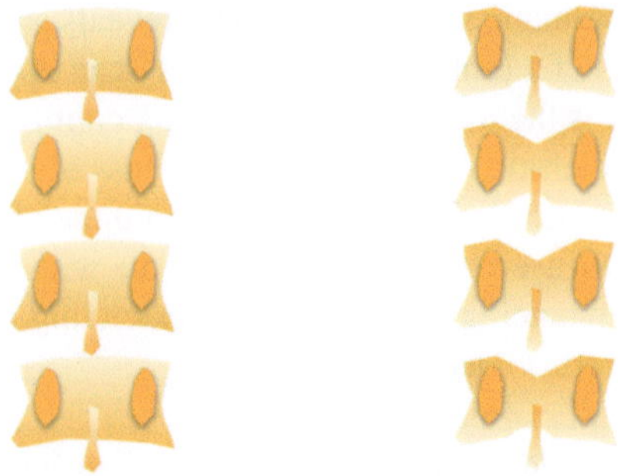
Normal coronal lumbar x-ray
Coronal lumbar x-ray showing H-shaped vertebra in sickle cell disease

Fig. 2.26 Illustration showing normal coronal lumbar X-ray compared to X-ray in a sickle cell disease patient showing the classic H-shaped vertebrae

affect long bones. X-rays may show patchy or diffuse sclerosis. It is caused by bone infarcts, osteopenia with vertebral compression fractures, and occasionally, tower vertebrae due to compensatory vertical growth. CT scans highlight mottled sclerosis in the medullary spaces and central endplate deformities, confirming the H-shaped vertebrae, as well as osteoporotic compression fractures (Fig. 2.26).

(RP)

Spine Neurophysiology, Electrodiagnostic, and Neuromonitoring

3

1. In the context of nerve conduction studies, which of the following changes is most indicative of demyelinating peripheral neuropathies?
   A. Decreased amplitude of action potentials
   B. Prolonged latency and decreased conduction velocity
   C. Increased amplitude with normal latency
   D. Normal conduction velocity with decreased amplitude
   Correct Answer: B
   Explanation:
   Demyelinating peripheral neuropathies disrupt normal nerve signal transmission. The most common feature is **slowed conduction velocity** and **prolonged latency**. This occurs due to damage to the myelin sheath, which impairs rapid impulse conduction. Amplitude reduction is not a primary feature since axons remain mostly intact. Instead, decreased conduction speed is the hallmark finding in nerve conduction studies.
   (SS, p. 169)
2. EMG is used to assess the following muscle characteristics:
   A. Insertional activity
   B. Motor unit action potential
   C. Rccruitments
   D. All of the above
   Correct Answer: D
   (SS, p. 169)
3. What do Motor Unit Action Potentials (MUAPs) represent in EMG?
   A. Brain signals during movement
   B. Single muscle fiber activity at rest
   C. Motor neuron and muscle fiber signals during contraction
   D. Sensory neuron response to stimulation
   Correct Answer: C
   Explanation:

K. F. AlAli, H. T. Hashim, *Spine Surgery and Peripheral Nerve Surgery*,
https://doi.org/10.1007/978-3-031-98543-0_3

MUAPs are electrical signals from a motor neuron and its muscle fibers during contraction. EMG detects these signals to assess neuromuscular function.

(SS, p. 169)

4. What do fibrillation potentials indicate in an EMG study?
   A. Complete nerve regeneration
   B. Motor axon loss
   C. Sensory nerve dysfunction
   D. Muscle hypertrophy

   Correct Answer: B

   Explanation:

   Fibrillation potentials signal motor axon loss and are seen in neuropathy, trauma, and muscle disorders. They do not indicate sensory dysfunction or muscle growth. Their presence confirms denervation, but their number does not reflect the severity of axonal loss.

   (SS, p. 171)
5. Why is the F-wave not highly reliable for diagnosing radiculopathy?
   A. It only detects sensory nerve damage.
   B. Most muscles are supplied by multiple roots, making localization difficult.
   C. It does not change after nerve injury.
   D. It is only abnormal in mild radiculopathy.

   Correct Answer: B

   Explanation:

   An **F-wave** occurs when a **supramaximal electrical stimulus** excites a **peripheral nerve**, sending an **antidromic signal** to the spinal cord. A small number of **anterior horn cells** are then activated, generating a **returning motor response** recorded in the muscle.

   It can be abnormal after nerve root injury, but since most muscles receive input from multiple roots, identifying one affected root is challenging. F-wave studies are more useful for detecting multiple root lesions or proximal neuropathies, like Guillain-Barré syndrome.

   (SS, p. 173)
6. Which of the following is **NOT** a common EMG finding in radiculopathy?
   A. Positive sharp waves
   B. Fibrillation potentials
   C. Fasciculation potentials
   D. Prolonged F-wave latency

   Correct Answer: C

   Explanation:

   Fasciculation potentials are associated with hyperexcitability of nerve and anterior horn cell diseases. Radiculopathy on EMG typically shows positive sharp waves and fibrillation potentials with prolonged F-wave latency due to nerve root irritation.

   (SS, p. 171)

7. Regarding EMG role in thoracic radiculopathy:
   7a. How can needle EMG help diagnose thoracic radiculopathy?
      A. By detecting fibrillations in abdominal wall muscles
      B. By measuring sensory nerve conduction in the thoracic spine
      C. By assessing reflex responses in the lower limbs
      D. By analyzing motor unit recruitment in the hands
   7b. Why is EMG not always conclusive in diagnosing thoracic radiculopathy?
      A. It cannot detect denervation in thoracic muscles.
      B. It cannot differentiate between compressive and diabetic thoracic radiculopathy.
      C. It is only useful for lumbar radiculopathy.
      D. It cannot detect fibrillations in paraspinal muscles.

   Correct Answers: 7a: A, 7b: B

   Explanation:

   EMG helps in the diagnosis of thoracic radiculopathy by recognizing fibrillations in the anterior abdominal wall and thoracic paraspinal muscles. However, it cannot differentiate between compressive and metabolic causes of radiculopathy. Sensory conduction tests are ineffective in diagnosing thoracic radiculopathy.

   (SS, p. 173)

8. What is the sensitivity range of EMG for detecting cervical radiculopathy?
   A. 10%–30%
   B. 25%–40%
   C. 50%–71%
   D. 80%–95%

   Correct Answer: C

   Explanation:

   EMG sensitivity for cervical radiculopathy is generally between 50% and 71%. For lumbosacral radiculopathy, reported sensitivity varies from 29% to 90%.

   (SS, p. 174)

9. One of the following explains the limitation of electrodiagnostic studies in patients with a history of laminectomy:
   A. Denervated paraspinal muscle
   B. Lack of spinous process
   C. Enhanced EMG sensitivity for radiculopathy
   D. Preservation of all motor unit potentials

   Correct Answer: A

   Explanation:

   Electrodiagnostic tests have limited usefulness after laminectomy. Paraspinal muscle changes are hard to assess since denervation signals may come from surgical trauma rather than nerve abnormalities.

   (SS, p. 175)

10. Which modality would be best suited during the intraoperative neuromonitoring (IONM) to evaluate the functional integrity of the dorsal columns of the spinal cord?
   A. H-reflex
   B. Transcranial motor evoked potentials (TcMEPs)
   C. Electromyography (EMG)
   D. Somatosensory evoked potentials (SSEPs)

   Correct Answer: D

   Explanation:

   SSEPs are used to monitor the dorsal column (medial lemniscus) pathway. It is responsible for proprioception and fine touch. EMG monitors muscle activity, and the H-reflex assesses reflex arcs and peripheral nerves.

   (SS, p. 169)
11. All of the following is correct about somatosensory-evoked potentials (SSEPs), EXCEPT:
   A. It is a modification of the basic EEG.
   B. It is a continuous monitoring.
   C. It assesses the direct spinal cord motor tracts.
   D. It monitors cortical responses to repetitive stimuli.

   Correct Answer: C

   Explanation:

   SSEP is continuous monitoring during spinal surgery. It is basically a modification of an EEG. It monitors cortical and subcortical responses to repetitive peripheral nerve stimulation cranially and caudally to the operative field. It gives direct monitoring to the spinal cord sensory tracts and indirect monitoring to the spinal cord motor tracts.

   (SS, p. 217)
12. All of the following can interfere with SSEPs, EXCEPT:
   A. Neuronavigation
   B. Halogenated anesthetic agents
   C. Nitrous oxide
   D. Hypertension

   Correct Answer: D

   Explanation:

   Any electrical power in the operating room can affect SSEP recordings, like neuronavigation. It can also be affected by halogenated anesthetic agents, nitrous oxide, hypothermia, and hypotension.

   (SS, p. 218)
13. What do transcranial electrical motor evoked potentials (TcMEPs) measure during spine surgery?
   A. Sensory nerve conduction in the spinal cord
   B. Electrical activity in the dorsal columns
   C. Motor pathways function by stimulating the motor cortex
   D. Reflex responses from peripheral nerves

   Correct Answer: C

   Explanation:

TcMEPs monitor the corticospinal tract, making it a complement to SSEPs. It is done by applying scalp electrodes to induce a high-voltage stimulus to stimulate specific areas of the motor cortex. Then the impulses go through cortical spine tracts and are recorded from electrodes placed in muscles in the upper and lower extremities. It can record compound muscle action potential (CMAP).

(SS, p. 218)

14. Why is EMG monitoring used during spinal procedures?
    A. To evaluate the functional status of individual nerve roots
    B. To monitor blood flow in the spinal cord
    C. To measure muscle strength during surgery
    D. To assess bone density around pedicle screws

    Correct Answer: A

    Explanation:

    EMG helps detect nerve root irritation or injury during spinal procedures. It ensures nerve integrity is maintained when inserting pedicle screws, manipulating nerve roots, or placing implants.

    (SS, p. 219)
15. When is free-running EMG most useful during spine surgery?
    A. Before surgery to map nerve pathways
    B. During pedicle screw insertion and nerve root manipulation
    C. After surgery, to check for nerve healing
    D. Only in cases of severe spinal cord injury

    Correct Answer: B

    Explanation:

    There are two types of EMG used in spine surgery monitoring. Free-running EMG (spontaneous EMG) detects nerve irritation in dynamic phases of surgery, such as screw placement or nerve root manipulation. Triggered EMG, or stimulus-evoked EMG, is used in static phases (after screw placement).

    (SS, p. 219)
16. What indicates a pedicle wall breach when testing with EMG?
    A. No response at any stimulation level
    B. Sudden loss of spinal reflexes
    C. Increased cerebrospinal fluid pressure
    D. Muscle contraction due to nerve root stimulation

    Correct Answer: D

    Explanation:

    If the pedicle wall is damaged, electrical current escapes through the breach when using an EMG probe and stimulates the nerve root, leading to muscle contraction. This response is detected on EMG and signals potential screw misplacement.

    (SS, p. 219)
17. Which nerve is monitored using SSEPs to detect brachial plexopathy due to arm positioning?
    A. Musculocutaneous nerve
    B. Ulnar nerve
    C. Tibial nerve

D. Radial nerve

Correct Answer: B

Explanation:

SSEPs of the ulnar nerve help detect brachial plexus compression caused by improper arm positioning during surgery. This helps prevent permanent nerve damage in the upper limb.

(SS, p. 219)

18. In the setting of acute spinal cord injury, which neuromonitoring finding is most predictive of a poor neurological outcome?
A. Absent TcMEPs
B. Preserved SSEPs
C. Decreased amplitude of EMG
D. Unchanged H-reflex

Correct Answer: A

Explanation:

The absence of TcMEPs is highly predictive of postoperative motor deficits, as it indicates a loss of motor pathway function. SSEPs may be preserved even with significant motor deficits, as they monitor different pathways.

(GB, p. 253)

19. What is the most common cause of false-negative SSEP findings during spinal surgery?
A. Technical error in electrode placement
B. Intraoperative hypothermia
C. Use of neuromuscular blocking agents
D. Use of inhalational anesthetics

Correct Answer: D

Explanation:

Inhalation anesthetics can severely affect the SSEP signals considerably, which leads to false negative results. It is important to communicate with the anesthesia team to maintain anesthesia that enables reliable SSEP monitoring.

(GB, p. 1732)

20. Which of the following is NOT a recommended practice for reducing the risk of false positives during EMG monitoring in spine surgery?
A. Minimizing the use of electrocautery near monitored muscles
B. Ensuring proper grounding of the patient
C. Using high-frequency filters to reduce electrical interference
D. Increasing the stimulus intensity to maximum levels

Correct Answer: D

Explanation:

Increasing stimulus intensity to maximum levels can increase the risk of false positives due to crosstalk and direct muscle stimulation. It is important to use an appropriate stimulus intensity that is sufficient to elicit a response without causing artifacts.

[71]

21. Which electrodiagnostic test is the most sensitive to recognizing earlier changes in the context of spondylotic cervical spondylotic myelopathy?
    A. SSEPs elicited by median nerve stimulation
    B. TcMEPs elicited by transcranial electrical stimulation
    C. Needle EMG of upper limb muscles
    D. Nerve conduction studies (NCS) of the median nerve

    Correct Answer: A

    Explanation:

    SSEPs are sensitive to recognizing subclinical changes in the dorsal columns that can be influenced early in cervical spondylotic myelopathy.

    (SS, p. 169)
22. What is the primary limitation of free-running EMG in detecting nerve root injury during spine surgery?
    A. It cannot differentiate between mechanical and thermal nerve root injury.
    B. It is highly sensitive to anesthetic agents.
    C. It only provides information about motor fibers.
    D. It is unable to detect injury until it has occurred.

    Correct Answer: D

    Explanation:

    Free-running EMG detects spontaneous muscle activity indicative of nerve irritation or injury, but does not predict or prevent injury.

    [72]
23. One of the findings in EMG is exclusive to severe spinal stenosis:
    A. Chronic denervation in lower limb muscles
    B. Reduced recruitment patterns
    C. Fibrillation potentials
    D. Normal findings at rest

    Correct Answer: C

    Explanation:

    In severe stenosis, fibrillation potentials and positive sharp waves are exclusive findings in EMG compared to mild or moderate spinal stenosis cases.

    [73]
24. What is the most common cause of intraoperative loss of SSEPs that is NOT due to a surgical event?
    A. Patient movement
    B. Anesthetic depth
    C. Electrode displacement
    D. Blood pressure changes

    Correct Answer: B

    Explanation:

    Anesthetic agents, particularly inhalational agents, can significantly affect SSEP amplitude and latency, leading to changes that are not related to surgical manipulation.

    (GB, p. 1732)

25. Which of the following complications is common when using transcranial electrical motor evoked potentials (TcMEPs)?
    A. Tongue or lip laceration
    B. Permanent nerve damage
    C. Sudden cardiac arrhythmia
    D. Loss of somatosensory function

    Correct Answer: A

    Explanation:

    TcMEPs produce positive electrical shocks to the motor cortex, resulting in muscle contractions. This can cause tongue or lip injuries.

    (SS, p. 219)
26. During surgery for an intramedullary spinal cord tumor, SSEPs suddenly disappear, but MEPs remain normal. What is the most likely cause?
    A. Anesthetic effects
    B. Dorsal column injury
    C. MEP technical issue
    D. Inadequate muscle relaxation

    Correct Answer: B

    Explanation:

    SSEPs monitor dorsal column function, while MEPs assess corticospinal tracts. A sudden loss of SSEPs with intact MEPs suggests isolated dorsal column damage. Anesthesia affects both signals, not just SSEPs. MEP issues or muscle relaxation problems would alter MEPs, not SSEPs alone.

    (GB, p. 253)
27. In intraoperative neuromonitoring (IONM), what does an increase in latency and a decrease in amplitude of SSEPs suggest?
    A. Normal variability
    B. Technical issue with the recording equipment
    C. Possible neurological injury
    D. Improved neurological function

    Correct Answer: C

    Explanation:

    An increase in latency and a decrease in amplitude of SSEPs may indicate a compromise of the sensory pathways, suggesting possible neurological injury.

    [74]
28. Which of the following is NOT a recommended intervention when a significant change in TcMEPs is observed intraoperatively?
    A. Increase mean arterial pressure (MAP)
    B. Administer corticosteroids
    C. Warm the patient to normothermia
    D. Immediate cessation of surgery

    Correct Answer: D

    Explanation:

    While cessation of surgery may be considered in some cases, the initial interventions typically include optimizing MAP, warming the patient, and

potentially administering corticosteroids to address reversible causes of the changes in TcMEPs.
(SS, p. 219)

29. Which of the following is the most appropriate electrodiagnostic study to assess chronic radiculopathy?
    A. Sensory Nerve Conduction Studies (NCS)
    B. Motor Nerve Conduction Studies (NCS)
    C. Somatosensory Evoked Potentials (SSEPs)
    D. Needle Electromyography (EMG)

    Correct Answer: D
    Explanation:
    EMG is most useful in detecting chronic radiculopathy, showing denervation in muscles innervated by the affected nerve root.
    (HS, p. 81)

30. In a patient with chronic radiculopathy, which of the following EMG findings is most consistent with reinnervation?
    A. Fibrillation potentials
    B. Polyphasic motor unit action potentials (MUAPs)
    C. Positive sharp waves
    D. Decreased recruitment pattern

    Correct Answer: B
    Explanation:
    Polyphasic MUAPs suggest reinnervation as axonal sprouting leads to more complex action potentials.
    (HS, p. 82)

31. Which nerve is most likely affected if EMG shows spontaneous activity in the peroneus longus muscle?
    A. L4
    B. L2
    C. L5
    D. L3

    Correct Answer: C
    Explanation:
    The peroneus longus muscle is innervated by the L5 nerve root, and spontaneous activity may suggest radiculopathy.
    (GB, p. 534)

32. In a patient with lumbar stenosis and radiculopathy, which electrodiagnostic finding is most likely?
    A. Normal nerve conduction studies (NCS) with abnormal EMG
    B. Abnormal NCS with normal EMG
    C. Decreased sensory nerve action potentials (SNAPs)
    D. Increased insertional activity in the paraspinal muscles only

    Correct Answer: A
    Explanation:

Nerve conduction studies are often normal in radiculopathy because they assess peripheral nerves, whereas EMG detects denervation in affected muscles.

(GB, p. 255)

33. Which of the following electrodiagnostic findings is typical in Guillain-Barré syndrome (GBS)?
    A. Decreased CMAP amplitude
    B. Normal conduction velocity
    C. Prolonged distal motor latency
    D. Reduced F-wave latency

    Correct Answer: C

    Explanation:

    GBS often presents with prolonged distal latencies due to demyelination, polyradiculopathy, and may have features of axonal degeneration in EMG.

    (NB, p. 423)
34. Which nerve conduction study finding is most characteristic of carpal tunnel syndrome?
    A. Increased conduction velocity across the wrist
    B. Decreased amplitude of CMAPs over the median nerve
    C. Increased F-wave latency in the ulnar nerve
    D. Prolonged distal latency of the median nerve sensory response

    Correct Answer: D

    Explanation:

    Carpal tunnel syndrome results in delayed conduction across the wrist, especially affecting sensory fibers. It causes prolonged median nerve sensory latencies with prolongation of motor distal latency.

    (GB, p. 548)
35. Which of the following is true regarding H-reflex testing?
    A. It is used to assess sensory fibers.
    B. It primarily evaluates the S1 nerve root.
    C. It is absent in all demyelinating conditions.
    D. It is more sensitive than F-wave testing.

    Correct Answer: B

    Explanation:

    The H-reflex assesses the S1 nerve root and is used to evaluate radiculopathies or sacral plexopathies.

    (SS, p. 172)
36. In a patient with L5 radiculopathy, which EMG finding is most characteristic?
    A. Normal motor unit potentials in the tibialis anterior
    B. Fibrillation potentials in the gluteus maximus
    C. Polyphasic motor unit potentials in the gastrocnemius
    D. Positive sharp waves in the tibialis anterior

    Correct Answer: D

    Explanation:

    Positive sharp waves and fibrillations are seen in denervated muscles, such as the tibialis anterior, in L5 radiculopathy.

    (SS, p. 174)

37. Which of the following best explains why needle EMG is useful in identifying acute denervation?
    A. It detects decreased conduction velocity
    B. It can identify fibrillations
    C. It measures compound motor action potentials.
    D. It evaluates distal motor latencies.

    Correct Answer: B

    Explanation:

    Fibrillations and positive sharp waves are characteristic of acute denervation on EMG. Early denervation might also induce motor unit potential (MUP) variation.

    (NB, p. 208)
38. In the comparison between EMG and NCS, which statement is CORRECT?
    A. NCS can detect muscle denervation earlier than EMG.
    B. EMG is primarily used to assess myelin integrity, while NCS evaluates muscle function.
    C. NCS is more useful than EMG for diagnosing radiculopathy.
    D. EMG is best for detecting radiculopathy, and NCS is best for entrapment neuropathy.

    Correct Answer: D

    (SS, p. 169)
39. Why are electrodiagnostic studies not indicated during the early phase of the injury?
    A. Axonal degeneration occurs gradually.
    B. NCS is always inaccurate for nerve injuries.
    C. Early nerve injuries heal too quickly for testing.
    D. EMG can detect denervation immediately after injury.

    Correct Answer: A

    Explanation:

    After nerve injury, Wallerian degeneration occurs distal to the lesion, but it takes 7–10 days to appear on nerve conduction studies (NCS). Fibrillation potentials on EMG also take about 10–14 days to develop. NCS is still reliable, but it must be done at the right time. Nerve healing does not occur too quickly, and EMG cannot detect immediate denervation.

    (SS, p. 169)
40. What EMG finding helps distinguish radiculopathy from peripheral nerve injury?
    A. Slow conduction velocity
    B. Loss of sensory nerve action potentials
    C. Abnormalities confined to a single myotome
    D. Decreased motor unit recruitment in all tested muscles

    Correct Answer: C

    Explanation:

    In radiculopathy, EMG changes show up in one myotome. Peripheral nerve injuries follow a specific nerve's path instead. Sensory nerve action potentials stay normal in radiculopathy. This happens because the lesion is before the dorsal root ganglion.

(SS, p. 171)

41. Why are paraspinal muscles important in diagnosing radiculopathy by EMG?
    A. They are always affected in radiculopathy.
    B. They help confirm radiculopathy when limb muscles are normal.
    C. They are the first muscles to show denervation.
    D. Their findings alone are enough for diagnosis.

    Correct Answer: B

    Explanation:

    Paraspinal muscles are only innervated by spinal nerve roots, not peripheral nerves. Their involvement confirms a radicular origin of the problem, but they may appear normal in chronic or cervical radiculopathies.

    (SS, p. 171)

4 Biologics in Spine Fusion Surgery

1. Which property of autograft bone makes it the gold standard for spinal fusion?
   A. Osteoconduction only
   B. Osteoinduction only
   C. Osteogenesis only
   D. All of the above
   Correct Answer: D
   Explanation:
   Autograft bone is bone taken from the patient and grafted in another site of the same patient (e.g., iliac crest graft) or grafted in the same site, called local autograft (e.g, laminectomy). Autograft bone is the only material that possesses all three essential properties required for successful spinal fusion.
   (SS, p. 243)
2. What is the primary advantage of using the iliac crest bone graft in spinal fusion?
   A. Minimal harvest-related morbidity
   B. High arthrodesis rates
   C. Osteogenic only properties
   D. Low cost
   Correct Answer: B
   Explanation:
   Iliac crest bone graft provides excellent osteoconductive, osteoinductive, and osteogenic properties, making it effective for high fusion rates.
   (SS, p. 243)
3. Which of the following is a limitation of using demineralized bone matrix (DBM) in spinal fusion?
   A. Lack of osteoinductive properties
   B. Lack of osteoconductivity
   C. Lack of osteogenesis
   D. All of the above
   Correct Answer: C

K. F. AlAli, H. T. Hashim, *Spine Surgery and Peripheral Nerve Surgery*,
https://doi.org/10.1007/978-3-031-98543-0_4

Explanation:

DBM has osteoinductive properties and is osteoinductive but lacks osteogenesis.

(SS, p. 243)

4. Which biologic agent should NOT be used in the anterior cervical spine due to its associated risks?
   A. Autograft
   B. Allograft
   C. Recombinant human bone morphogenetic protein-2 (rhBMP-2)
   D. Ceramic-based graft

   Correct Answer: C

   Explanation:

   rhBMP-2 carries significant risks in the anterior cervical spine, such as swelling and dysphagia.

   (SS, p. 250)
5. Which material is most commonly used as an osteoconductive scaffold in spinal fusion?
   A. Demineralized bone matrix
   B. Allograft
   C. Ceramic-based bone graft
   D. Bone marrow aspirate

   Correct Answer: C

   Explanation:

   Cement itself is used as a bone graft extender and not as a substitute for bone graft. Ceramic-based grafts are a cement extender with osteoinductive materials.

   They provide an osteoconductive matrix that supports bone growth.

   (SS, p. 249)
6. Which method helps increase the yield of osteogenic cells from bone marrow aspirate (BMA)?
   A. Reducing aspirate volume to below 2 mL
   B. Using the iliac crest only as the aspiration site
   C. Adding demineralized bone matrix to the aspirate
   D. Using an allograft to dilute the aspirate

   Correct Answer: A

   Explanation:

   Keeping the aspirate volume below 2 mL reduces dilution with peripheral blood, increasing the concentration of osteogenic precursor cells.

   (BS, p. 797)
7. Which of the following is a recognized advantage of using an allograft in spinal fusion?
   A. High osteoinductive properties
   B. Low risk of disease transmission
   C. Absence of harvest-related morbidity
   D. Unlimited osteogenic potential

   Correct Answer: C

Explanation:

Allografts eliminate the need for bone harvest from the patient, avoiding the morbidity associated with autograft harvest.

(BS, p. 797)

8. One of the following is the possible explanation why allografts have low osteoinductivity:
   A. Processing technique of allografts
   B. Higher concentration of bone morphogenetic proteins
   C. Immune response to allograft
   D. All of the above

   Correct Answer: A

   Explanation:

   Allografts undergo significant processing techniques to reduce immunogenicity and minimize infections. This can lead to low osteoinductivity.

   (BS, p. 797)
9. One of the following is correct about allograft osteoconductivity:
   A. Low osteoconductivity
   B. High osteoconductivity
   C. Absence of osteoconductivity
   D. Variable osteoconductivity depending on the manufacturer.

   Correct Answer: B

   (BS, p. 797)
10. Which of the following has shown a significantly higher fusion rate in lumbar interbody fusion compared to iliac crest bone graft?
    A. Recombinant human BMP-2
    B. Ceramic-based graft
    C. Allograft
    D. Bone marrow aspirate

    Correct Answer: A

    (BS, p. 799)
11. What is the primary mechanism through which recombinant human BMP-2 promotes spinal fusion?
    A. Osteoconduction
    B. Osteogenesis
    C. Osteoinduction
    D. Cartilage formation

    Correct Answer: C

    Explanation:

    rhBMP-2 stimulates the transformation of mesenchymal stem cells into osteoblasts. This promotes bone formation through osteoinduction.

    (BS, p. 799)
12. Which property is NOT a characteristic of a successful bone graft material in spine fusion?
    A. Osteogenesis
    B. Osteoconduction
    C. Osteodestruction

D. Osteoinduction

Correct Answer: C

Explanation:

Successful bone graft materials should promote osteogenesis, osteoconduction, and osteoinduction, but not osteodestruction, which would harm bone tissue.

(SS, p. 243)

13. Which of the following best describes osteoconduction?
    A. The ability of a graft to act as a scaffold for bone growth
    B. The process by which uncommitted stem cells differentiate into bone-forming cells
    C. The provision of living osteoblasts to the fusion site
    D. The ability to provide structural support in spine fusion

    Correct Answer: A

    Explanation:

    Osteoconduction refers to when the graft acts as a scaffold or matrix to provide a framework for new bone growth (Table 4.1).

    (SS, p. 243)
14. All of the following are potential allograft harvesting sites, EXCEPT??
    A. Ilium
    B. Fibula
    C. Ribs
    D. Clavicle

    Correct Answer: D

    (SS, p. 243)

Table 4.1 Outlining the differences between **osteoinduction**, **osteoconduction**, **osteogenesis**, and other related terms

Term	Definition	Key Function	Examples
Osteoinduction	Undifferentiated stem cells are stimulated to become osteoblasts (bone-forming cells)	Initiates bone formation by inducing the differentiation of progenitor cells into osteogenic cells	Bone Morphogenetic Proteins (BMPs), Demineralized Bone Matrix (DBM)
Osteoconduction	Scaffold or matrix provides a framework for new bone growth	Serves as a scaffold for the migration and attachment of bone-forming cells	Ceramic-based grafts, allograft
Osteogenesis	The formation of new bone by living cells, such as osteoblasts	Provides the local fusion bed with bone-forming cells to directly create new bone	Autograft (e.g., iliac crest bone graft)
Osteopromotion	The enhancement of bone healing without directly inducing bone formation itself	Enhances the activity of other osteoinductive materials but does not induce bone formation	Enamel matrix proteins, certain growth factors
Osteolysis (-destruction)	The pathological destruction or absorption of bone tissue	Leads to the loss of bone density or volume, often due to inflammatory reactions	Infection-related bone resorption

15. Which of the following is true regarding the use of ceramic-based bone grafts in spinal fusion?
    A. They provide osteoinductive and osteogenic properties.
    B. They offer excellent mechanical strength and resist resorption.
    C. They act as an osteoconductive scaffold.
    D. They are always superior to autografts.

    Correct Answer: C

    Explanation:

    Ceramic-based grafts are commonly used for their osteoconductive properties, but they lack the osteoinductive and osteogenic properties of autografts.

    (BN, p. 797)
16. Which of the following describes the role of growth factors in biologics for spine fusion?
    A. They provide a mechanical framework for bone growth.
    B. They stimulate the local blood supply at the fusion site.
    C. They enhance cellular processes such as osteogenesis and angiogenesis.
    D. They degrade bone matrix to allow new bone growth.

    Correct Answer: C

    Explanation:

    Growth factors like bone morphogenetic proteins (BMPs) promote bone healing. They stimulate osteogenesis and angiogenesis at the fusion site.

    (BS, p. 124)
17. How does nicotine negatively affect bone healing and graft incorporation?
    A. It enhances osteoblast function.
    B. It reduces fracture end resorption.
    C. It induces calcitonin resistance.
    D. It accelerates graft revascularization.

    Correct Answer: C

    Explanation:

    Nicotine impairs bone healing by inducing calcitonin resistance, inhibiting osteoblast function, delaying revascularization, and increasing fracture end resorption.

    (BS, p. 125)
18. Which of the following is a known risk associated with recombinant human bone morphogenetic protein-2 (rhBMP-2) in spinal fusion?
    A. It selectively enhances only cortical bone healing without affecting trabecular bone.
    B. Increased risk of cancer.
    C. It reduces the likelihood of postoperative radiculopathy and nerve irritation.
    D. It prevents ectopic bone formation in soft tissues adjacent to the fusion site.

    Correct Answer: B

    (SS, p. 250)

19. What is the primary function of bone marrow aspirate in spine fusion?
    A. To provide an osteoconductive matrix
    B. To enhance osteogenesis through stem cell differentiation
    C. To replace damaged intervertebral discs
    D. To increase the mechanical stability of the spine

    Correct Answer: B

    Explanation:

    Bone marrow aspirate provides osteogenic potential through its population of mesenchymal stem cells, which can differentiate into osteoprogenitor cells and support bone formation.

    (BS, p. 797)
20. Which type of graft material is designed to improve the fusion rate beyond what autograft alone can achieve?
    A. Enhancer
    B. Extender
    C. Substitute
    D. Composite graft

    Correct Answer: A

    (SS, p. 243)
21. Which of the following is CORRECT about graft extenders' function in spinal fusion?
    A. They replace autograft completely while maintaining fusion rates.
    B. They enhance osteogenesis by directly stimulating bone formation.
    C. They extend autograft volume over more levels without lowering fusion success.
    D. They are only used in combination with allografts, not autografts.

    Correct Answer: C

    (SS, p. 243)
22. Which graft material is intended to provide an alternative to autograft while ensuring similar or superior fusion success?
    A. Enhancer
    B. Extender
    C. Substitute
    D. Demineralized bone matrix

    Correct Answer: C

    Explanation:

    Graft materials are classified based on their function in spinal fusion. **Extenders** are used with autografts to spread a smaller volume over more levels without reducing fusion success. **Enhancers** work alongside autografts to improve the fusion rate beyond what autografts alone achieve. **Substitutes** serve as alternatives to autografts, aiming to match or surpass their fusion success.

    (SS, p. 243)

Spine Degenerative Disease

5

Lumbar and Thoracic Degenerative Disc Diseases

1. In lumbar degenerative disc disease, which of the following imaging findings is most indicative of disc dehydration?
   A. Loss of signal intensity on T2-weighted MRI
   B. Loss of signal intensity on T1-weighted MRI
   C. Loss of disc height on plain radiographs
   D. Modic changes on MRI
   Correct Answer: A
   Explanation:
   In T2-weighted MRI, loss of signal intensity indicated loss of water content of the nucleus pulposus.
   (DI, p. 1093)
2. Which structure is most likely to cause spinal stenosis leading to neurogenic claudication?
   A. Posterior longitudinal ligament
   B. Ligamentum flavum
   C. Intervertebral disc
   D. Facet joint
   Correct Answer: B
   Explanation:
   Lumbar spinal stenosis is often caused by the hypertrophy and infolding of the **ligamentum flavum**, which leads to compression of neural elements. Facet joint hypertrophy and disc herniation can also cause lumbar stenosis in some cases.
   (GB, p. 1328)

K. F. AlAli, H. T. Hashim, *Spine Surgery and Peripheral Nerve Surgery*,
https://doi.org/10.1007/978-3-031-98543-0_5

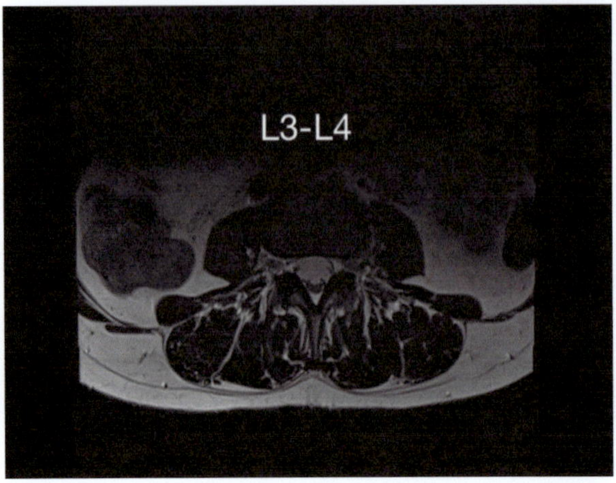

Fig. 5.1 Case 3 MRI

3. 42-year-old patient with a 4-month history of low back pain radiating to left anterior thigh, knee, and medial shin. He reports difficulty climbing stairs. MRI is shown (Fig. 5.1):
   Which major muscle is likely affected?
   A. Quadriceps muscle
   B. Hamstring muscle
   C. Adductor longus
   D. All of the above are affected.

   Correct Answer: A

   Explanation:

   The MRI showed L3–L4 far lateral disc herniation at the left, compressing the L3 (exiting nerve root). The quadriceps muscle is innervated mostly by the L3 nerve and is affected in this patient, which explains the difficulty climbing the stairs (extending the knee) (Fig. 5.2).

4. Regarding the far-lateral disc herniation

   4a. The most common site for a far-lateral disc herniation is:
   A. L1–L2
   B. L2–L3
   C. L4–L5
   D. L5–S1

   4b. All of the following are correct about extraforaminal disc herniation (far lateral), EXCEPT:
   A. The nerve root involved is usually the one exiting at that level.
   B. The straight leg raising sign is positive in 85–90%.
   C. The dorsal root ganglion may be compressed directly.
   D. Pain is usually reproduced by lateral bending to the side of the herniation.

   Correct Answers: 4a: C, 4b: B

   Explanation:

   Far-lateral disc herniation (extra-foraminal) represents 5–10% of all lumbar disc herniations. The L3–L4 and **L4–L5 levels** are the most

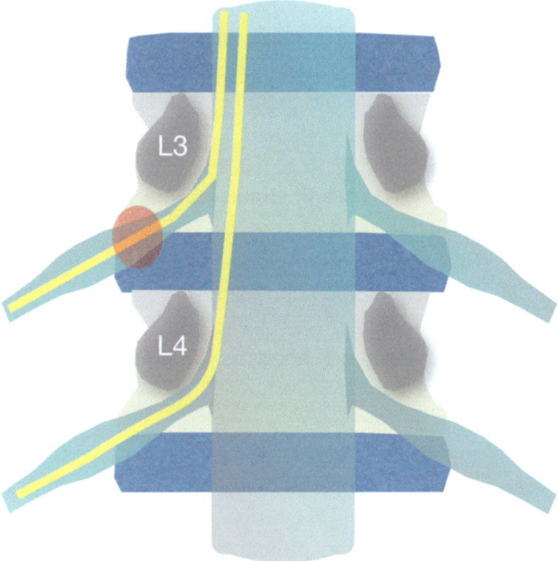

Fig. 5.2 Illustration showing L3 exciting nerve root is affected by L3–L4 far lateral disc herniation (red circle)

common sites for far-lateral disc herniation. L5–S1 level is the second most common level. The **straight leg raising test** is typically not positive in this type of herniation.

(GP, p. 1264) (SSW, p. 1736)

5. Which of the following proteins is primarily involved in the matrix breakdown and inflammation observed in degenerative disc disease?
   A. Collagen
   B. Aggrecan
   C. Matrix metalloproteinases (MMPs)
   D. Proteoglycans
   Correct Answer: C
6. What is the primary mechanism behind the pain experienced in lumbar facet joint syndrome?
   A. Compression of nerve roots
   B. Inflammatory cytokine release
   C. Stretching of Ligamentum flavum
   D. Mechanical stress on the facet joint capsule
   Correct Answer: D
7. Which of the following is NOT a component of the Wiltse classification for lumbar spondylolisthesis?
   A. Dysplastic
   B. Isthmic
   C. Degenerative
   D. Dysmorphic
   Correct Answer: D

Explanation:

The Wiltse classification for lumbar spondylolisthesis: Dysplastic (Type I), Isthmic (Type II), Degenerative (Type III), Traumatic (Type IV), Pathologic (Type V), and Postsurgical (Type VI). Dysmorphic is not a recognized classification within this system.

(SS, p. 232)

8. Which of the following interventions has shown the best evidence for long-term improvement in lumbar spinal stenosis with neurogenic claudication?
   A. Epidural steroid injections
   B. Physical therapy and exercise
   C. Laminectomy/lumbar decompression
   D. Radiofrequency ablation

   Correct Answer: C

   Explanation:

   Lumbar decompression has been shown to offer the best evidence for long-term improvement in patients with lumbar spinal stenosis with neurogenic claudication for pain, disability, and quality of life. The SPORT trial compares surgical versus nonsurgical treatment for lumbar spinal stenosis. Over a two-year follow-up, patients who underwent surgery showed significantly greater improvements in pain relief and physical function compared to those treated nonsurgically. However, many patients in the nonsurgical group ultimately shifted to surgery due to persistent symptoms. Despite high crossover rates between groups, surgery consistently provided better outcomes in terms of bodily pain and disability. The study supports surgery as a more effective long-term treatment for spinal stenosis in appropriate candidates.

   [4]

9. Which of the following is NOT a recognized radiographic sign of instability in degenerative lumbar spondylolisthesis?
   A. Translation greater than 4 mm on dynamic X-rays
   B. Angular motion greater than 10 degrees on flexion-extension films
   C. Presence of a vacuum sign in the disc space
   D. Disc height loss with associated Modic 1 changes

   Correct Answer: C

   Explanation:

   While translation greater than 4 mm, angular motion greater than 10 degrees, and disc height loss with Modic changes are recognized signs of instability in degenerative lumbar spondylolisthesis, the presence of a vacuum sign is not considered a sign of instability but rather a sign of disc degeneration. Other radiographic signs of instability are increased sagittal translation (thresholds between $\geq$3 and 5 mm, slip percentage of $\geq$8% and severe facet joint degeneration with effusion and > 1 mm articular gap.

   (**PR:** degenerative spinal instability)

10. In the treatment of lumbar disc herniation, which of the following factors is most predictive of a favorable outcome after microdiscectomy?
    A. Presence of Modic changes
    B. Preoperative opioid use
    C. Degree of disc protrusion
    D. The duration of symptoms is less than six months

Correct Answer: D

Explanation:

Rihn et al., in an analysis of the as-treated SPORT data, found that symptom duration influenced the outcomes of lumbar disc herniation treatment. Patients who had symptoms for more than 6 months before seeking treatment experienced significantly worse outcomes with nonoperative treatment compared to those whose symptoms lasted less than 6 months.

(RS, p. 849)

11. A 59-year-old male patient with chronic lower back pain and intermittent bilateral leg pain, worsens with standing and walking, but improves when sitting or leaning forward. On examination, there is no significant motor weakness, but she has diminished lumbar range of motion and positive straight-leg raise bilaterally. MRI and CT are shown (Fig. 5.3):

11a. What is the diagnosis?
   A. L4–L5 degenerative spondylolisthesis
   B. L4–L5 isthmic spondylolisthesis
   C. L4–L5 high-grade spondylolisthesis
   D. L4–L5 spondylolysis with stenosis

11b. Which of the following is the most likely mechanism contributing to her condition?
   A. Pars interarticularis defect
   B. Facet joint osteoarthritis
   C. Congenital hypoplasia of the posterior elements
   D. High-energy trauma

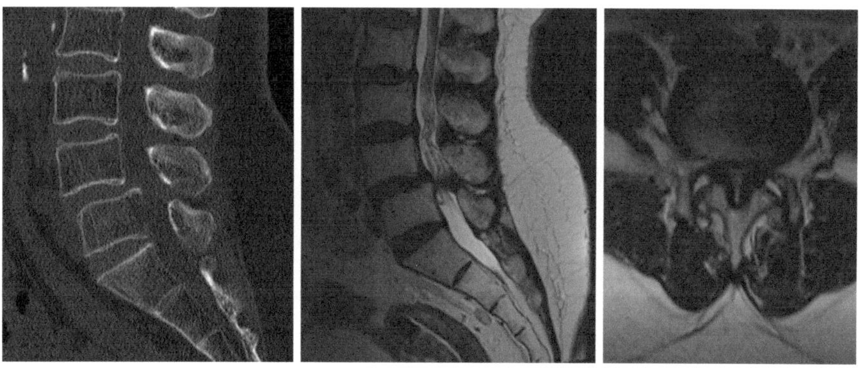

Fig. 5.3 Case 11 MRI (on right) and CT (on left)

11c. One of the following is CORRECT about the natural history of this condition:

A. The majority of patients usually require surgery.
B. Progression often decreases with age.
C. Further degenerative changes, like facet joint arthritis, often worsen the condition over time.
D. All of the above are correct.

Correct Answers: 11a: A, 11b: B, 11c: B

Explanation:

This case shows L4–L5 low-grade spondylolisthesis with the axial MRI showing severe facet arthritis and stenosis, so the diagnosis is degenerative spondylolisthesis. This type of spondylolisthesis commonly occurs at the L4–L5 level and is related to facet joint osteoarthritis (see axial MRI). It can be associated with spinal stenosis due to facet and flavum ligaments hypertrophy and degenerative disc disease. It typically affects elderly females.

Degenerative spondylolisthesis typically progresses slowly, with most patients experiencing stable or mild progression over time, yet most are treated conservatively. 10–15% require surgery and typically have severe lumbar stenosis with neurogenic claudication, who have failed 3–6 months of conservative management.

[62]

12. In lumbar disc herniation, the presence of which reflex would suggest an S1 radiculopathy?

A. Patellar reflex
B. Plantar reflex
C. Ankle jerk reflex
D. All of the above

Correct Answer: C

Explanation:

The **ankle jerk reflex** (Achilles reflex) is mediated by the S1 nerve root. The patellar reflex corresponds to L4, and the plantar reflex is not specific to radiculopathies. (GB, p. 1252)

13. A patient with lumbar spinal stenosis and degenerative spondylolisthesis is scheduled for surgery. Which of the following factors is most predictive of the need for fusion in addition to decompression?

A. Age over 65
B. Instability on flexion-extension radiographs
C. Presence of back pain
D. Single-level stenosis

Correct Answer: B

Explanation:

Surgical fusion is indicated for patients with persistent pain, progressive spondylolisthesis, instability signs like translation on flexion-extension radiographs, or neurologic symptoms who fail conservative management.

(RS, p. 554)

14. Which of the following is NOT a feature of Modic Type I changes on MRI?
    A. Hypo-intensity on T1-weighted MRI
    B. Hyperintensity on T2-weighted MRI
    C. Presence of fibrovascular tissue within the bone marrow
    D. Reflects advanced disc degeneration

    Correct Answer: D

    Explanation:

    Modic Type I changes are characterized by T1 hypointensity and T2 hyperintensity, indicating bone marrow edema and inflammation. These changes are associated with active inflammation rather than advanced disc degeneration.

    (**SS**, p. 460)
15. One of the following can describe annular tears (fissures) in intervertebral discs:
    A. Separations between annular fibers
    B. Avulsions of fibers from their vertebral body insertions
    C. Breaks through fibers that extend radially, transversely, or concentrically
    D. All of the above

    Correct answer: D

    (GB, p. 1227)
16. In the Oswestry disability index score for low back pain, 41–60% disability is described as:
    A. Pain and difficulty with sitting, lifting, and standing. The patient may be disabled from work.
    B. Pain is the main problem, as other patients' life is affected
    C. Back pain impinges on all aspects of the patient's life.
    D. Patients are either bedbound or are exaggerating their symptoms.

    Correct Answer: B

    Explanation:

    The Oswestry Disability Index (ODI) is an outcome score for low back pain. A score of 41–60% is classified as severe disability. At this level, pain is the primary issue, but other aspects of life, such as activities of daily living, are also affected. Patients can still function but face significant challenges in managing pain (Table 5.1).

    (GB, p. 1228)
17. The Lasègue's sign (ipsilateral straight leg raising) test has
    A. Sensitivity of 40%, Specificity 80%
    B. Sensitivity of 80%, Specificity 80%
    C. Sensitivity of 80%, Specificity 40%
    D. Sensitivity of 40%, Specificity 40%

    Correct Answer: C

    Explanation:

    The Lasègue's sign, also known as the straight leg raising (SLR) test, is used to diagnose lumbar disc herniation. It has a high sensitivity of 80%. It is good at detecting. It has lower specificity (40%), indicating a moderate rate of false positives.

    (GB, p. 1252)

Table 5.1 Oswestry Disability Index (ODI) score table

Score	Interpretation
0–20%	Minimal disability: Can cope with most daily activities
21–40%	Moderate disability: Pain and difficulty with sitting, lifting, and standing. May be disabled from work
41–60%	Severe disability: Pain is the main issue, but other areas are affected
61–80%	Crippled: Back pain impacts all aspects of life
81–100%	Patients are either bedbound or exaggerating symptoms

18. The femoral stretch test is usually positive in the compression of the following nerve root(s)
    A. L1 and L2
    B. L1, L2, and L3
    C. L1, L2, L3, and L4
    D. L1, L2, L3, L4, and L5

    Correct Answer: C

    Explanation:

    The femoral nerve stretch test, or reverse straight-leg raise, targets the L2, L3, and L4 nerve roots. Performed with the patient prone or in a lateral position. The test involves extending the hip and flexing the knee. It is considered positive if it elicits radicular pain in the anterior thigh.

    (SS, p. 56)
19. The following findings in clinical examination may indicate non-organic low back pain.
    A. Waddle sign
    B. Abductor sign
    C. Fares sign
    D. Hashim sign

    Correct Answer: A

    Explanation:

    Waddell described five categories of tests to help evaluate the potential psychological or socioeconomic factors contributing to low back pain. These tests do not indicate malingering but highlight nonorganic components to the pain. The presence of three or more positive signs is considered significant. The tests include:

    Superficial tenderness, where pain is reported with light touch in a non-anatomic distribution.

    Simulation, where pain is elicited during maneuvers that should not cause discomfort.

    Distraction, where a test is positive when the patient is focused but negative when distracted.

    Regionalization involves findings that do not align with neuroanatomy.

    Overreaction, where the patient responds disproportionately during the examination.

    (SS, p. 56)

20. All of the clinical findings can be found in cauda equina syndrome, EXCEPT:
    A. Bladder and/or bowel dysfunction
    B. Reduced sensation in the perineal region
    C. Babinski sign
    D. New onset of sexual dysfunction

    Correct Answer: C

    Explanation:

    Cauda equina syndrome has characteristic clinical features. Sphincter disturbances are common. Urinary retention is the most common sphincter symptom and occurs in about 90% of cases. This can be evaluated through post-void residual measurements or a cystometrogram. Urinary or fecal incontinence may present in cases of overflow. Anal sphincter tone is diminished in 60–80% of patients. Sensory deficits, particularly saddle anesthesia (around the anus, genitals, and buttocks), occur in about 75% of cases. Motor weakness often involves multiple nerve roots and can progress to paraplegia if untreated. Low back pain or sciatica, which is usually bilateral, and bilateral absence of the Achilles reflex are also noted. Sexual dysfunction is usually a late-detected symptom.

    Babinski sign is an upper motor neuron sign, like in spinal cord compression.

    (GB, p. 1254)
21. According to the available evidence, the best timing for surgical treatment of cauda equina syndrome is:
    A. Within 24 h
    B. Within 48 h
    C. Within 72 h
    D. None of the above

    Correct Answer: B

    Explanation:

    Severe retrospective studies suggest that surgery within 48 h offers a better outcome than delays beyond this window. Meta-analyses indicate that outcomes may worsen with prolonged delays.

    (**GB,** p. 1255)
22. Regarding arachnoiditis:

    22a. One of the following is a risk factor for post-discectomy arachnoiditis:
    A. Epidural hematoma
    B. Post-op discitis
    C. Patients with a tendency to develop hypertrophic scars (keloids)
    D. All of the above

    22b. All of the following are MRI patterns indicating arachnoiditis, EXCEPT:
    A. Central adhesion, where nerve roots clump into cords
    B. Empty thecal sac
    C. Nerve roots symmetrically dispersed and floating freely in CSF
    D. Thecal sac filled with inflammatory tissue

    Correct Answers: 22a: D, 22b: C

Explanation:

Arachnoiditis is an inflammatory condition affecting the lumbar nerve roots and involves fibrosis across all three meningeal layers. Risk factors include spinal anesthesia, spinal meningitis (pyogenic, syphilitic, or tuberculous), neoplasms, older myelographic contrast agents, trauma (especially **post-surgical**), **hemorrhage**, and idiopathic causes. Radiographically, arachnoiditis can resemble tumors, making diagnosis complex. MRI shows three common patterns: central adhesion (nerve roots clumping into cords), the "empty thecal sac" pattern (roots adhering to the meninges), or thecal sac filled with inflammatory tissue with no CSF signal. Acute cases may show enhancement on MRI, but chronic cases typically do not. Myelograms may reveal complete blocks or nerve root clumping.

(GB, p.1259)

23. One of the following is a limitation in the SPORT trial for surgical versus non-surgical therapy for lumbar spinal stenosis:
    A. High value of intention-to-treat analysis
    B. High rates of nonadherence
    C. High power ratio
    D. Follow-up rate of 85%

    Correct Answer: B

    Explanation:

    The SPORT trial compares surgical versus nonsurgical treatment for lumbar spinal stenosis. Patients who underwent surgery showed significantly greater improvements in pain relief and physical function compared to those treated nonsurgically in over 2 years of follow-up. Many patients in the nonsurgical group ultimately opted for surgery due to persistent symptoms **(high rates of nonadherence**). Despite high crossover rates between groups, surgery consistently provided better outcomes in terms of bodily pain and disability. The study supports surgery as a more effective long-term treatment for spinal stenosis in appropriate candidates. [4]

24. All of the following are correct regarding neurogenic vs vascular claudication, EXCEPT:
    A. Neurogenic claudication is described as tiredness, heaviness, and discomfort in the lower extremities with ambulation.
    B. Vascular claudication is described as cramping or tightness in the calf associated with ambulation.
    C. In neurogenic claudication, patients experience relief of symptoms with activities performed in extension.
    D. In vascular claudication, symptoms are not affected by posture.

    Correct Answer: C

    Explanation:

    Neurogenic claudication presents with tiredness, heaviness, and discomfort in the lower extremities during walking. Symptoms vary daily or even within the same walk. Forward flexion, like leaning forward or cycling, provides relief. Walking downhill or standing worsens symptoms.

In contrast, vascular claudication presents as cramping or tightness in the calf during walking. Symptoms occur at a consistent distance. Unlike neurogenic claudication, posture does not affect symptoms. Both walking uphill, downhill, and cycling aggravate vascular claudication.

(SS, p. 467)

25. The most common physical examination finding in lumbar spine stenosis is:
    A. Normal examination
    B. Reproduction of pain with lumbar extension
    C. Weakness of the extensor hallucis longus muscle
    D. Sensory deficits over the lower extremities

    Correct Answer: A

    Explanation:

    Physical examination of lumbar spine stenosis usually reveals normal findings or subtle positive findings, such as non-dermatomal sensory deficits, reproduction of pain with lumbar extension, or mild weakness of the extensor hallucis longus muscle.

    (SS, p. 477)

26. All of the following are positive predictors for the outcome of surgical treatment of lumbar spine stenosis, EXCEPT:
    A. Female sex
    B. Younger age
    C. Less comorbidity
    D. Severe canal stenosis

    Correct Answer: A

    Explanation:

    Positive predictors for surgical outcomes in lumbar spine stenosis include younger age, male patients, less comorbidity, and severe canal stenosis.

    (UP)

27. The most commonly affected muscle in upper lumbar disc herniation (L1–L4) is:
    A. Psoas
    B. Sartorius
    C. Quadriceps femoris
    D. Tibialis antcrior

    Corrcct Answcr: C

    Explanation:

    The quadriceps femoris can be affected in upper lumbar disc herniations. It is innervated by the femoral nerve, which originates from L2, L3, and L4

    (GB, p. 1263)

28. The overall lumbar interbody fusion rates for transforaminal lumbar interbody fusion (TLIF) are approximately:
    A. 30%
    B. 50%
    C. 60%
    D. 90%

    Correct Answer: D

Explanation:

The transforminal lumbar interbody fusion (TLIF) has a high rate of fusion that can reach 90%.

[5]

29. In thoracic disc herniation, which imaging modality is necessary to determine the surgical approach?
    A. A thoracic anteroposterior (AP) view X-ray to measure the Cobb angle
    B. CT scan
    C. MRI T1 without contrast
    D. Flexion-extension thoracic X-ray

    Correct Answer: B

    Explanation:

    CT scans are useful in evaluating calcification in thoracic disc herniations, which is crucial for planning the surgical approach. Calcified thoracic disc herniation is found in 65% of patients considered for surgery. Calcified herniated thoracic discs are more challenging to remove via posterior or lateral approach than non-calcified discs. Thoracotomy is usually the surgical approach of choice for calcified herniated thoracic discs.

    (GB, p. 1271)
30. The following surgical approach is unacceptable in thoracic disc herniation:
    A. Thoracic laminectomy
    B. Transpedicular approach
    C. Lateral Extracavitary
    D. Costotransversectomy

    Correct Answer: A

    Explanation:

    Thoracic laminectomy is generally considered an unacceptable surgical approach for thoracic disc herniations due to its high risk of neurological complications, including paraplegia, stemming from excessive spinal cord retraction.

    (RS, p. 796)
31. Which molecular change is linked to intervertebral disc degeneration?
    A. More aggrecan
    B. Fewer matrix metalloproteinases (MMPs)
    C. Increased IL-1β & TNF-α
    D. More type II collagen

    Correct Answer: C

    Explanation:

    Inflammatory cytokines (IL-1β, TNF-α) accelerate disc degeneration by breaking down the matrix.

    (RS, p. 813)
32. A 55-year-old patient presents with chronic lower back pain radiating to the left leg. MRI shows Modic Type II changes at the L4–L5 vertebral endplates. What do these Modic Type II changes indicate?
    A. Fibrovascular bone marrow changes
    B. Fatty replacement of bone marrow

C. Sclerotic bone formation
D. Normal aging process

Correct Answer: B

Explanation:

Modic changes are MRI findings that reflect specific changes in the vertebral endplates and bone marrow. It is commonly associated with disc degeneration. **Modic Type I** indicates active inflammation and bone marrow edema, showing low signal on T1 and high signal on T2-weighted images. **Modic Type II** reflects **fatty replacement of bone marrow**, appearing as high signal on both T1 and T2. **Modic Type III** represents sclerotic bone changes, with low signal on both T1 and T2.

(GB, p. 1335)

33. Which of the following is the clinical significance of the findings in the following MRI? (Fig. 5.4)

A. Represents fat deposition and is typically asymptomatic
B. Indicates bone marrow edema and is associated with acute low back pain
C. Sign of disc calcification and long-standing degenerative disease
D. Represents fibrous tissue replacement and is associated with chronic symptoms

Correct Answer: B

Explanation:

The MRI shows typical Modic type 1 at L5–S1 disc level with hyperintensity in T2 and hypointensity in T1. This indicates active inflammation with bone marrow edema and is associated with acute low back pain.

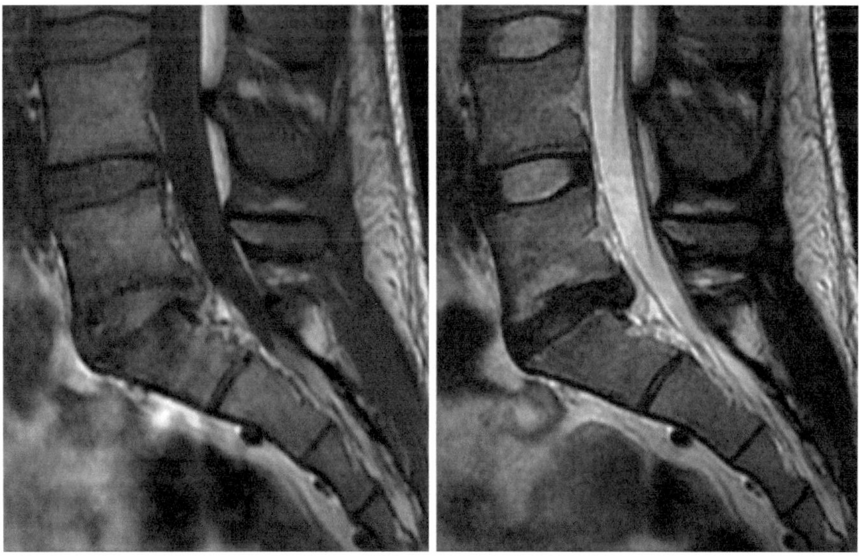

Fig. 5.4 Case 33 MRI

34. In the context of lumbar degenerative disc disease, which surgical approach is most appropriate for direct visualization and removal of a centrally located disc herniation at L5–S1 in a patient with high iliac crests?
    A. Posterior lumbar interbody fusion (PLIF)
    B. Anterior lumbar interbody fusion (ALIF)
    C. Transforaminal lumbar interbody fusion (TLIF)
    D. Lateral lumbar interbody fusion (LLIF)
    Correct Answer: B
    Explanation:
    ALIF is the most appropriate approach for removing centrally located disc herniation at L5–S1 in patients with high iliac crests.
    (BS, p. 740)
35. Which of the following genetic polymorphisms has been associated with an increased risk of lumbar disc degeneration?
    A. COL1A1 gene polymorphism
    B. Vitamin D receptor gene polymorphism
    C. TNF-α gene polymorphism
    D. MMP-2 gene polymorphism
    Correct Answer: B
    Explanation:
    Studies link lumbar disc degeneration to gene polymorphisms in aggrecan, collagen IX, MMP-3, and vitamin D receptor. These genes affect disc metabolism and degeneration. Vitamin D receptor polymorphism is strongly linked to lumbar disc disease.
    (RS, p. 85)
36. Which of the following statements is true regarding the natural history of lumbar degenerative disc disease?
    A. Most patients will require surgical intervention within 2 years
    B. Disc degeneration always leads to chronic pain
    C. Disc herniations tend to resorb over time
    D. Physical therapy has no role in management
    Correct Answer: C
    Explanation:
    Despite the treatment type, most of the herniated lumbar discs resorb within time. This has been shown in several studies on follow-up MRIs.
    [11]
37. Which of the following radiographic signs is most indicative of instability in lumbar degenerative disc disease requiring surgical fusion?
    A. Disc height loss greater than 50%
    B. Facet joint effusion on MRI
    C. Spondylolisthesis greater than 3 mm on flexion-extension films
    D. Presence of Schmorl's nodes
    Correct Answer: C

Explanation:

In lumbar degenerative disc disease, instability is best detected on **flexion-extension radiographs**, where a **spondylolisthesis of greater than 3 mm** suggests dynamic instability. This finding is a strong indicator that surgical fusion may be necessary to stabilize the segment. Other indicators of instability may include facet joint effusion, but spondylolisthesis on flexion-extension views is considered the most reliable.

(SS, p. 510)

38. A 50-year-old male with a history of lumbar degenerative disc disease undergoes MRI, which reveals a high-intensity zone (HIZ) in the annulus fibrosus at L4–L5. What does this HIZ most likely represent?
   A. Nucleus pulposus herniation
   B. Annular tear with granulation tissue
   C. Vertebral endplate fracture
   D. Normal aging change

   Correct Answer: B

   Explanation: An annular tear, also known as an annular defect or high-intensity zone (HIZ), refers to the disruption of the concentric collagen fibers comprising the annulus fibrosus.

   (DI, p. 392)

39. 12. Which cytokine is primarily involved in the pain generation associated with degenerative disc disease due to its role in nociceptor sensitization?
   A. Interleukin-6 (IL-6)
   B. Tumor necrosis factor-alpha (TNF-α)
   C. Interleukin-10 (IL-10)
   D. Transforming growth factor-beta (TGF-β)

   Correct Answer: B

   Explanation:

   TNF can independently trigger spontaneous electrical activity in A-delta and C nociceptors, leading to pain signals interpreted by the brain.

   (RS, p. 124)

40. A patient with degenerative lumbar scoliosis presents with neurogenic claudication. Which of the following is the most appropriate surgical treatment?
   A. Decompression alone without fusion
   B. Decompression with limited fusion at the apex
   C. Decompression with long-segment fusion
   D. Anterior lumbar interbody fusion only

   Correct Answer: C

   Explanation:

   In degenerative lumbar scoliosis with neurogenic claudication, long-segment fusion is often best. It relieves nerve compression and stabilizes the spine. This helps prevent deformity progression.

   (SS, p. 488)

41. Which of the following clinical signs is most characteristic and can help in localizing the level of the lesion in thoracic disc herniations?
    A. Lhermitte's sign
    B. Hoffmann's sign
    C. Brown-Séquard syndrome signs
    D. Abdominal reflex asymmetry

    Correct Answer: D

    Explanation:

    Abdominal reflex asymmetry is a key clinical sign used in the diagnosis of thoracic disc herniation. The asymmetry occurs when the abdominal muscles fail to contract evenly in response to stimulation. It indicates possible spinal cord compression at the thoracic level. Imaging is required to confirm the diagnosis.

    (SS, p. 53)

Cervical Degenerative Disease

42. Which is the most common site for cervical disc herniation?
    A. C3–C4
    B. C4–C5
    C. C5–C6
    D. C6–C7

    Correct Answer: D

    Explanation:

    C6–C7 level is the most common level involved with herniation, causing compression of the C7 root. C5–C6 is the second most common location, compressing the C6 root.

    (DI, p. 397)

43. In cervical spondylotic myelopathy, which clinical sign is most indicative of upper motor neuron involvement?
    A. Hyporeflexia
    B. Babinski sign
    C. Fasciculations
    D. Lhermitte's sign

    Correct Answer: B

    Explanation:

    A **Babinski sign** is indicative of **upper motor neuron involvement** and is commonly observed in patients with cervical spondylotic myelopathy. The presence of a positive Babinski sign, where the big toe moves upward when the sole of the foot is stroked, reflects corticospinal tract dysfunction.

    (GB, p. 1298)

44. Based on the following T2 axial MRI of C6–C7 level, which feature in the MRI suggests the possibility of approaching the herniated disc via posterior foraminotomy (Fig. 5.5)?

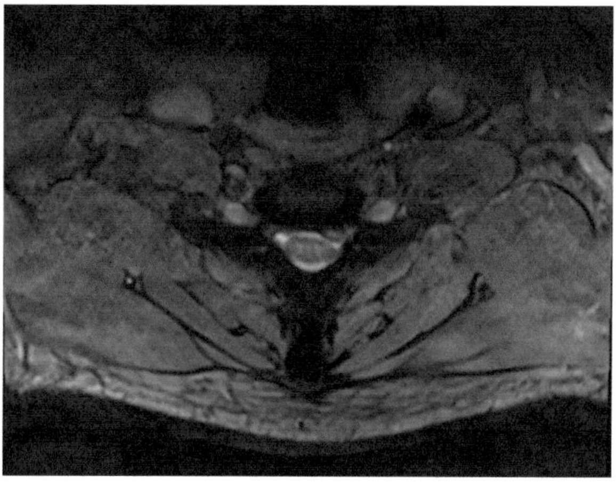

Fig. 5.5 Case 44 MRI

A. Lateral disc herniation
B. No significant central canal stenosis
C. High T2 signal in the herniated fragment
D. All of the above

Correct Answer: D

Explanation:

A cervical foraminotomy is indicated for patients with monoradiculopathy caused by posterolateral **soft** disc sequestration or small lateral osteophytic spurs. It is unsuitable for central or broad-based disc herniations or spinal canal stenosis. This approach is ideal for individuals like professional speakers or singers, where avoiding recurrent laryngeal nerve injury is critical. It is also preferred for treating lower or upper cervical nerve root compression in patients with short, thick necks, where an anterior approach is more challenging. Additionally, it is recommended for patients who wish to avoid fusion surgery.

(GB, p. 1292)

45. Which of the following cervical spine segments is least likely to be affected by degenerative changes?

A. C1–C2
B. C2–C3
C. C3–C4
D. C4–C5

Correct Answer: A

Explanation:

Atlantoaxial degeneration refers to arthritis affecting the atlantodens and atlanto-axial facet joints, which are critical for cervical spine rotation, contributing up to 70% of total movement. The incidence of atlantoaxial degeneration is unclear; however, clinically, it is the lowest level seen in the spine practice.

[12]

46. In cervical spondylotic myelopathy, which of the following is NOT a typical finding on MRI?
    A. T2-weighted MRI high signal
    B. Facet joint hypertrophy
    C. Disc-osteophyte complex formation
    D. Spinal cord enhancement
    Correct Answer: D
    Explanation:
    In cervical spondylosis, T1 MRI shows subarachnoid space effacement and cord compression. Disc herniations, osteophytes, and bulges are common. T2 MRI reveals space narrowing from disc-osteophyte complexes and ligament thickening. Intramedullary T2 hyperintensity suggests myelomalacia, demyelination, or edema. T2 GRE highlights uncovertebral and facet joint hypertrophy with foraminal narrowing. Post-gadolinium T1 may show cord enhancement in a horizontal linear pattern; however, it is not a typical finding. (DI, p. 455)
47. Based on AO Spine guidelines for cervical degenerative myelopathy in 2017:
    47a. Which of the following factors is emphasized as critical in determining the management approach for patients with degenerative cervical myelopathy?
    A. Patient age and comorbidities
    B. Severity of myelopathy symptoms
    C. Duration of symptoms
    D. MRI findings alone
    47b. For patients with mild degenerative cervical myelopathy, the guideline suggests:
    A. An initial trial of structured nonoperative management
    B. Immediate surgical decompression for all cases
    C. Nonoperative management only if radiographic findings are absent
    D. Delayed surgical intervention regardless of symptom progression
    47c. In patients with radiographic evidence of cervical cord compression but no myelopathy symptoms, the guideline recommends:
    A. Immediate surgical decompression to prevent myelopathy
    B. Routine follow-up with an MRI every six months
    C. Observation and counseling on potential symptom progression
    D. Initiation of prophylactic physical therapy
    47d. In the guideline, the severity of cervical spondylotic myelopathy is categorized according to:
    A. Oswestry Disability Index (ODI)
    B. Nurick grading system
    C. SF-36 physical health score
    D. Modified Japanese Orthopaedic Association (mJOA) score
    Correct Answers: 47a: B, 47b: A, 47c: C, 47d: D
    Explanation:
    The study by Fehlings et al. provides evidence-based guidelines for the management of degenerative cervical myelopathy (DCM. Severity is

categorized using the modified Japanese Orthopaedic Association (mJOA) score: mild (≥15), moderate [12–14], and severe (≤11). Surgical decompression is strongly recommended for moderate to severe cases and for mild cases with symptom progression or significant impact on quality of life. MRI is considered the diagnostic gold standard. Both anterior and posterior approaches are effective, with the choice depending on patient-specific factors. Early treatment improves functional outcomes, highlighting the importance of timely diagnosis.

[61]

48. A patient with cervical radiculopathy has a large disc herniation at C6–C7. What is the most likely nerve root affected?
    A. C5
    B. C6
    C. C7
    D. C8

    Correct Answer: C

    Explanation:

    In the cervical spine, nerve roots exit above their corresponding vertebrae, so a C6–C7 disc herniation will affect the C7 root.

    (GB, p. 1296)

49. Which statement best describes the K-line as a radiographic parameter of clinical significance in the assessment of cervical deformity?
    A. A positive K-line indicates a higher risk of neurological deterioration after laminoplasty.
    B. A negative K-line suggests a favorable outcome for anterior decompression and fusion.
    C. A positive K-line is associated with a lower risk of axial neck pain postoperatively.
    D. A negative K-line contraindicates the use of cervical disc arthroplasty.

    Correct Answer: B

    Explanation:

    The K-line is a radiographic tool drawn on a lateral cervical X-ray, connecting the midpoints of the spinal canal at C2 and C7. A **negative K-line** suggests that posterior surgeries like laminoplasty are NOT recommended, and anterior decompression and fusion are preferred due to the location of the ossification in relation to the spinal cord (Fig. 5.6).

    (SW, p. 1664)

50. In the context of cervical ossification of the posterior longitudinal ligament (OPLL), which surgical approach is associated with a higher risk of cerebrospinal fluid (CSF) leak?
    A. Anterior cervical discectomy and fusion
    B. Posterior cervical laminectomy and fusion
    C. Laminoplasty
    D. Anterior cervical corpectomy and fusion

    Correct Answer: D

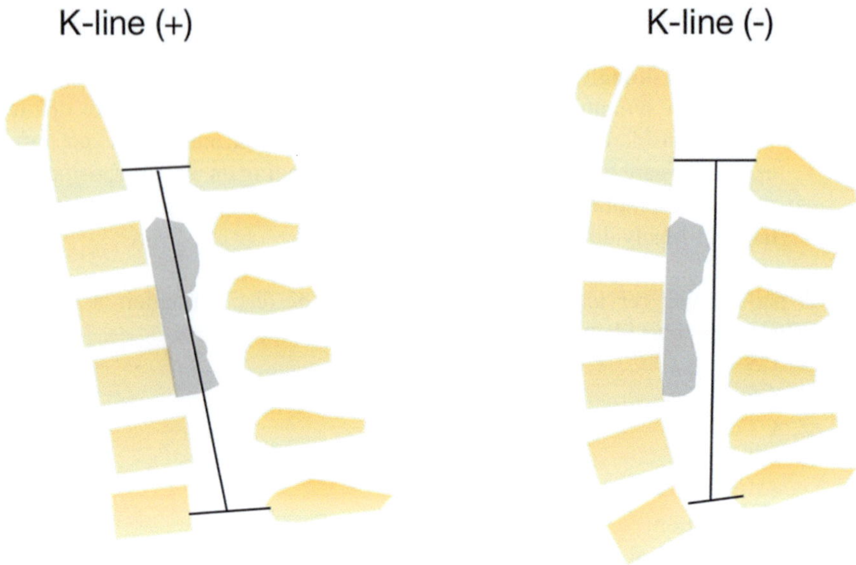

Fig. 5.6 The K-line is a line connecting midpoints between spinal canals of C2 to C7. If the ossified posterior longitudinal ligament (grey part) lies posterior to the line, the k-line is positive, and vice versa

Explanation:

In cervical degenerative disease with OPLL, anterior cervical corpectomy has the highest risk of CSF leak or incidental durotomy, with incidence ranging from 12.5% to 32%, making cervical corpectomy CSF leak risk far more common than after other general spinal operations (0%–8.3%). [13]

In cases of cervical degenerative disc disease without OPLL, posterior laminectomy has the highest risk of CSF leak (Table 5.2) [14].

51. Which of the following factors is MOST predictive of pseudarthrosis after anterior cervical discectomy and fusion (ACDF)?
 A. Use of allograft bone
 B. Smoking status
 C. Multilevel fusion
 D. Posterior surgical approach

Correct Answer: B

Explanation:

Smoking status is one of the most significant risk factors for pseudarthrosis after anterior cervical discectomy and fusion (ACDF). Nicotine impairs the healing process by reducing blood flow and osteoblastic activity, which are crucial for bone fusion.

(GB, p. 1289)

Table 5.2 Incidence of durotomy/CSF leak

Surgical approach	Incidence of durotomy/CSF leak
ACDF	0.1–0.3%
Corpectomy	0.5–2%
Laminectomy	3–8%
Laminoplasty	1–4%

52. The Torg-Pavlov ratio is used to assess cervical spinal canal stenosis. What is the critical value below which the spinal canal is considered stenotic?
    A. 0.80
    B. 0.70
    C. 0.90
    D. 1.00

    Correct Answer: A

    Explanation:

    The Torg-Pavlov ratio is used to assess cervical spinal stenosis. It is calculated by dividing the sagittal diameter of the spinal canal by the sagittal diameter of the vertebral body. A ratio below **0.80** is considered indicative of cervical stenosis (Fig. 5.7).

    (GB, p. 1302)
53. In the management of cervical degenerative disc disease, which of the following is NOT a typical indication for foraminotomy?
    A. Symptomatic lateral disc herniation
    B. Progressive myelopathy
    C. Unilateral radiculopathy due to foraminal stenosis
    D. Medial soft disc herniation

    Correct Answer: B

    Explanation:

    Foraminotomy is often recommended for those with unilateral radiculopathy resulting from foraminal stenosis or lateral disc herniation. However, it is often not advised for progressing myelopathy, a disease that normally requires more severe decompression.

    (SSW, p. 1598)
54. Which of the following factors is NOT considered a relative contraindication for cervical disc arthroplasty?
    A. Advanced spondylosis
    B. Ossification of the posterior longitudinal ligament (OPLL)
    C. Segmental instability
    D. Young age of the patient

    Correct Answer: D

    (SSW, p. 1640)
55. The following is from the 2014 North American Spine Society Coverage Committee regarding cervical laser discectomy:
    A. It is not indicated at this time due to a lack of high-quality clinical trials.
    B. It is indicated by a small central disc herniation.
    C. There is conflicting evidence regarding its indication.

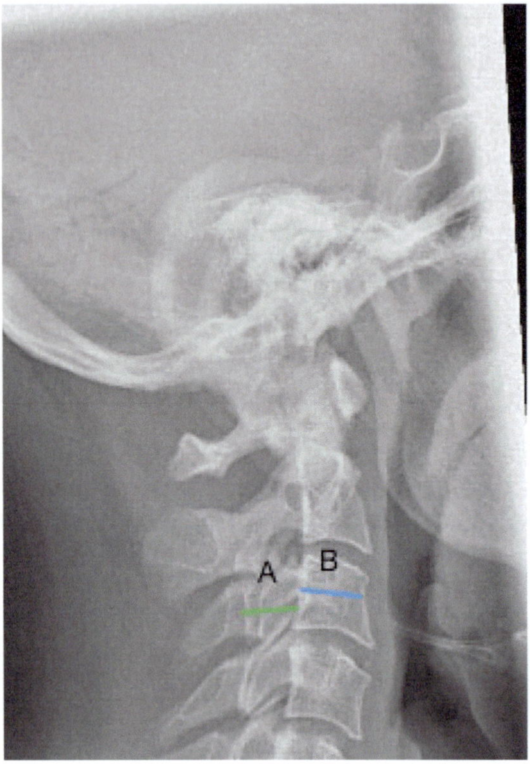

Fig. 5.7 The Torg-Pavlov ratio calculated by dividing the sagittal diameter of the spinal canal (**a**) by the sagittal diameter of the vertebral body (**b**)

D. None of the above

Correct Answer: A

Explanation:

According to the 2014 North American Spine Society (NASS) Coverage Committee, **laser spine surgery is not indicated**. This is due to the lack of high-quality clinical trials supporting its efficacy in both cervical and lumbar spine surgeries.

(GB, p. 1257)

56. All of the following can be found in the clinical examination of C4–C5 disc herniation, EXCEPT:

A. Diminished reflex of the deltoid

B. Diminished reflex of the pectoralis

C. Deltoid muscle weakness

D. Pectoralis major muscle weakness

Correct Answer: D

Explanation:

A C4–C5 disc herniation usually affects the C5 nerve root, which supplies the deltoid muscle weakness. The pectoralis reflex is useful to assess C4–C5 level and above. **Pectoralis major muscle weakness** is associated with C6 and below.

(GB, p. 1280)

57. The following cervical disc herniation can produce pain simulating myocardial infarction (pseudo-angina):
   A. C4–C5
   B. C5–C6
   C. C6–C7
   D. C7–T8
   Correct Answer: B
   Explanation:
   A disc herniation at the **C5–C6** level can sometimes produce pain that mimics myocardial infarction (pseudo-angina) due to the compression of the C6 nerve root, which can refer pain to the chest.
   (GB, p. 1280)
58. One of the following is correct about Spurleng's sign in cervical disc herniation examination:
   A. Radicular pain is reproduced when the examiner exerts downward pressure on the vertex while tilting the head towards the symptomatic side
   B. Radicular pain is reproduced when the examiner exerts downward pressure on the vertex while tilting the head away from the symptomatic side.
   C. Radicular pain is reproduced when the examiner exerts upward pressure on the vertex while tilting the head towards the symptomatic side.
   D. Radicular pain is reproduced when the examiner exerts upward pressure on the vertex while tilting the head away from the symptomatic side.
   Correct Answer: A
   Explanation:
   Spurling's sign is positive when radicular pain is reproduced by the examiner applying downward pressure on the vertex while tilting the head toward the symptomatic side. This maneuver narrows the intervertebral foramen and increases the disc bulge.
   (GB, p. 1282)
59. The anterior cervical discectomy and fusion (ACDF) was first described by:
   A. Anderson
   B. Cloward
   C. Penfield
   D. Yasargil
   Correct Answer: B
   (SSW, p. 1595)
60. Which of the following findings is most predictive of symptom improvement following anterior cervical discectomy and fusion (ACDF) for cervical degenerative disc disease?
   A. Degree of disc height loss on imaging
   B. Presence of myelomalacia on MRI
   C. Correlation of clinical symptoms with radiographic findings
   D. Duration of symptoms is less than six months
   Correct Answer: C

Explanation:

One of the most important factors in predicting symptom improvement after ACDF is the **correlation of clinical symptoms with radiographic findings**.

(SSW, pp. 1595–1603)

61. Which statement best describes the role of apoptosis in intervertebral disc degeneration?
    A. Apoptosis is decreased. This leads to the accumulation of senescent cells.
    B. Increased apoptosis causes a loss of disc cellularity.
    C. Apoptosis does not play a significant role in disc degeneration.
    D. Apoptosis affects only the annulus fibrosus, not the nucleus pulposus.

    Correct Answer: B

    Explanation:

    Apoptosis plays a key role in intervertebral disc degeneration. It reduces the number of disc cells. This leads to a loss of disc cellularity. The process weakens the disc's structure and function.

    (SSW, p. 1672)

62. Which statement is true about cervical disc arthroplasty compared to ACDF for single-level cervical degenerative disc disease?
    A. Cervical disc arthroplasty has a higher rate of pseudarthrosis.
    B. ACDF preserves motion at the operated level.
    C. Cervical disc arthroplasty causes less adjacent segment degeneration over time.
    D. ACDF has lower reoperation rates at the index level.

    Correct Answer: C

    Explanation:

    Cervical disc arthroplasty causes less adjacent segment degeneration over time.

    ACDF reduces motion at the operated level. This can speed up degeneration at adjacent levels.

    (SSW, p. 1601)

63. In cervical spondylotic myelopathy, which MRI finding best predicts poor neurological recovery after surgery?
    A. Signal changes in the cord on T2-weighted images
    B. Ventral cord compression from osteophytes
    C. Sagittal canal diameter less than 10 mm
    D. Posterior cord compression from ligamentum flavum hypertrophy

    Correct Answer: A

    Explanation:

    T2 signal changes indicate myelomalacia. This suggests irreversible spinal cord damage. Patients with these changes often have worse recovery after surgery.

    (SSW, p. 1653)

64. When considering anterior cervical corpectomy and fusion (ACCF) versus multilevel ACDF for multilevel cervical spondylotic myelopathy, which of the following is an advantage of ACCF?
   A. Lower risk of dysphagia
   B. Reduced operative time and blood loss
   C. Higher fusion rates due to a larger surface area
   D. Less risk of graft subsidence

   Correct Answer: C

   Explanation:

   An advantage of anterior cervical corpectomy and fusion (ACCF) over multilevel anterior cervical discectomy and fusion (ACDF) is that ACCF provides a **larger surface area for fusion**. This increased surface area contributes to **higher fusion rates**, which is a key benefit of ACCF when managing extensive spondylotic disease. In contrast, multilevel ACDF may offer a lower risk of graft subsidence but often does not match the fusion rates achieved by ACCF due to the smaller contact area available for fusion.

   (**SSW**, p. 1654)

Cervical Spine Trauma

6

1. Question: Which of the following statements about a hangman fracture is FALSE?
   A. A hangman fracture involves a fracture of the pars interarticularis of the C2 vertebra on both sides.
   B. The most common cause of a hangman fracture is hyperextension and distraction.
   C. Neurological impairment is seen in the majority of patients with a hangman fracture.
   D. Treatment options for a hangman fracture can include a cervical collar, halo immobilization, or surgical fixation, depending on the severity and stability of the fracture.

   Correct Answer: C

   Explanation:

   Most of the patients with a hangman fracture present only with neck pain. Neurological impairment is seen in only about 5% of patients.

   (GP, p. 1166)

2. A 34-year-old presented with neck pain after a motor vehicle crash. A CT cervical scan is seen below (Fig. 6.1):

   2a. The classification of this type of fracture is called:
   A. Anderson and D'Alonzo classification
   B. Anderson and Copper classification
   C. Anderson and Anderson junior classification
   D. Anderson classification

   2b. One of the following is FALSE about Type I of this fracture:
   A. It is an avulsion injury
   B. Can be associated with craniocervical junction injury
   C. Nonunion is common
   D. Treatment is with a collar

K. F. AlAli, H. T. Hashim, *Spine Surgery and Peripheral Nerve Surgery*,
https://doi.org/10.1007/978-3-031-98543-0_6

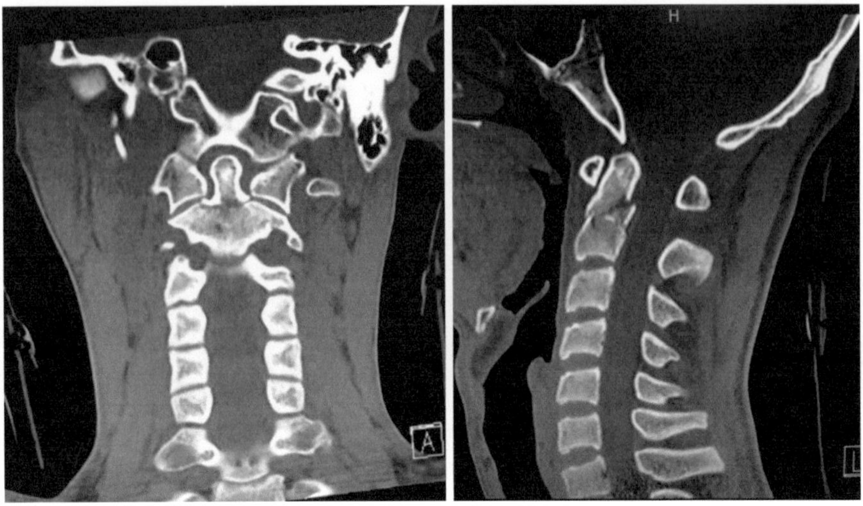

Fig. 6.1 A 34-year-old presented with neck pain after a motor vehicle crash

2c. Which of the following scenarios is most likely to result in a Type II fracture?

A. A 25-year-old football player who was struck in the face by another player
B. A 70-year-old individual experiences a low-speed car accident with a sudden deceleration.
C. A 45-year-old unrestrained driver in a high-speed car crash
D. A 30-year-old with a motorbike accident and thrown onto his shoulders

2d. The natural history of Type II fracture without surgical treatment has demonstrated a nonunion rate of:

A. More than 90%
B. 25–85%
C. 5–20%
D. Less than 5%

2e. Which of the following factors contributes to nonunion in type II fractures?

A. Female gender
B. Comminution of the fracture
C. Displacement > 5 mm
D. Delayed diagnosis and treatment (>2 weeks)

2f. Type III fracture can be mistaken for Type II in the imaging. Which of the following can be used to differentiate between the fractures?

A. MRI of the cervical spine
B. Dynamic flexion and extension cervical radiograph
C. Bone scan
D. Coronal view cervical CT scan

Correct Answers: 2a: A, 2b: C ,2c: B, 2d: B, 2e:D, 2f: A

Explanation:

The CT shows an odontoid C2 fracture.

C2 odontoid fracture represents 15% of cervical fractures and is usually a flexion injury. In younger adults, it is usually a result of high-impact injuries such as motor vehicle crashes, falls from heights, skiing accidents, or diving head-first into shallow water. In the elderly, it can result from a minor fall and is usually associated with head injury.

It is classified by Anderson & D'Alonzo into three types (Fig. 6.2)

Type I: Rare avulsion injury of the tip of the odontoid process from the alar ligament. Usually stable but can be associated with craniocervical junction injury. Treatment is with a collar, and nonunion is rare due to the rich blood supply in that region.

Type II: most common type, where the fracture is through the avascularized neck of the odontoid (seen in the CT of the case). Commonly seen in elderly patients due to low-energy trauma such as falls or low-speed car accidents.

Type II odontoid fracture is a fracture at the neck of the odontoid process where the bone is narrow, and yet vascularization is poor. This leads to a higher rate of nonunion if treated conservatively. The nonunion rates vary in the literature but ranging from 25–85%. The risk factors of nonunion are: older age, comminution of the fracture, displacement > 5 mm, delayed diagnosis and treatment (>2 weeks)

Treatment is highly debated, but usually surgical fusion. Radiographic (usually MRI) of the ligamentous injury (transverse ligament) is essential for the choice of the surgical approach (anterior odontoid screw vs posterior C1–C2 fusion)

Type III: fracture through the body of C2 and might involve the superior articular process. It can be easily mistaken as type II on sagittal cervical CT; therefore, coronal cervical CT is essential, where the fracture can be seen involving the C2 body (Fig. 6.2).

Type III fractures have lower nonunion rates, ranging between 15% and 40% if treated conservatively. A non-displaced fracture is treated with external cervical immobilization.

(GB, pp. 1171–1175), [1]

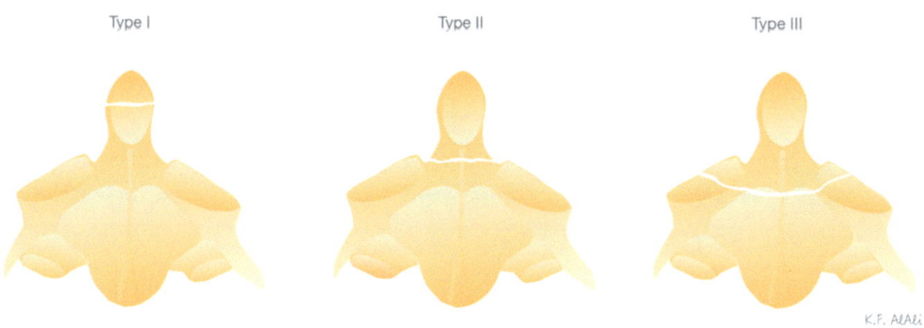

Fig. 6.2 Type of C2 odontoid fractures

3. A patient is diagnosed with a type I odontoid fracture after a fall. What is the most common mechanism of this injury?
   A. Flexion injury
   B. Hyperextension injury
   C. Rotational injury
   D. Axial loading injury
   Correct Answer: B
   Explanation:
   Type I odontoid fractures are a rare and results from an avulsion of the odontoid tip caused by traction on the alar ligament. Initially described with an angulated orientation, these fractures were considered stable but are often not isolated and may indicate atlantooccipital dislocation. Additionally, they can signal potential disruption of the transverse ligament, which may lead to atlantoaxial instability.
   (DI, p. 255)
4. One of the following clinical signs is more indicative of an occipitocervical dislocation?
   A. Severe neck pain without neurological deficit
   B. Upper limb weakness with preserved lower limb motor function
   C. Horner syndrome.
   D. Lower cranial nerve palsies
   Correct Answer: D
   Explanation:
   Lower cranial nerves are close to the occipitocervical junction, where significant displacement can cause direct injury or compression. Other common presentations are respiratory failure and motor deficit.
   (DI, p. 234)
5. A 42-year-old patient was involved in a motor vehicle crash. A CT scan is shown (Fig. 6.3):
   5a. The possible mechanism of this type of fracture is
   A. Extension
   B. Fexion

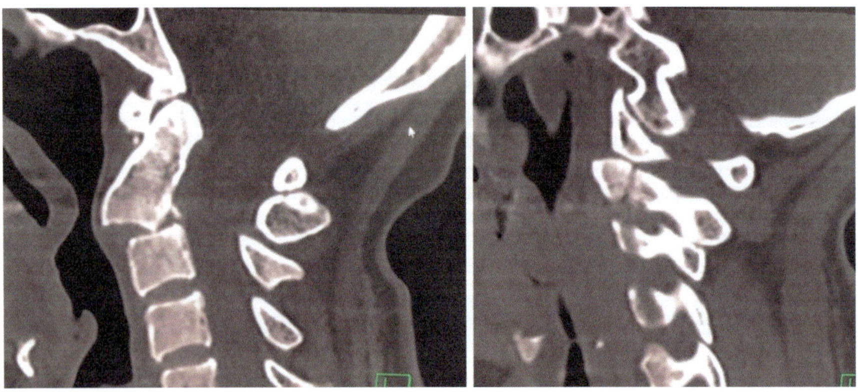

Fig. 6.3 A 42-year-old patient involved in a motor vehicle crash

C. Distraction
D. All of the above are possible mechanisms

5b. According to Levine's classification of this type of fractures (modified Effendi system), Type IA is:
A. Vertical pars fracture with ≤ 3 mm subluxation posterior to the vertebral body
B. Unparalleled bilateral pars fracture
C. Vertical pars fracture with disruption of C2–C3 disc and posterior longitudinal ligament
D. Oblique pars fracture

5c. According to Levine's classification of this type of fracture (modified Effendi system), the type of fracture seen in the CT scan is likely:
A. Type I
B. Type II
C. Type IIA
D. Type III

5d. All of the following are Effendi types of this fracture that are indicated for surgery, EXCEPT:
A. Type IA fracture with fracture line through the transverse foramen
B. Type II with subluxation ≥ 10° of angulation
C. Type II with > 5 mm subluxation
D. Type III without neurological deficit

5e. The recommended surgical approach for a surgically indicated type of this fracture is:
A. C1–C2 fusion
B. C1–C3 fusion
C. C2–C3 fusion
D. Occiput–C2 fusion

Correct Answers: 5a: D, 5b: B, 5c: D, 5d: A, 5d: C

Explanation:

The case showed C2 pars artciualris fracture, Hangman's fracture.

Hangman's fracture is a traumatic spondylolisthesis of the axis. The mechanism of injury can be extension, flexion, distraction, axial loading, or all combined.

It is classified based on Levine's classification of hangman's fractures (modified Effendi system) (Fig. 6.4):

Type I hangman's fracture of C2 pars: Vertical pars fracture with ≤ 3 mm subluxation of the posterior to the vertebral body.

Type IA: also known as atypical hangman's fracture. It is a bilateral C2 pars fracture where the two lines of the fractures are not parallel and may pass through the foramen transversarium on one side.

Both Type I and IA are treated with a rigid cervical collar for 8–12 weeks.

Type II: Vertical pars fracture with disruption of C2–C3 disc and posterior longitudinal ligament. Usually treated with cervical traction in extension + halo vest immobilization for 3 months, unless more than 5 mm subluxation

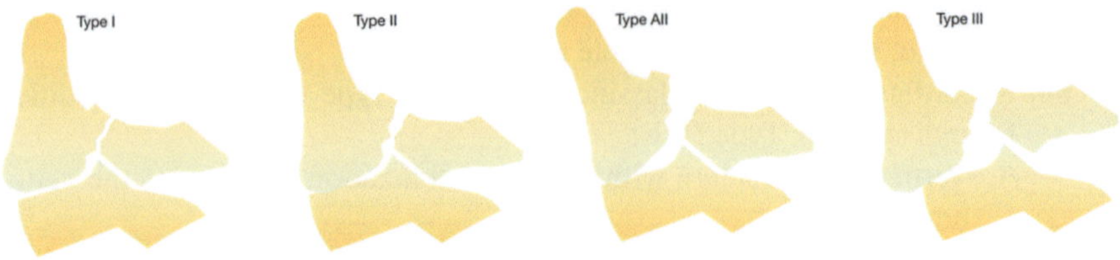

Fig. 6.4 Levine classification of hangman's fractures

or more than 10° of angulation, then surgery is a preferred choice (C2–C3 posterior fusion).

Type IIA: Oblique pars fracture. Traction is risky and causes severe overdistraction. Treatment with a halo vest immobilization for 3 months.

Type III: Type II + bilateral C2–C3 facet capsule disruption. The anterior longitudinal ligament may be injured. All were treated with C2–C3 posterior fusion.

This CT scan showed significant angulation and translation of C2 over C3, and that occurs with bilateral disruption of the C2–C3 facet, so the correct answer is type III (Fig. 6.4).

(GB, p. 1167)

6. Regarding occipital condyle fracture:

6a. The possible mechanism of injury is:

A. Hyperextension with axial loading
B. Low-impact rotational stress
C. High-energy blunt injury
D. Direct impact on the neck

6b. Which ligament is usually injured in a Type III occipital condyle fracture:

A. Lateral band of the cruciate ligaments
B. Alar ligament
C. Superior band of cruciate ligaments
D. Apical ligament

Correct Answers: 6a: C, 6b: B

Explanation:

Occipital condyle fracture is usually caused by blunt, high-energy trauma to the head and neck. Clinical presentation usually just head and/or neck pain; however, neurological deficit can occur, specifically lower cranial nerve palsies (30%). CT is the gold standard with coronal and sagittal reconstruction. MRI is essential to assess alar ligaments and tectorial membranes injury is expected.

Occipital condyle fractures classification (Anderson and Montesano):

Type I: Comminuted fractures caused by axial loading, usually stable. Treatment with a collar for 6–8 weeks

Type II: Occipital condyle fracture with extension to skull base, usually stable. Treatment with a collar for 6–8 weeks

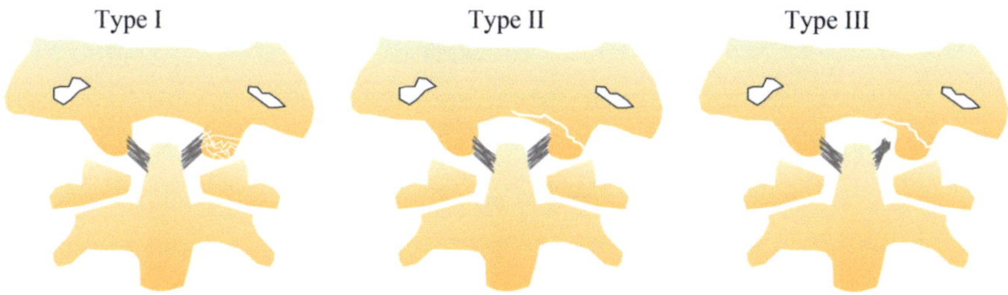

Fig. 6.5 illustration showing the sccipital condyle fractures classification by Anderson and Montesano

Type III: avulsion fracture due to with the alar ligament rupture, usually causes occipitocervical instability and requires occipitocervical fixation (Fig. 6.5). There is recent evidence (2024) that type III fractures can be treated with just a cervical collar [53].

(DI, p. 226)

7. Traction in cervical spine fracture with Gardner Wells tongs can be increased as follows:
   A. 2–5 lb per level
   B. 5–10 lb per level
   C. 10–15 lb per level
   D. 15–20 lb per level

   Correct Answer: B

   Explanation:

   Cervical spine traction is used to realign some type of cervical fracture. The initial weight is determined by three times the cervical levels above the fracture or 10–20 pounds. Then the weight can be increased by 5–10 pounds per level every 15 min. While doing this, regular cervical X-ray, neurological exam, and maybe neuromonitoring are done. If neurological deficit or over distraction is seen, the procedure must be halted.

   (GB, p. 1147, 1190)

8. Which type of occipitocervical dislocation cannot be detected by the powers ratio?
   A. Type 1
   B. Type 2
   C. Type 3
   D. All of the above

   Correct Answer: B

   Explanation:

   Power's ratio, which is calculated using the basion and the opisthion of the foramen magnum on imaging, is useful in detecting certain types of occipitocervical dislocation, primarily anterior-posterior dislocations (Fig. 6.6). However, Type 2 dislocations, which involve vertical displacement, cannot be reliably detected by Power's ratio because the ratio focuses on anterior or posterior displacement rather than vertical displacement. Vertical displacements

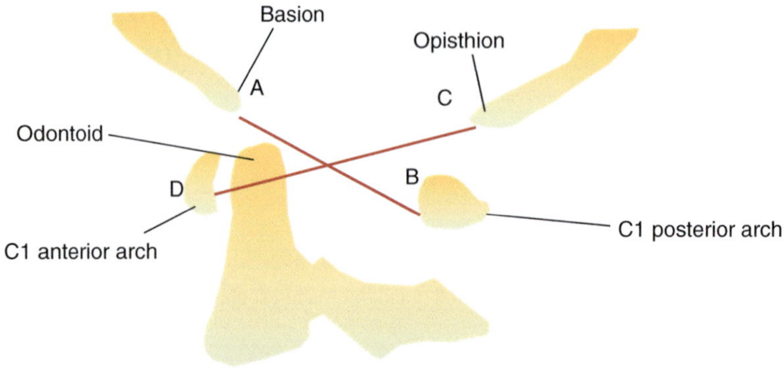

Fig. 6.6 Illustration of how the power ratio is calculated

require alternative imaging assessments, such as basion-dens interval or direct CT findings.

The power's ratio is calculated as ratio is measured as the ratio of the distance in the midsagittal plane between (AB/CD):

- Basion (A) and the posterior spinolaminar line of the atlas (B) and
- Opisthion (C) and the anterior arch of the atlas (D)

Normal values are <1 on CT or X-ray.

(RP)

9. The Traynelis Classification of the Occipitocervical Instability is based on:
   A. Degree of the dislocation
   B. Morphology of the dislocation
   C. Direction of the dislocation
   D. Which occipitocervical is ligament

   Correct Answer: C

   Explanation:

   The Traynelis classification system is used to categorize occipitocervical dislocations (Fig. 6.7). It divides the injury into three types based on the direction of the dislocation: anterior (Type I), vertical (Type 2), and posterior (Type 3). Each type of dislocation describes the movement of the occipital condyles in relation to the atlas (GB, p. 1155)

10. Which classification system is most commonly used for subaxial cervical spine injuries and taking into consideration neurological status?
    A. Allen and Ferguson classification
    B. Roy-Camille classification
    C. Subaxial Injury Classification (SLIC)
    D. AO Spine classification

    Correct Answer: C

    Explanation:

    Subaxial injury classification (SLIC) is one of the most used classifications for subaxial cervical fractures, which include C3–C7 vertebrae. It is based on three parameters:

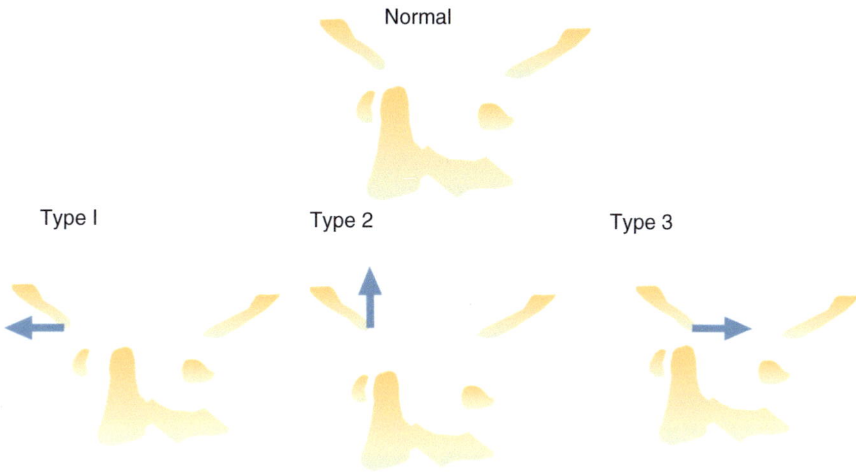

Fig. 6.7 Traynelis' classification of occipitocervical dislocations

Fracture morphology, discoligamentous complex integrity, and Neurological status (Table 6.1).

Each category is scored, and the total SLIC score aids in treatment decisions, particularly surgical interventions.

Treatment Recommendation:

- Total SLIC Score 0–3: Non-surgical management (conservative)
- Total SLIC Score ≥4: Surgical management (surgical stabilization)

(GB, p. 1181) [54]

11. All of the following structures are part of the discoligamentous complex (DLC) in the SLIC classification system EXCEPT:
    A. Anterior longitudinal ligament
    B. Ligamentum flavum
    C. Spinous processes
    D. Facet capsule

    Correct Answer: C

    Explanation:

    The discoligamentous complex consists of the anterior longitudinal ligament, posterior longitudinal ligament, ligamentum flavum, facet capsule, interspinous and supraspinous ligaments. The strongest component of the posterior DLC is the facet capsule. It is challenging to assess discoligamentous complex radiographically. MRI is the preferred imaging, specifically T2 with fat suppression (T2 STIR).

    (GB, p. 1182)

12. A 52-year-old male presented with neck pain after a motor vehicle crash. Examination revealed right triceps weakness and diminished sensation at the middle finger. Cervical CT is shown below (Fig. 6.8):

Table 6.1 Subaxial Injury Classification (SLIC) system

Parameter	Classification	Points
Injury morphology	Compression fracture	1
	Burst fracture	2
	Distraction injury (e.g., hyperflexion or hyperextension)	3
	Translation/rotation (e.g., fracture-dislocation)	4
Integrity of the Discoligamentous Complex (DLC)	Intact	0
	Indeterminate/disruption suspected	1
	Disrupted	2
Neurological status	Intact	0
	Nerve root injury (radiculopathy)	1
	Complete cord injury	2
	Incomplete cord injury	3
	Continuous cord compression (in the setting of ongoing cord compression with intact neurology)	+1

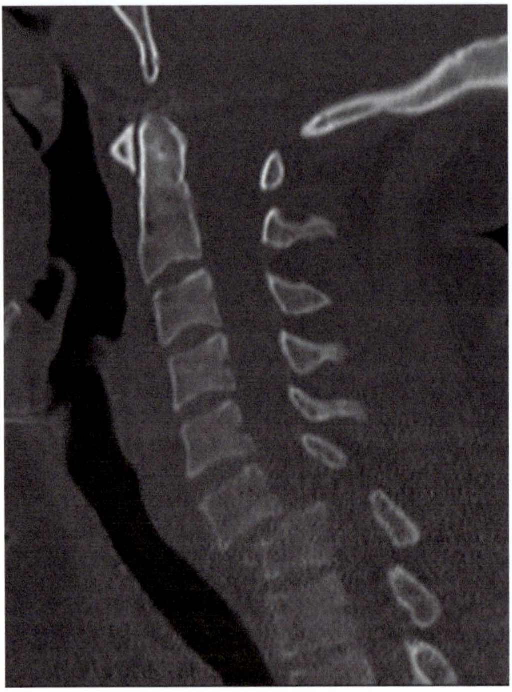

Fig. 6.8 A 52-year-old male presented with neck pain after a motor vehicle crash

12a. Based on the CT scan, is this injury unilateral or bilateral, and why?

A. Unilateral because the translation is not complete
B. Unilateral because it is at a lower cervical level
C. Bilateral because the translation is almost 50%
D. Bilateral because of the anterior fracture of the body of the lower vertebra

12b. What is the SLIC score for this patient?

A. 4
B. 5
C. 6
D. 7

12c. Axial CT cut is done through the fracture site. Identify labels A and B (Fig. 6.9):

A. A: Inferior facet of C6, B: superior facet of C7
B. A: Superior facet of C6, B: inferior facet of C7
C. A: pars articularis of C6, B: inferior facet of C7
D. A: Lateral mass of C6, B: superior facet of C7

12d. The best management strategy for this patient is:

A. Cervical traction is contraindicated in this type of fracture
B. Cervical traction, then C5–C7 anterior cervical discectomy and fusion (ACDF)
C. Cervical traction, then C5–C7 lateral mass fusion
D. B or C

Correct Answers: 12a: C, 12b: D, 12c: A, 12d: D

Explanation:

The case shows C6–C7 translation and C7 body compression fracture. The translation is 50% or slightly more, which indicates **bilateral** facet dislocation. To score this patient according to the SLIC score: morphology – translation, 4 points; DLC—disrupted, 2 points; C7 nerve root injury, 1 point. The total of

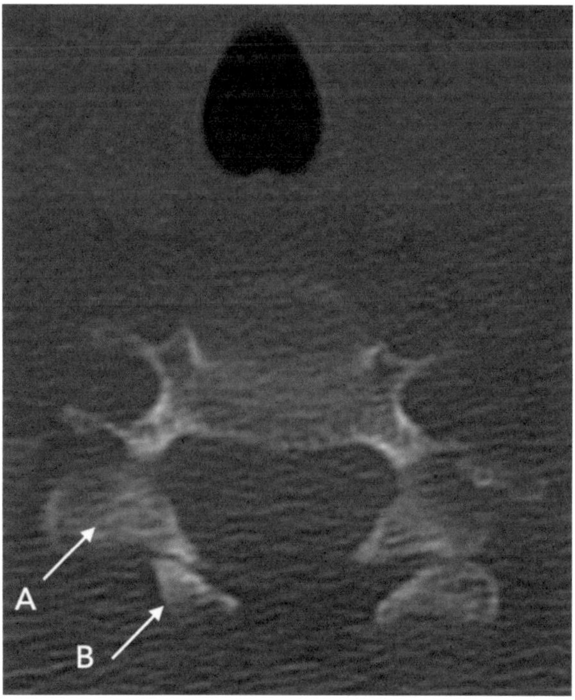

Fig. 6.9 Axial CT cut is done through the fracture site

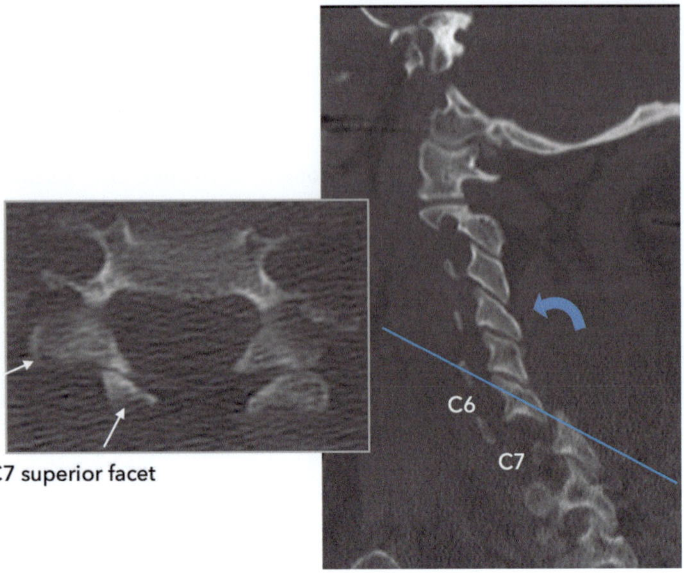

Fig. 6.10 Axial CT (left) showing cross section through the C6–C7 with classic "naked facet" sign where the inferior C6 facet is naked and the superior C7 facet appears posterior to the C6 facet. The sagittal CT scan (right) shows how the C6 inferior facet "jumped" (curved arrow) over and landed anterior to the superior facet of C7. The blue line represents the cross-sectional view seen in the axial CT cut

SLIC is 7. According to the SLIC, a score equal to or more than 4 is surgical. The translation needs reduction by **cervical traction**. Cervical traction can be done manually or with a weight. It should be monitored by serial cervical X-ray and or serial neurological examination. Once fracture is reduced, **C6–C7 ACDF and/or C6–C7 lateral mass screws** are done (Fig. 6.10).

The axial CT scan showed a classic "naked facet" sign where the inferior C6 facet is naked, with the superior C7 facet appearing posterior to the C6 facet, because this injury is a complete locked facet where the C6 inferior facet "jumped" over the C7 inferior facet. (GB, p. 1186)

13. Which of the following best describes the difference in neurological outcomes between unilateral locked facet and bilateral locked facet injuries?
    A. Unilateral injuries frequently result in complete quadriplegia, while bilateral injuries are more likely to present with root deficits only.
    B. Unilateral injuries have a higher incidence of incomplete cord injuries compared to bilateral injuries.
    C. Bilateral injuries are more likely to result in complete quadriplegia, while unilateral injuries often lead to root deficits or are neurologically intact.
    D. Both injuries have a similar distribution of complete and incomplete spinal cord injuries.

    Correct Answer: C

Bilateral facet injuries are more likely to result in complete quadriplegia, while unilateral injuries often lead to root deficits or are neurologically intact.

(GB, p. 1187)

14. What is the most common surgical approach for treating unilateral cervical locked facets if surgical intervention is required?
    A. Posterior open reduction and lateral mass screw fixation
    B. Anterior cervical discectomy and fusion (ACDF)
    C. Cervical disc arthroplasty
    D. Combined anterior and posterior approach (360° fusion)

    Correct Answer: B

    Explanation:

    Treatment of unilateral facet injury is controversial. The treatment may include a collar, halo vest with reduction, and surgical fusion. If nonsurgical treatment is chosen, close follow-up is required, and fusion is advised if instability develops. Surgical treatment includes ACDF or lateral mass fusion.

    (GB, pp. 1189–1190)
15. A hyperextension injury of the cervical spine is most likely to result in which of the following fracture patterns?
    A. Burst fracture
    B. Flexion teardrop fracture
    C. Hangman's fracture
    D. Laminar fracture

    Correct Answer: D

    Explanation:

    Laminar fracture is usually caused by hyperextension injury and may result in a floating lateral mass. Hangman's fracture is also caused by hyperextension injury, but it also requires axial loading. Cervical burst fracture requires axial loading or vertical compression.

    (GB, p. 1165, 1182).
16. What has been observed regarding the timing of surgical decompression following spinal cord injury in terms of motor score improvement?
    A. Motor score improvement decreases as time to decompression increases beyond 24 h.
    B. Motor score improvement is the same regardless of when decompression occurs.
    C. Motor score improvement is greater in the lower extremities than in the upper extremities with early decompression.
    D. Decompression in less than 24 h or within 24–48 h leads to favorable outcomes.

    Correct Answer: A

    Explanation:

    The timing of decompression surgery for spinal cord injury has always been a topic of discussion. Theoretically, early decompression restores blood flow to salvageable spinal cord tissue. Before 2012, studies in humans have shown mixed results, and the optimal timing of surgery remains debated. In 2012, the STASCIS trial [58] enrolled 313 patients, with 182 undergoing early surgical decompression (less than 24 h) and 131 undergoing late surgical decompression (more than 24 h). Of the 222 patients with follow-up available at 6 months post injury, 19.8% of patients undergoing early surgery showed a ≥2 grade improvement in ASIA impairment scale compared to 8.8% in the late decompression group (significant). They concluded that decompression surgery for cervical spinal cord injury within 24 h is safe and can cause motor improvement.

[52]

17. The presence of which imaging finding on CT scan is most indicative of a traumatic disc herniation in the setting of cervical spine trauma?
    A. Prevertebral soft tissue swelling
    B. Widened interspinous distance
    C. Focal kyphosis
    D. Anterior subluxation of the vertebral body

    Correct Answer: A

    Explanation:

    Prevertebral soft tissue swelling is the most indicative of a traumatic disc herniation on CT scan in the setting of cervical spine trauma. This swelling reflects an inflammatory response or hemorrhage from ligamentous or bony injury, which can often precede more overt signs like disc herniation or vertebral dislocation. Early recognition of this finding on CT is an indication for MRI.

    (DI, p. 291)
18. Which of the following is NOT a component of the Canadian C-spine rule?
    A. Age over 65 years
    B. Dangerous mechanism of injury
    C. Paresthesias in the extremities
    D. Low risk factors allow a safe assessment of the range of motion

    Correct Answer: C

    Explanation:

    The Canadian C-spine rule helps to identify patients at high risk for cervical spine injury after trauma, with factors like age over 65, dangerous mechanism of injury, and low risk factors for safe assessment of neck motion. Paresthesias in extremities are part of the high-risk factors but not independently listed in the rule (Table 6.2).

Table 6.2 Canadian C-spine rule table

Step	Criteria	Answer	Action
1. High-risk factors	Age ≥ 65 years Dangerous mechanism Numbness or tingling in the extremities	Yes No	C-Spine immobilization Go to step 2
2. Low-risk factors allow a safe range of motion assessment	Simple rear-end MVC (motor vehicle collision) Ambulatory at any time No neck pain at the scene No midline C-spine tenderness	Yes No	Go to step 3 C-Spine immobilization
3. Voluntary neck rotation	Patient is able to actively rotate neck 45° left and right	Yes	No C-spine immobilization
		No	C-Spine Immobilization

Dangerous mechanism: Fall from elevation ≥3 feet/5 stairs, axial load to head (e.g., diving), high-speed motor vehicle crash (>100 km/h), rollover, ejection, motorized recreational vehicles, bicycle collision with an object.

19. All of the following criteria are critical in the NEXUS cervical spine rule to clear the cervical spine after trauma, EXCEPT:
    A. No posterior midline cervical spine tenderness
    B. No evidence of intoxication
    C. No chest or abdominal injuries
    D. No focal neurological deficit

    Correct Answer: C

    Explanation:

    The NEXUS cervical spine clearance rule is another system used to clear the cervical spine after trauma. It is based on identifying low-risk criteria. If all these criteria are met, cervical spine radiography is not needed. Associated chest or abdominal injuries are not among these criteria (Table 6.3).

    (SS, p. 520)
20. In comparison between NEXUS and the Canadian C-spine rule in clearing the cervical spine after trauma, one of the following is CORRECT:
    A. The Canadian C-spine rule has higher sensitivity and specificity for cervical spine injury.
    B. The NEXUS criteria have higher sensitivity and specificity for cervical spine injury.
    C. Both have the same sensitivity and specificity for cervical spine injury.
    D. The Canadian C-spine rule is more sensitive but less specific.

    Correct Answer: A

    Explanation:

    In a prospective cohort multicenter study, NEXUS and the Canadian C-spine rule were compared in clearing cervical spine injury. The Canadian C-spine rule were found more sensitive than the NEXUS low risk criteria (99.4% versus 90.7%, $P < 0.001$) and more specific (45.1% versus 36.8%, $P < 0.001$) for injury and would have resulted in lower cervical spine imaging rates (55.9% versus 66.6%, $P < 0.001$).

    [53]
21. Regarding the Jefferson fracture:

    21a. What is the most common mechanism of injury for a Jefferson fracture?
    - A. Flexion
    - B. Extension
    - C. Axial loading
    - D. Lateral bending

Table 6.3 The NEXUS low-risk criteria table

Cervical spine radiography is indicated unless all of the following are met:
No posterior midline cervical spine tenderness
No evidence of intoxication
A normal level of alertness
No focal neurologic deficit
No painful, distracting injuries

21b. Type II Landells classification of Jefferson fracture is:

A. Fracture involving one side of the anterior arch and the contralateral side of the posterior arch
B. Fracture involving one side of the anterior arch and the ipsilateral side of the posterior arch
C. Fracture involving both sides of the anterior arch and both the contralateral sides of the posterior arch
D. All of the above

21c. Regarding the stability of the Jefferson fracture, which state is CORRECT:

A. Type I can be stable or unstable.
B. Type II is always unstable.
C. Type III is always unstable.
D. Stability depends on the integrity of the transverse ligament of the atlas.

21c. All of the following are surgical options for an unstable Jefferson fracture, EXCEPT:

A. C1 wiring
B. C1–C2 fusion
C. Occipito-cervical fusion
D. C1 direct fracture screw placement

Correct Answers: 21a: C, 21b: D, 21c: D, 21d: A

Explanation:

Jefferson fracture is a fracture of the C1 ring, typically resulting from axial loading or compression, which causes the C1 ring to burst outward. This is common in situations like diving accidents, where a direct axial force is applied to the head. IT is usually a stable fracture. The stability depends on the integrity of the transverse ligament of the atlas (aka. Transverse atlantal ligament (TAL))

There are two classification systems, Jefferson and Landells. Landells classifies Jefferson into three types:

Type I: The fracture involves either the anterior ring or the posterior ring. Usually, stable.

Type II: The fracture involves both the anterior ring and posterior ring. There are three patterns: fracture involving one side of the anterior arch and the contralateral side of the posterior arch, one side of the anterior arch and the ipsilateral side of the posterior arch, or involving both sides of the anterior arch and both sides of the posterior arch. Can be stable and unstable

Type III: fracture of the lateral mass. Can be stable and unstable.

The surgical options of the unstable fractures include C1–C2 fusion for unilateral or anterior ring fractures, occipito-cervical fusion for multiple rings fracture and/lateral mass fractures, C1 direct fracture screw placement usually done posteriorly (Fig. 6.11).

(SS, p. 537) (GB, p. 1164)

22. A 62-year-old patient presented after a fall in the bathroom with bilateral upper extremity weakness, more at the hands. He also reported slight weakness in his legs with paresthesia more in the upper extremities than lower extremities. Neurological examination reveals impaired motor strength in the upper

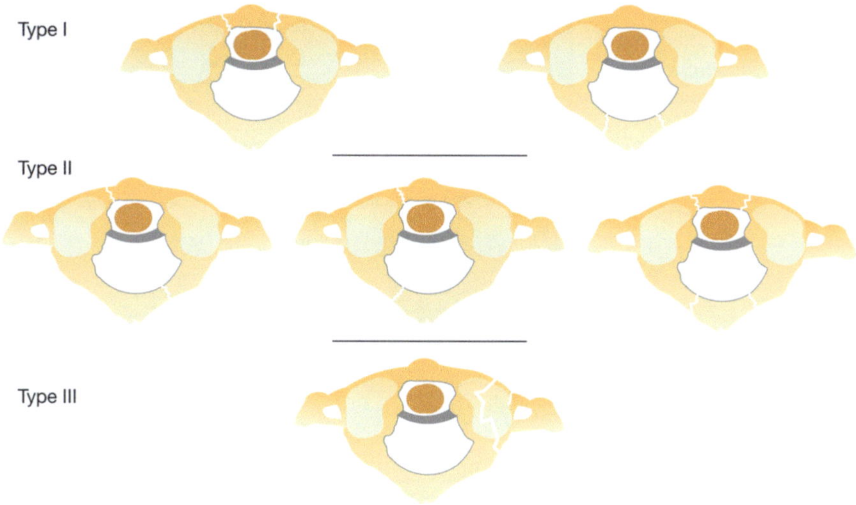

Fig. 6.11 Landell's classification of Jefferson fracture

extremities, particularly in the distal muscles of the hands, while the lower extremities have near-normal strength. MRI of the cervical spine is shown (Fig. 6.12):

22a. Which of the following is CORRECT regarding the pathophysiology of this condition?

A. The injury is primarily to the posterior columns.
B. The injury is primarily to the medial portion of the corticospinal tracts.
C. The injury is primarily to the lateral portion of the corticospinal tracts.
D. The injury is primarily to the medial parts of the posterior columns and corticospinal tracts.

22b. Which of the following is NOT a typical feature of this condition?

A. Greater motor impairment in the upper extremities than in the lower extremities
B. Bladder dysfunction
C. Preservation of proprioception
D. Hyperreflexia below the level of injury

Correct Answers: 22a: B, 22b: D

Explanation:

Central cord syndrome (CCS) presents with a variety of symptoms, often following a hyperextension injury, particularly in individuals with preexisting cervical stenosis. While this classic mechanism is seen in a minority of cases, around 60% of acute traumatic CCS patients have associated fracture subluxations or acute disc herniations. A hallmark of CCS is bilateral weakness, with more pronounced deficits in the **arms** than the legs, often accompanied by bladder dysfunction and variable sensory loss. Some patients may experience symptoms like "**burning hands**: despite normal neurological exams. The ASIA motor score for upper extremities should be at least ten points lower than for the lower extremities.

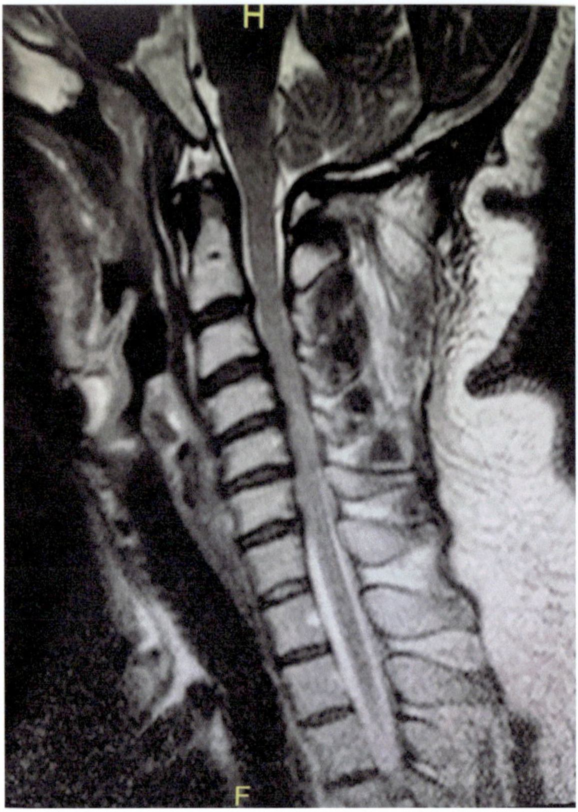

Fig. 6.12 A 62-year-old patient presented after a fall in the bathroom with bilateral upper extremity weakness, more at the hands

Treatment:

Monitoring and Stabilization: Continuous cardiac, hemodynamic, and respiratory monitoring, with maintenance of mean arterial pressure (MAP) at 85–90 mm Hg in the first week post-injury to support spinal cord perfusion.

Early Intervention: Prompt reduction and stabilization of fracture-dislocation injuries.

Surgical Decompression: Recommended for cases with focal, anterior spinal cord compression. Timing of surgery:

- **Immediate**: Emergency surgery for progressive neurological decline.
- **Early (<24 h)**: For spinal instability or significant deficits.
- **Elective (2–3 weeks)**: For patients with improving symptoms, typically without urgent signs of compression (Fig. 6.13).

(DI, p. 346; GB, p. 1132)

23. One of the following is CORRECT about traumatic cervical spondyloptosis?
    A. It is caused by low-energy trauma
    B. It is usually present with neck pain without neurological deficit
    C. It involves the complete displacement of one vertebral body over another
    D. All of the above are correct

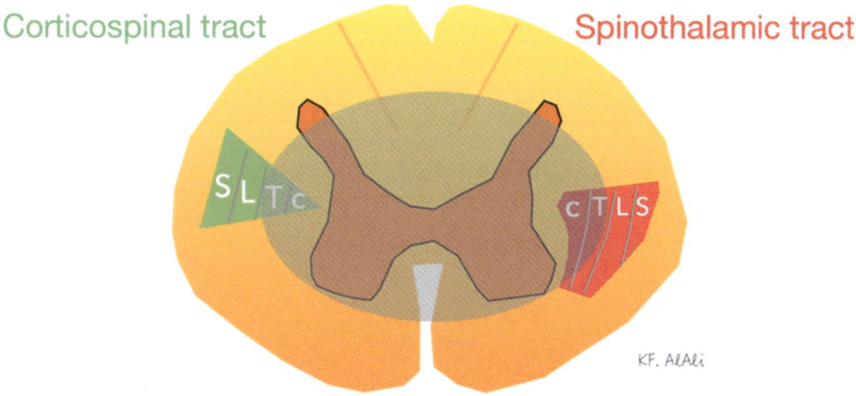

Fig. 6.13 Cross section of cervical spinal cord showing the area affected in central cord syndrome injury affecting medial parts of corticospinal and spinothalamic tracts (gray shadow). *C* cervical, *L* lumbar, *T* thoracic, *S* sacral

Correct Answer: C

Explanation:

Cervical spondyloptosis is rare, where there is 100% listhesis. It prominently affects lower cervical spine levels. It is a highly unstable injury that requires cervical reduction and surgical stabilization, preferably combined anterior and posterior approach.

[3]

24. A 31-year-old who is 3 months post odontoid screw for type II odontoid fracture presented with severe neck pain. The flexion and extension radiographs are shown. What is the appropriate management?
    A. Pain medication and physiotherapy
    B. Revision odontoid screw
    C. C1–C2 instrumentation and fusion
    D. Repeat the dynamic study in 6–9 months to assess fusion

    Correct Answer: C

    Explanation:

    This case showed instability of the atlantoaxial confirmed by abnormal atlantodental interval (ADI) on flexion X-ray. The atlantoaxial instability in type II odontoid fracture is usually due to disruption of the transverse atlantal ligament (TAL), which is confirmed by MRI initially. Type II odontoid fracture with intact TAL can be treated with odontoid screw, however when TAL is disrupted C1–C2 fixation is indicted. In this case, TAL disruption was missed initially, and the patient developed symptoms due to untreated atlantoaxial instability (Fig. 6.14).

    (GB, p. 1173)
25. The Vaccaro modification to the AO classification of upper cervical injuries includes which additional feature?
    A. Vertebral artery injury
    B. Occipital condyle avulsion

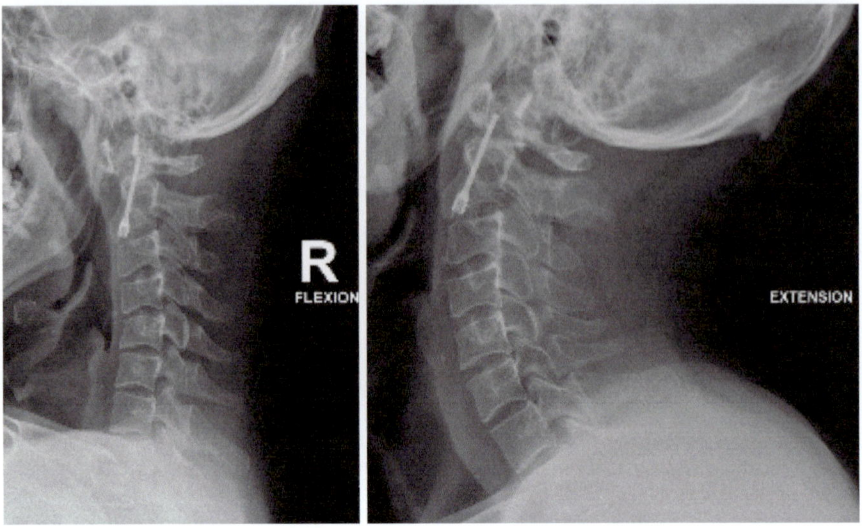

Fig. 6.14 Case 25 X-ray

C. Horizontal atlantoaxial dislocation
D. Transverse atlantal ligament injury

Correct Answer: D

Explanation:

The new AO Spine Upper Cervical Classification System (UCCS)—2022, proposed by Vaccaro et al., differs from previous systems by offering a comprehensive framework that covers all upper cervical injuries, including the occipital condyles, C1, and C2, in a unified classification. It introduces a hierarchical A/B/C system based on injury severity, stability, and **ligamentous involvement** (transverse atlantal ligament), which was absent in earlier models. Additionally, the system incorporates modifiers for fracture complexity and patient-specific factors, enhancing its ability to guide treatment and prognosis more effectively than prior classifications.

[15]

26. Which of the following is the most significant prognostic factor for neurological recovery after a cervical spinal cord injury?
A. Age of the patient
B. Initial ASIA (American Spinal Injury Association) Impairment Scale grade
C. Presence of a cervical collar on arrival
D. Time to surgical decompression

Correct Answer: B

Explanation:

The ASIA Impairment Scale (AIS) evaluates the severity of spinal cord injury and serves as a strong predictor of recovery outcomes.

(RS, p. 1315)

27. A 34-year-old was involved in a motor vehicle crash and has a C4–C6 unilateral facet fracture. Axial CT scan at the level of the injury is seen below (Fig. 6.15):

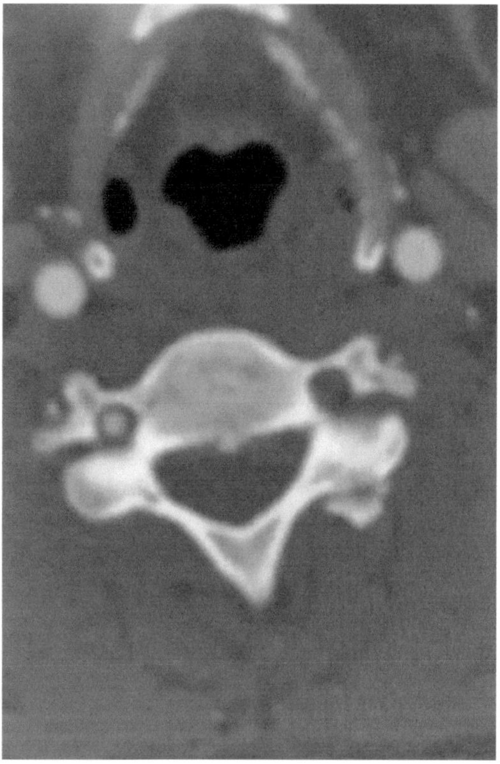

Fig. 6.15 A 34-year-old involved in a motor vehicle crash has a C4–C6 unilateral facet fracture

27a. Which of the following is the most common clinical presentation of the condition seen in the CT scan?

A. Nuchal rigidity
B. Tinnitus
C. Neck pain
D. Ataxia

27b. This type of condition commonly occurs at:

A. C1–C2
B. C2–C3
C. C3–C4
D. C4–C5

27c. One of the following treatment options for this condition is CORRECT:

A. Antiplatelets
B. Anticoagulation
C. Both A and B are valid options
D. Posterior lateral mass fusion

Correct Answers: 27a: C, 27b: A, 27c: C

Explanation:

The CT scan showed the absence of contrast at the left transverse foramen, indicating traumatic vertebral artery dissection.

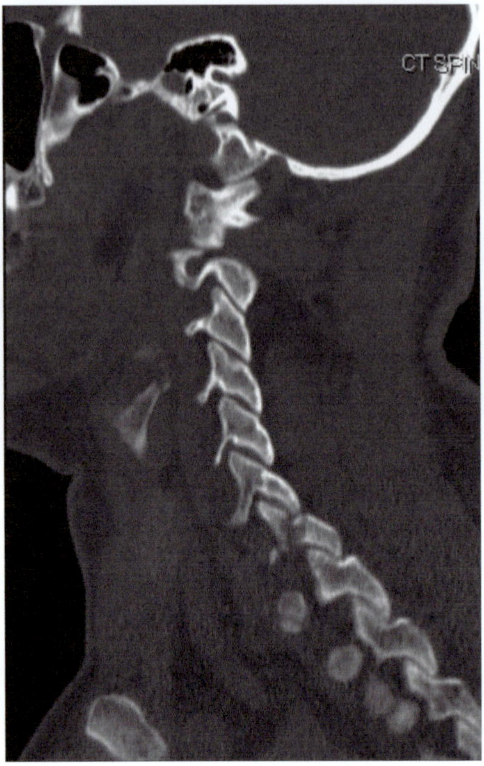

Fig. 6.16 A 45-year-old involved in a motor vehicle crash. He has only neck pain without neurological deficit. The CT scan showed a unilateral finding on the left

Traumatic vertebral artery dissection occurs more at the C1–C2 junction, where the vertebral artery is more mobile and adjacent to bony prominences. Dissection can extend intracranially, and a Fusiform aneurysm can occur along the dissection. Clinical presentation is commonly neck pain. More severe presentations can occur, like neck hematoma or intracranial bleeding.

Treatment includes antithrombotic treatment using either antiplatelet or anticoagulation. There is no clear guideline about the proper choice of treatment.

28. A 45-year-old was involved in a motor vehicle crash. He has only neck pain without neurological deficit (Fig. 6.16). The following is a CT scan that showed a unilateral finding in the left. Which of the following is correct regarding this type of injury?
    A. There is a high risk of vertebral artery injury at this level,
    B. Treatment without evidence of dislocation or subluxation remains controversial.
    C. Plain cervical spine X-rays are sufficient for the diagnosis.
    D. Usually, the finding in the CT scan is bilateral.

    Correct Answer: B

    Explanation:

    The CT showed a unilateral superior C7 facet fracture. In most of the patients, the vertebral artery does not pass through the C7 transverse foramen, making vertebral artery injury unlikely.

Isolated cervical spine facet fractures are frequently missed. Computed tomography (CT) is the primary imaging technique for detecting these injuries. Management of unilateral cervical facet fractures without dislocation or subluxation is debated, as existing evidence on treatment approaches remains limited and of low quality.

[16]

29. A 45-year-old patient presents with a nondisplaced unilateral C6 facet fracture following a motor vehicle accident. CT shows no evidence of listhesis or dislocation. Which of the following is most predictive of failure of nonoperative management?
   A. Fracture height involving 30% of the lateral mass
   B. Use of a rigid cervical collar for 6 weeks
   C. Presence of acute radiculopathy
   D. Age over 50 years

   Correct Answer: C

   Explanation:

   Risk factors for unsuccessful nonoperative management for a nondisplaced unilateral cervical facet fracture include comminution of the articular mass or facet joint, presence of acute radiculopathy, high BMI, listhesis greater than 2 mm, fragment diastasis, acute disc injury, bilateral fractures, and fractures impacting over 40% of the lateral mass height or reducing its absolute height to 1 cm.

   [16]

30. Regarding the AO Spine Subaxial Cervical Classification:

   30a. According to the AO Spine Subaxial Cervical Classification, which of the following statements best describes a Type A2 injury?
   A. A single endplate compression fracture without posterior vertebral body wall involvement
   B. A pincer fracture involving both endplates without posterior vertebral body wall involvement
   C. A burst fracture with posterior vertebral wall involvement affecting one endplate
   D. A translational injury requiring surgical stabilization

   30b. The following fracture type is considered a flexion-distraction injury:
   A. A4
   B. B1
   C. B2
   D. B3

   30c. The following modifications (M) are included in the classification, EXCEPT:
   A. Ligamentous injury
   B. Disc herniation
   C. Vertebral artery injury
   D. Facet joint involvement

   Correct Answers: 30a: B, 30b: C, 30c: D

Explanation:

AO Spine Subaxial cervical injuries classification system:

- **Type A:** Includes minor fractures (e.g., lamina, spinous process) treated nonoperatively with a cervical orthosis. Subtypes A1 (single endplate compression) and A2 (coronal split) are usually managed with a rigid orthosis, while A3 and A4 (burst fractures with posterior wall involvement) often need surgery.
  Type A2: a coronal split or pincer fracture involving both endplates without involvement of the posterior wall of the vertebral body.
- **Type B:** Involves distraction injuries. B1 (posterior osseous injury) may be treated nonoperatively if neurologically intact, while B2 (flexion-distraction) and B3 (anterior tension band disruption) generally require surgery.
- **Type C:** Highly unstable translational injuries necessitating surgical stabilization.
- **Type F:** Facet-specific injuries, graded F1–F4, range from stable unilateral nondisplaced fractures to dislocated facets, with treatment varying from rigid collars to surgical reduction and fusion.

Clinical modifiers (M1-M4) account for additional factors like ligamentous injury, disc herniation, and vertebral artery injury.

(SS, p. 9)

31. In the initial management of an unconscious patient with suspected cervical spine injury, which of the following is the most appropriate first imaging modality?
    A. Plain radiographs (AP, lateral, odontoid)
    B. CT scan of the cervical spine
    C. MRI of the cervical spine
    D. Flexion-extension X-rays

    Correct Answer: B

    Explanation:

    CT scans are the gold standard for initial evaluation of cervical spine trauma, providing excellent detail on bone injuries and detecting fractures that might be missed on plain radiographs. It is recommended to do thin slice cuts (1 mm or less) with axial, sagittal, and coronal views reconstructions.

    (SS, p. 521)

32. What is the most appropriate management for a stable type III odontoid fracture in an elderly patient?
    A. Conservative management with a rigid cervical collar
    B. Halo-vest immobilization
    C. C1–C2 posterior fusion
    D. Odontoid screw fixation

    Correct Answer: A

    Explanation:

    In type III odontoid fracture, approximately 90% of cases heal with external immobilization (and analgesics) if maintained properly for 8–14 weeks. The halo-vest brace is likely the most effective option, achieving close to a 100% fusion rate in one study. With a rigid collar, the fusion rate is around 50–70%;

if chosen, patients should undergo frequent cervical spine X-rays to monitor for potential nonunion. Even though the halo-vest brace has a better fusion rate than a rigid collar, its complications are a concern in elderly patients, making the rigid collar a better option.

(GB, p. 1174)

33. Which of the following clinical signs is most indicative of an unstable cervical spine injury?
    A. Neck pain without neurological deficits
    B. Loss of sensation in a dermatomal pattern
    C. Inability to rotate the neck
    D. Step-off deformity or palpable misalignment of the vertebrae

    Correct Answer: D

    Explanation:

    A step-off deformity or palpable vertebral misalignment suggests an unstable cervical spine injury, often indicative of ligamentous or significant bony disruption and displacement.

    (SS, p. 66)

34. A 33-year-old male was involved in a motor vehicle crash, and CT shows C5–C6 locked facet. What is the most appropriate initial treatment in the emergency department?
    A. C5–C6 ACDF
    B. Closed reduction with traction
    C. MRI of the cervical spine to assess ligamentous injury
    D. Cervical collar with observation

    Correct Answer: B

    Explanation:

    Bilateral locked cervical facet injury is usually treated with fixation either anterior (ACDF) or posterior (lateral mass fixation). Before the fixation, cervical traction is needed to restore alignment. It is indicated in a locked facet when the patient is awake with or without neurological deficit (Table 6.4).

    (EM, p. 260)

35. A 45-year-old man is involved in a motor vehicle collision. He reports neck pain and stiffness. Examination reveals reduced range of motion and point tenderness but no neurological deficits. Flexion-extension X-rays show no abnormalities.

    35a. What is the appropriate next step in management?
    A. Perform an MRI to rule out soft tissue injury
    B. Prescribe NSAIDs and encourage early return to activities
    C. Recommend a soft cervical collar for 2 weeks
    D. Administer trigger point steroid injections

    35b. After 7 months, the patient presents to the clinic with chronic neck pain and headache. MRI and X-ray cervical spine are all unremarkable except for decreased cervical lordosis. What is the initial step in the management that could have prevented the chronic symptoms of the patient?
    A. Early return to activities
    B. Soft cervical collar for 2 weeks

Table 6.4 Procedure: cervical traction with Gardner-Wells tongs

Aspect	Details
Pin placement	1 cm above the pinna, aligned with the external auditory meatus, and below the skull's equator.
Risk of incorrect pin placement	Pins placed too anteriorly risk damaging the temporalis muscle, superficial temporal artery, and vein. Pins above the skull equator may pull out with traction
Preparation	Prep with povidone-iodine or alcohol. If awake, apply local anesthesia (0.5% Marcaine with epinephrine)
Pin tightening	Tighten pins sequentially from side to side for even tension until the spring-loaded indicator shows 1 mm, equal to ~30 lb of force
Moment applied	Anterior pin applies flexion moment; posterior pin applies extension moment to the cervical spine
Traction setup	Rope is tied to an S hook, passed over a fulcrum at the bed's top, and weighted on the other end as needed
Initial weight	Start with ~10–13 lbs (average head weight), increasing gradually as needed
Monitoring	Regularly assess neurologic function during weight increases

C. Trigger point steroid injections
D. Extensive physiotherapy immediately after the injury

35c. What is the natural history of this condition?
A. Most of the patients develop cervical degenerative disc disease
B. Neurological symptoms persist in the majority of cases beyond 5 years.
C. Most patients develop chronic myelopathy within 1 year.
D. 50% of the patients recovered within 3 months, and most within 2 years

Correct Answers: 35a: B, 35b: A, 35c: D

Explanation:

Whiplash injury is a traumatic injury to the soft tissues of the cervical spine, usually caused by hyperflexion, hyperextension, or rotational forces. It usually occurs without fractures or discherniation. Clinical presentation includes delayed symptoms of neck pain, headaches, and/or cognitive impairment.

Whiplash injury grades:

Grade 0: No complaints or signs. Often do not require imaging.

Grade 1: Neck pain or stiffness without objective signs. Often do not require imaging.

Grade 2: Symptoms with reduced range of motion or tenderness. C-spine X-rays, potentially with flexion-extension views

Grade 3: Symptoms with neurological deficits (e.g., weakness, sensory loss). C-spine X-rays, potentially with flexion-extension views, and manage as a spinal cord injury

Grade 4: Includes fracture/dislocation (excluded from classic whiplash definition). Managed for potential spinal cord injuries.

Whiplash injury is usually self-limiting and resolves within weeks. Immediate range of motion exercises, early return to activities, and optional NSAIDs or analgesics for $\leq$ 3 weeks are advised. Prolonged cervical collars (>72–96 h), bed rest, and unproven therapies (e.g., muscle relaxants, homeopathy) are all discouraged.

About 50% of the patients recovered within 3 months, and most (82%) within 2 years.

(GB, pp. 119–120)

36. 16. The best imaging MRI sequence to assess ligamentous injury in cervical spine trauma is:
   A. T1-weighted MRI
   B. T2-weighted MRI
   C. Short Tau Inversion Recovery (STIR) MRI
   D. T1-weighted MRI

   Correct Answer: C

   Explanation:

   STIR MRI is highly sensitive to soft tissue and ligamentous injuries, providing excellent contrast for detecting edema and hemorrhage in ligaments following trauma while suppressing far, making it the preferred sequence for cervical ligamentous assessment.

   (DI, p. 237)

37. Which of the following cervical spine fractures carries the worst prognosis for neurological recovery?
   A. Hangman's fracture
   B. Odontoid fracture
   C. Jefferson fracture
   D. Flexion teardrop fracture

   Correct Answer: D

   Explanation:

   Flexion teardrop fracture is described by Schneider and Kahn. This injury results from hyperflexion or axial loading at the vertex with the neck flexed, which flattens the cervical lordosis. It involves two forces: anterior column compression and tension on the posterior ligaments. In severe cases, all ligaments, facet joints, and intervertebral discs may be disrupted, with $\geq$ 3 mm of posterior vertebral displacement into the spinal canal, often causing instability.

   This injury is seen in approximately 5% of patients with cervical spine trauma on X-ray, and patients are frequently **quadriplegic**, although some may retain intact function or present with anterior cervical cord syndrome.

   Treatment depends on the integrity of the ligaments and spinal canal compression, but usually, surgical fixation is advisable:

   - **If MRI shows intact ligaments and discs (which is unlikely)**, A halo brace may be used, followed by flexion-extension X-rays post-removal to check for residual instability.
   - **If ligamentous or disc injury is present**, Surgical stabilization is advised, with posterior fusion sufficient if the injury is posterior without anterior canal compromise. When there is anterior canal compression, anterior decompression and fusion are performed first, followed by posterior fusion with lateral mass screws and rods.

   (GB, p. 1184)

38. A 55-year-old male presents with a flexion teardrop fracture at C5 following a car accident. Which spinal ligament is most likely to be disrupted in this injury?
    A. Anterior longitudinal ligament
    B. Posterior longitudinal ligament
    C. Interspinous ligament
    D. Ligamentum flavum

    Correct Answer: A

    Explanation:

    A flexion teardrop fracture is characterized by a fragment of the anteroinferior aspect of the vertebral body being separated due to a flexion and axial loading mechanism. This unstable type of fracture is typically associated with disruption of the anterior longitudinal ligament (A), as this ligament is avulsed by the fragment of the vertebral body that is displaced anteriorly.

    While other ligaments, such as the posterior longitudinal ligament (B), interspinous ligament (C), and ligamentum flavum (D), may also be damaged due to the high-energy nature of the trauma and the associated instability, the anterior longitudinal ligament is the most directly implicated in the mechanism of a flexion teardrop fracture.

    Therefore, the most likely ligament to be disrupted in a flexion teardrop fracture at C5 is the A. Anterior longitudinal ligament.

    (DI, p. 273)
39. Which of the following best describes the differences between cervical extension teardrop fracture and cervical flexion teardrop fracture?
    A. Extension teardrop fractures typically happen at C5–C7, and flexion teardrop fractures typically occur at C2–C4.
    B. Flexion teardrop fractures are typically stable with minimal ligament involvement, while extension teardrop fractures are highly unstable.
    C. Flexion teardrop fractures cause posterior displacement and spinal canal compromise, while extension teardrop fractures usually have minimal or no spinal canal compromise.
    D. Flexion teardrop fractures affect only the posterior longitudinal ligament, while extension teardrop fractures affect both anterior and posterior longitudinal ligaments.

    Correct Answer: C

    Explanation:

    The differences between flexion and extension cervical teardrop fractures are summarized in the following table (Table 6.5 and Fig. 6.17):

    (GB, p. 1185)
40. A 65-year-old man presents with a hyperflexion injury, resulting in an unstable flexion teardrop fracture at C5 with anterior cord compression. What surgical approach is preferred?
    A. Posterior cervical fusion
    B. Anterior cervical discectomy and fusion
    C. Combined anterior-posterior fusion
    D. Halo traction

    Correct Answer: C

Table 6.5 Differences between extension and flexion cervical teardrop fractures

Feature	Flexion teardrop fracture	Extension teardrop fracture (avulsion fracture)
Mechanism of injury	Hyperflexion with axial loading	Hyperextension
Common location	Typically occurs in the lower cervical spine (C5–C7)	Common in the upper cervical spine (C2–C4)
Primary ligament disrupted	Anterior longitudinal ligament (ALL)	Anterior longitudinal ligament (ALL), but milder damage
Vertebral body involvement	Fracture with a displaced triangular fragment anteriorly	Small, triangular fragment anteriorly without displacement
Spinal canal compromise	Significant due to posterior vertebral body displacement	Minimal or no spinal canal compromise
Neurological impact	Often severe, including potential quadriplegia	Usually mild or no neurological deficits
Stability	Highly unstable, involving multiple ligament disruptions	Typically stable, minimal ligament disruption
Imaging findings	Large teardrop fragment with posterior displacement	Small teardrop fragment with little or no displacement
Treatment approach	Surgical decompression and stabilization are often required	Conservative treatment, such as immobilization
Prognosis	Poorer prognosis due to high risk of spinal cord injury	Generally good prognosis

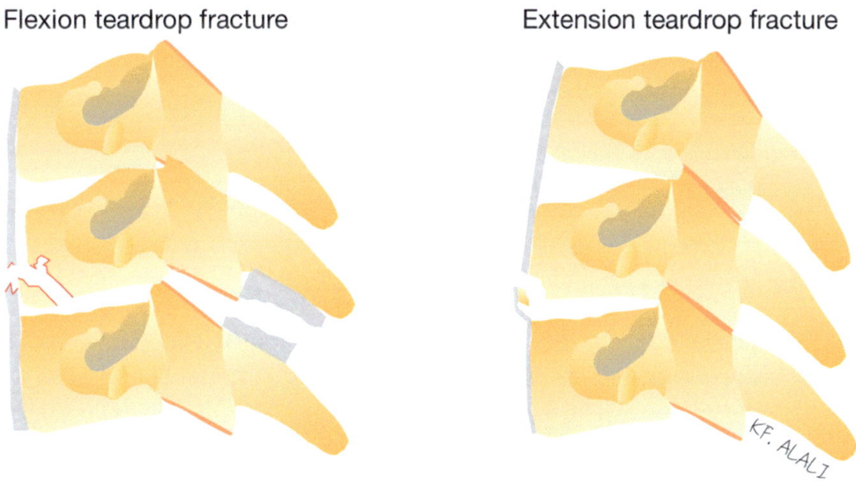

Fig. 6.17 Illustration of cervical flexion teardrop fracture vs extension teardrop fracture

Explanation:

A flexion teardrop fracture is usually a highly unstable fracture. It is typically associated with disruption of the anterior longitudinal ligament, as this ligament is avulsed by the fragment of the vertebral body that is displaced anteriorly. Anterior decompression and fusion are performed first, followed by posterior fusion with lateral mass screws and rods.

(GB, p. 1184)

41. The following are contraindications for cervical traction, EXCEPT:
    A. Atlantooccipital dislocation
    B. Type II hangman's fracture
    C. Elderly patients
    D. Age < 3 years old

    Correct Answer: B

    Explanation:

    Traction may be indicated in Type II hangman's fractures for initial stabilization. Contraindications of cervical traction are:

    - Atlantooccipital dislocation
    - Types IIA or III hangman's fracture (p. 1011)
    - Skull defect or fracture at the anticipated pin site
    - Age $\leq$ 3 years (use with caution in other pediatric age groups)
    - Very elderly patients
    - Demineralized skull like osteogenesis imperfecta
    - Associated rostral cervical injury
    - Movement disorders

    (GB, p.1147)

42. In cases of atlanto-occipital dissociation, which of the following is the most specific diagnostic feature on imaging?
    A. Widened atlantodental interval (ADI)
    B. Increased distance between the occiput and C1
    C. Lateral displacement of C1 lateral masses
    D. Presence of a teardrop fracture

    Correct Answer: B

    Explanation:

    Various methods have been developed to diagnose atlanto-occipital dissociation (AOD) radiographically. None are entirely reliable. Measurements on CT scans are more precise than those on plain radiographs. Some of the commonly used measurements (Fig. 6.18):

    - **Basion-Axial Interval (BAI)**: This measurement represents the distance from the basion to the upper margin of the posterior axial line (PAL) on C2. It is effective for detecting both anterior and posterior AOD. Normal BAI values on plain X-ray are $\leq$ 12 mm in adults and up to 12 mm in pediatric cases. On CT, it may be used, but reliability is limited.
    - **Basion-Dental Interval (BDI)**: This interval is the distance from the basion to the tip of the odontoid and is useful for identifying distracted AOD. Normal BDI values on X-ray for adults are $\leq$12 mm. In children under 13, BDI is unreliable due to varying ossification ages and fusion stages of the

Fig. 6.18 Atlanto-occipital dissociation (AOD)

odontoid. For adults on CT, the normal BDI should be <8.5 mm, while for pediatric patients, it should be <10.5 mm.

- **The condylar-C1 Interval (CCI)** or **condylar gap**, measures the distance between the occipital condyle and the superior articular surface of C1. On plain X-ray, the interval should be ≤2 mm in adults and ≤5 mm in pediatric patients. On CT, the normal value for adults is <1.4 mm. For pediatric patients, it should be <2.5 mm.
- **Power's ratio. See question 8's answer.**

  (GB, p. 1153)

43. What is the most appropriate management for a patient with atlantoaxial instability and neurological deficits following trauma?
    A. Halo-vest immobilization
    B. Surgical stabilization with C1–C2 fusion
    C. Cervical collar immobilization
    D. Closed reduction followed by bracing

    Correct Answer: B

    Explanation:

    Atlantoaxial instability is caused by ligamentous injury, yet surgical stabilization is indicated. The etiologies of traumatic atlantoaxial instability: unstable odontoid fractures, odontoid nonunion, unstable os odontoideum. The non-traumatic etiologies are: rheumatoid arthritis, congenital malformations, Down syndrome, and ankylosing spondylitis.
44. What is the primary feature that differentiates a stable from an unstable cervical spine fracture?
    A. Normal neurological exam
    B. Intact posterior ligamentous complex
    C. Fracture of all columns
    D. Pain that resolves with rest

    Correct Answer: B

    Explanation:

    Cervical spine stability depends on the integrity of the posterior ligamentous complex (PLC). The PLC includes the following structures (Fig. 6.19):

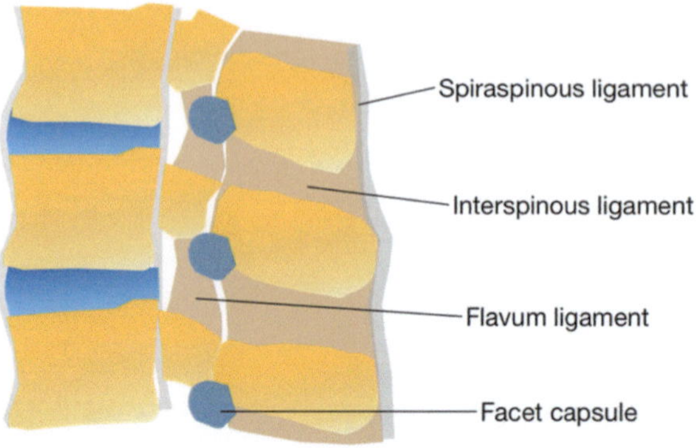

Fig. 6.19 Illustration of mid-sagittal view of cervical spine showing posterior ligamentous complex

- **Supraspinous ligament** connects the tips of the spinous processes from C7 vertebra to L4.
- **Interspinous ligament** connects between adjacent spinous processes and limits flexion.
- **Ligamentum flavum** is a thick ligament that connects the laminae of adjacent vertebrae from their ventral sides.
- **Facet joint capsules** engulf the facet joints and provide additional stability, preventing rotational forces.

  (GB, p. 1201)

45. What is the recommended time frame for performing early decompression surgery in patients with acute spinal cord injury to maximize potential neurological and functional recovery?
    A. Within 12 h of injury
    B. Within 24 h of injury
    C. Within 48 h of injury
    D. Within 72 h of injury

    Correct Answer: B.

    Explanation:

    Fehling et al. [6] conducted a study comparing the results of early (less than 24 h) and delayed decompression surgery for spinal cord injury and central cord syndrome.

    Method: A multidisciplinary panel evaluated the evidence and ranked the strength of the recommendations using evidence grading.

    Key Recommendations: Early surgery is recommended as an option for adult spinal cord injury and central cord syndrome patients due to potential neurological and functional benefits.

    Outcomes: Early decompression shows possible motor improvement at 6–12 months, with functional gains in ASIA score.

    Complications did not significantly differ between early and late surgery groups. [6]

46. In a patient with a type II odontoid fracture and nonunion after conservative treatment, what surgical option provides the most direct stabilization?
    A. Posterior C1–C2 fusion
    B. Anterior odontoid screw fixation

C. Occipitocervical fusion
D. Halo vest placement
Correct Answer: B
Explanation:
Anterior odontoid screw provides direct stabilization for the fracture without adding fusion to the other vertebrae like in C1–C2 fusion (Table 6.6).

Table 6.6 Procedure: anterior odontoid screw placement

Steps	Details
Preoperative assessment	**Imaging**: AP, lateral, and open-mouth odontoid views, plus thin-cut CT **Challenges**: Any deformity of body figure that may obstruct screw trajectory like short neck, barrel chest, or kyphotic alignment; scout CT views can help assess possible instrument paths **Contraindications**: severe osteopenia, chronic nonunion, posterior displacement, complex fracture patterns, irreducible canal compromise, or fracture patterns that extend from posterior-superior to anterior-inferior (see below) 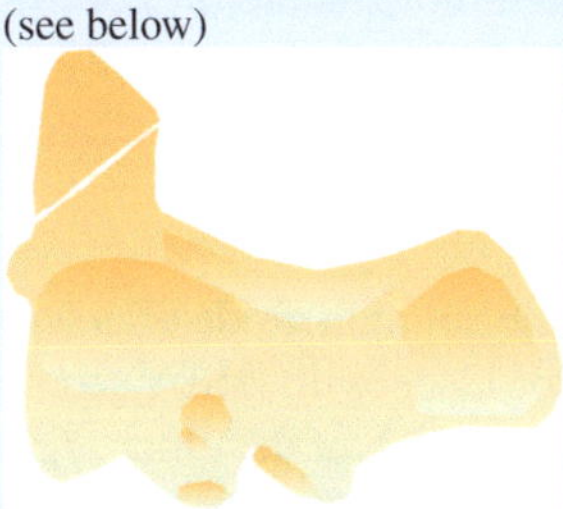 Posterior-superior to anterior-inferior fracture is contraindicated
Positioning	**Setup**: supine on a radiolucent table with a shoulder roll for neck extension, which aids in achieving the proper screw trajectory **Stabilization**: Gardner-Wells tongs with 10 lbs of traction stabilize the head and assist with fracture reduction, or a Mayfield head clamp if the fracture is reduced **Fluoroscopy**: AP and lateral fluoroscopy
Surgical technique	**Approach**: standard anterior cervical approach **Instrumentation**: K-wire is inserted to mark the trajectory, using AP and lateral fluoroscopy for guidance. Avoid advancing the K-wire past the cortex initially to prevent penetration of the brainstem **Screw Placement**: a cannulated screw is placed over the K-wire, achieving bicortical purchase when feasible
Instrumentation details	**Measurement**: screw length is measured using the K-wire for bicortical purchase, which helps compress the fracture site without exceeding safe depths **Guidewire technique**: During drilling, slightly retract the K-wire to avoid pushing it into the brainstem. Drilling is completed under biplanar fluoroscopy, and a partially threaded screw is passed over the K-wire to compress the fracture **Verification**: Fluoroscopic views confirm depth and positioning
Postoperative management	**Stabilization**: cervical collar for 6–12 weeks **Early Mobilization**: Encourage early movement to aid recovery **Follow-Up Imaging**: CT: immediate post op and 6–12 months post-op should show fracture healing and preservation of C1–2 motion without translation

47. Which of the following is most likely affected in anterior cord syndrome?
    A. Pain and temperature sensation
    B. Vibration and proprioception
    C. Motor deficit in bilateral upper extremities
    D. It will cause Horner's syndrome.

    Correct Answer: A

    Explanation:

    Anterior cord syndrome is a type of incomplete spinal cord injury. It is characterized by bilateral motor paralysis as well as loss of pain and temperature perception below the level of the injury. Proprioception and touch are typically retained.

    (SS, p. 9)
48. Using the ASIA score, which of the following best describes the motor level of a spinal cord injury?
    A. The last spinal level with normal light touch sensation.
    B. The lowest spinal segment with a motor score of 3 or greater
    C. The uppermost spinal segment with a motor score of 4 or greater
    D. The last spinal level with normal pain sensation.

    Correct Answer: B

    Explanation:

    The lowest segment with a muscle strength grade of at least three is regarded as being at the motor level in accordance with ASIA scoring guidelines, provided that the muscle strength grade in each of the other segments above is five.

    (SS, p. 519)
49. Using the ASIA score, which of the following best describes the sensory level of a spinal cord injury?
    A. The first spinal level with abnormal sensation.
    B. The lowest spinal level with no light touch and pinprick sensation in the lower extremities.
    C. The last spinal level with normal sensation is light touch and pinprick
    D. The last level of the spine with normal motor function and sensation

    Correct Answer: C

    Explanation:

    The ASIA sensory level in spinal cord injury is defined as the lowest spinal level or segment in both light touch and pinprick sensations are intact. (SS, p. 519)

Thoracic, Lumbar Sacral Spine Trauma and Spinal Cord Injury

7

1. A 35-year-old male falls from a height and presents with severe back pain but no neurological deficits. CT scan reveals a burst fracture of L1 with retropulsion of bone fragments into the spinal canal, causing 30% canal compromise. According to the Thoracolumbar Injury Classification and Severity Score (TLICS), which management option is most appropriate?
   A. Conservative management with a thoracolumbosacral orthosis (TLSO)
   B. Posterior short-segment fixation without decompression
   C. Posterior decompression and instrumented fusion
   D. Bed rest and analgesia without bracing

   Correct Answer: C

   Explanation:

   The Thoracolumbar Injury Classification and Severity (TLICS) score is a widely used system for evaluating thoracolumbar spine injuries and determining the most appropriate treatment. It is based on three critical factors: the morphology of injury, the patient's neurological condition, and the condition of the posterior ligamentous complex (PLC). Compression fractures receive 1 point, burst fractures score 2 points, and translational or rotational injuries score 3 points. Neurological assessment assigns points for an intact nervous system (0), nerve root injury (2), incomplete spinal cord injury (3), and complete spinal cord injury (2), with cauda equina syndrome receiving the highest score of 3. The PLC is scored as intact (0), indeterminate (2), or disrupted (3).

   A score below 3 indicates that management is not surgical, and a score of 5 or higher generally implies that surgery is necessary. A score of 4 requires careful clinical analysis for proper decision.

   By using this scoring system, it is possible to establish consistent treatment decisions for injuries in the thoracolumbar spine.

   [44]

K. F. AlAli, H. T. Hashim, *Spine Surgery and Peripheral Nerve Surgery*,
https://doi.org/10.1007/978-3-031-98543-0_7

2. Which of the following thoracic spine fractures is most commonly associated with intra-abdominal injuries due to the mechanism of trauma?
   A. Compression fracture of T6
   B. Flexion-distraction injury at T12–L1
   C. Burst fracture of T4
   D. Fracture-dislocation at T10–T11

   Correct Answer: D

   Explanation:

   Fracture-dislocation represents a severe spinal injury characterized by the disruption of all three columns of the spine. It involves force applied transversely at vector causes a shearing injury, potentially combined with flexion and/or rotation.

   This includes damage to the anterior longitudinal ligament (ALL), posterior longitudinal ligament (PLL), facet capsule ligamentous complex, and the interspinous and supraspinous ligaments. The involvement of these critical stabilizing structures highlights the severity and instability of the injury. It is usually associated with head injury and thoraco-abdominal injuries.

   (DI, p. 299)
3. A 45-year-old woman presents with low back pain and lower extremity weakness after a fall. Imaging reveals a transverse fracture through the L1 vertebral body extending into the posterior elements, with widening of the interspinous distance. Which injury mechanism is most consistent with these findings?
   A. Axial compression
   B. Flexion-compression
   C. Flexion-distraction (Chance fracture)
   D. Extension

   Correct Answer: C

   Explanation:

   Flexion-distraction is also known as chance fracture. It is disruption of the middle and posterior column with compression to the anterior column. It also can be associated with intraabdominal or thoracic injury; however, it is more common in Fracture-dislocation injury (Fig. 7.1).

   (DI, p. 299)

   It is crucial to differentiate between fracture-dislocation and flexion-detraction fractures.

   The following table explains the differences (Table 7.1):
4. A patient with a sacral fracture exhibits loss of bowel and bladder function, saddle anesthesia, and weakness in lower extremity muscles innervated by sacral nerve roots. Which type of sacral fracture is most likely responsible for these findings?
   A. Zone I fracture
   B. Zone II fracture
   C. Zone III fracture
   D. Transverse fracture of the distal sacrum

   Correct Answer: C

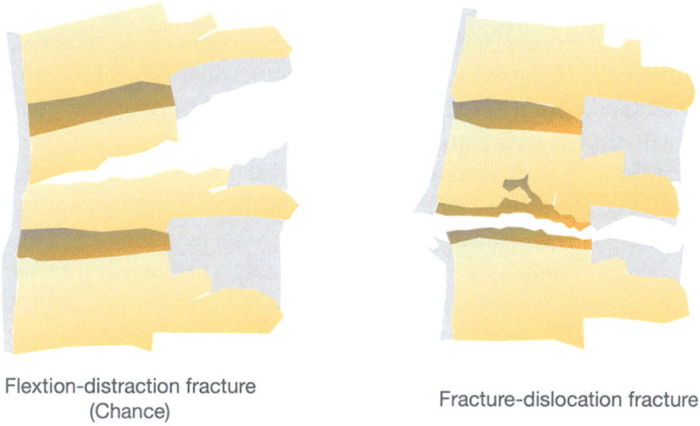

Fig. 7.1 Flexion-distraction fracture vs fracture-dislocation injury

Table 7.1 Differences between spine fracture-dislocation and flexion-distraction fracture

Feature	Fracture-dislocation	Flexion-distraction (chance fracture)
Mechanism of injury	High-energy trauma with rotational or shearing forces	Hyperflexion forces causing failure of posterior elements
Columns involved	Disruption of all three columns (anterior, middle, and posterior)	Primarily affects the middle and posterior columns
Ligamentous injury	Disruption of ALL, PLL, interspinous, supraspinous, and zygapophyseal ligaments	Failure of posterior ligaments, including interspinous and supraspinous ligaments. Usually, undisrupted ALL
Fracture pattern	Often involves vertebral body, pedicles, and posterior elements with displacement	May show fractures of posterior elements (e.g., spinous process, lamina) without significant displacement
Alignment	Significant vertebral displacement and malalignment	Minimal displacement, with kyphotic angulation common
Neurological involvement	Frequently associated with spinal cord or nerve root injury	Neurological injury less common but possible
Radiographic features	Malalignment, widening of interspinous distances, and vertebral body fractures	Widened interspinous space, horizontal fractures of posterior elements
CT findings	Complete disruption of vertebral alignment and possible facet dislocations	Horizontal or oblique fracture lines through posterior elements, often sparing the vertebral body except for compression and loss of height
MRI findings	Disruption of all ligamentous structures with evidence of cord compression or injury	Hyperintensity in posterior ligaments and edema in adjacent tissues

Explanation:

Sacral fractures are classified into three zones based on the anatomical region of involvement and the associated clinical implications. Zone I fractures involve the ala of the sacrum, sparing the central canal and neural foramina, and are occasionally linked with partial L5 root injury, often due to entrapment between an upwardly migrated fracture fragment and the transverse process of the L5 vertebra. Zone II fractures affect the region of the sacral foramina but spare the central canal. These vertical fractures may involve unilateral L5, S1, and/or S2 nerve roots, occasionally causing sciatica, though bladder dysfunction is rare. Zone III fractures involve the sacral canal and are frequently associated with sphincter dysfunction, saddle anesthesia, and, in bilateral cases, root injuries. Zone III fractures are further subdivided into vertical and transverse types. Vertical fractures are often linked to pelvic ring fractures, while transverse fractures, though rare, usually result from a high-impact force and can lead to significant neurological deficits, including bowel and bladder incontinence (Fig. 7.2).

(GB, p. 1216)

5. A 25-year-old male presents to the emergency department after a motorcycle accident. He has a T3 spinal cord injury confirmed by MRI. His systolic blood pressure is 80 mmHg despite no significant blood loss on imaging or examination. Heart rate is 50 bpm, and he demonstrates flaccid paralysis below the T3 level with absent reflexes. Which of the following mechanisms most accurately explains the patient's hemodynamic status?
   A. Loss of parasympathetic tone
   B. Increased venous return due to loss of skeletal muscle tone
   C. Sympathetic interruption
   D. Direct injury to the bulbocavernosus reflex arc

   Correct Answer: C

   Explanation:

   The patient's hemodynamic findings (hypotension and bradycardia) are indicative of **neurogenic shock** in the context of a T3 spinal cord injury. Neurogenic shock results from disruption of the sympathetic nervous system, which causes **Vasodilation**: Loss of sympathetic tone leads to unopposed parasympathetic activity and systemic vascular resistance reduction, resulting in **hypotension**.

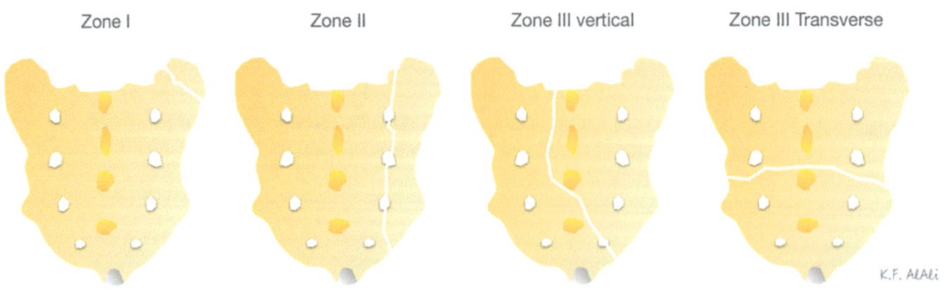

Fig. 7.2 Classification of sacral fractures

Bradycardia: Unopposed vagal tone due to lack of sympathetic innervation results in a slow heart rate.

The findings of flaccid paralysis and absent reflexes are features of **spinal shock**, which coexists but does not explain the hemodynamic instability.

(GB, p. 1119)

6. A 45-year-old male presents with sudden onset of bilateral lower extremity paralysis and a loss of pain and temperature sensation below the level of T6. CT scan reveals a dislocated bone fragment compressing the anterior spinal cord. Which of the following findings is most likely preserved in this patient?
   A. Pain sensation in the lower extremities
   B. Two-point discrimination in the lower extremities
   C. Motor function in the upper extremities
   D. Temperature sensation above T6

   Correct Answer: B

   Explanation:

   The anterior spinal cord compression with clinical picture (loss of pain and temperature sensation indicate anterior cord syndrome. Anterior cord syndrome spares posterior column functions, such as two-point discrimination and joint position sense, while impairing motor and spinothalamic tract functions below the lesion.

   (GB, p. 1135)

7. A 30-year-old patient with quadriplegia secondary to anterior spinal artery syndrome is being evaluated for recovery potential. Which of the following findings on clinical examination would most strongly suggest a poor motor prognosis?
   A. Return of sensation to light touch in the lower extremities
   B. Absence of proprioception below the lesion
   C. Complete loss of voluntary motor function after 6 months
   D. Persistent hyperreflexia below the lesion after 3 months

   Correct Answer: C

   Explanation:

   Anterior cord syndrome:

   Also known as anterior spinal artery syndrome, anterior cord syndrome occurs due to infarction in the territory supplied by the anterior spinal artery. It is more common than central cord syndrome and can result from anterior spinal artery occlusion or anterior cord compression, such as by a dislocated bone fragment or herniated disc. Patients typically present with paraplegia or quadriplegia (if the lesion is above C7) and dissociated sensory loss below the lesion, including loss of pain and temperature sensation (spinothalamic tract) while preserving posterior column functions like two-point discrimination and joint position sense. It is critical to roll out non-surgical condition such as anterior spinal artery occlusion from surgical causes like cord compression. This requires evaluating the CT and the MRI. Anterior cord syndrome has a poor motor recovery rate, with only 10–20% regaining functional motor control. Persistent motor deficits after 6 months strongly suggest poor prognosis. Sensory recovery, such as touch or proprioception, may occur independent of motor recovery.

   (GB, p. 1135).

Surgical treatment is indicated for cord compression or spinal instability. Prognosis is poor, with only 10–20% regaining functional motor control, though some sensory recovery may occur to help prevent complications like burns or ulcers.

8. A 35-year-old male is brought to the emergency department following a high-speed motor vehicle collision. He is found to have a significant T12 vertebral body fracture on initial imaging. The patient is also intoxicated, with a Glasgow Coma Scale (GCS) score of 13. No other injuries are immediately noted on physical examination. What is the most appropriate next step in managing this patient?
   A. Focused imaging of the thoracolumbar spine to evaluate the extent of the T12 fracture
   B. Obtain an MRI of the thoracolumbar spine to assess ligamentous injury at T12
   C. Perform imaging of the entire spinal axis to rule out additional fractures
   D. Immediate surgical stabilization of the T12 fracture

   Correct Answer: C

   Explanation:

   Imaging the entire spinal axis (usually CT scan) is crucial when a significant spine fracture is identified in one region, as there is a 5–20% likelihood of a concurrent fracture in another region. The risk of missing additional spine fractures is heightened in patients with head injuries, intoxication, drug use, or polytrauma, underscoring the importance of comprehensive spinal imaging in such cases.

   (SS, p. 557)

9. A 40-year-old female presents after a stab wound to her back at upper thoracic spine. On examination, she has weakness and spasticity in her right lower limb, with absent proprioception and vibration sensation on the same side. She also reports loss of pain and temperature sensation on her left side below the T6 level. Which of the following best explains her clinical findings?
   A. Complete transection of the spinal cord at the T6 level
   B. Hemisection of the spinal cord at the T6 level
   C. Anterior spinal artery syndrome at the T6 level
   D. Central cord syndrome at the T6 level

   Correct Answer: B

   Explanation:

   Brown-Séquard syndrome results from a hemisection of the spinal cord accounts for 2–4% of traumatic spinal cord injuries. It is often caused by penetrating trauma but can also arise from conditions such as radiation myelopathy, spinal epidural hematoma, large cervical disc herniation, tumors, AVMs, spondylosis, or spinal cord herniation. Ipsilateral motor weakness, spasticity, and loss of proprioception and vibration are due to damage to the corticospinal tract and dorsal column, respectively. Contralateral loss of pain and temperature sensation occurs due to disruption of the spinothalamic tract, which crosses shortly after entering the spinal cord. Despite its severity, Brown-Séquard syndrome has a favorable prognosis, with approximately 90% of patients regaining independent ambulation and sphincter control (Fig. 7.3).

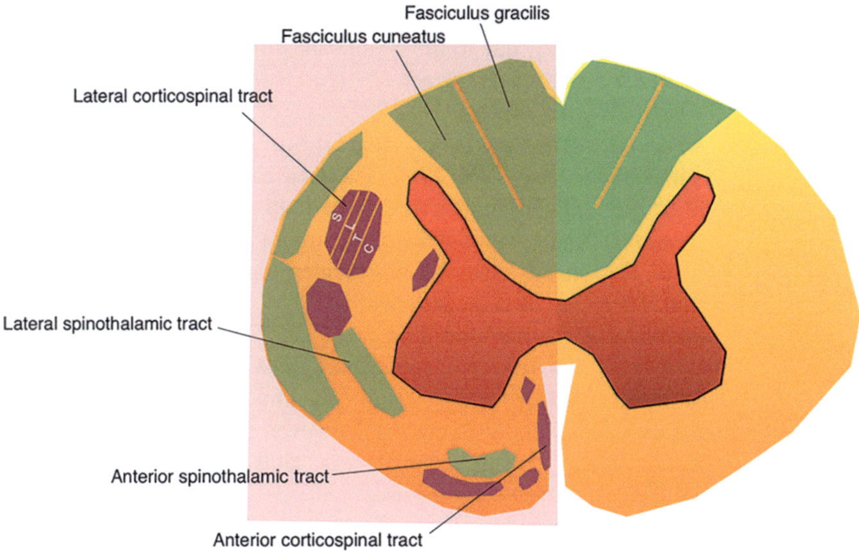

Fig. 7.3 Affected spinal tracts in Brown-Séquard syndrome

10. One of the following is correct regarding the evidence of the use of high methylprednisolone in spinal cord injury:
    A. NASCIS II and NASCIS III are high quality randomized clinical trials with few limitations.
    B. 2017 Guidelines by the American Association of Neurological Surgeons/ Congress of Neurological Surgeons Joint Guidelines Committee strongly advised the use of high methylprednisolone in spinal cord injury of cervical region.
    C. American Spinal Injury Association (ASIA) and International Spinal Cord Society (ISCoS) recommend the use of high methylprednisolone with caution.
    D. 2021 World Federation of Neurosurgical Societies (WFNS) Guidelines discourage the routine use of high methylprednisolone.

    Correct Answer: D

    Explanation:

    The use of methylprednisolone in the treatment of acute spinal cord injury has been a subject of intense debate for many years. The key findings and guidelines offer information on its effectiveness and flaws:

    NASCIS Trials:

    National Acute Spinal Cord Injury Study (NASCIS) II and III are randomized controlled trials (RCTs) conducted in the 1990s to evaluate the efficacy of high-dose methylprednisolone in SCI.

    Limitations: While these trials demonstrated some improvements in motor recovery when methylprednisolone was given within a predetermined time frame (8 h after injury), they faced criticism for methodological shortcomings, such as small sample numbers, inconsistent dosing protocols, and incomplete data retention. Additionally, due to the significant limitations and substandard quality of the trials. Thus, **A** is incorrect.

2017 AANS/CNS Guidelines:

The **American Association of Neurological Surgeons (AANS)/Congress of Neurological Surgeons (CNS)** 2017: The lack of substantial evidence to back the routine use of SCI is emphasized in the CNS guideline. However, they describe its use as an option within 8 h of being injured, taking into account the benefits against the serious risks of gastroenterology-related bleeding and hyperglycemia. Therefore, **B is incorrect**.

ASIA and ISCoS Recommendations:

The **American Spinal Injury Association (ASIA)** and the **International Spinal Cord Society (ISCoS)** emphasize the potential for methylprednisolone to offer minor benefits in motor recovery. However, they recommend its use only with caution, under specific circumstances. Thus, **C is incorrect**, as they do not strongly advocate for its routine use.

2021 WFNS Guidelines:

The **World Federation of Neurosurgical Societies (WFNS)** issued guidelines in 2020 explicitly discouraging the routine use of high-dose methylprednisolone in SCI. They highlight the lack of definitive evidence supporting its benefits and underline the significant risks associated with its use. This aligns with answer **D**, which is correct.

Conclusion:

The use of high dose methylprednisolone in SCI is controversial due to weak evidence of its benefits and high risk for complications. **The use of it as a routine practice is generally discouraged by current guidelines**, such as those from WFNS, which advocate for careful and individual decision-making in accordance with the clinical situation.

[45–47]

11. A patient presents with an L4 burst fracture with significant canal compromise but intact neurological function. According to the Load Sharing Classification, which of the following fracture characteristics would necessitate combined anterior and posterior surgical approaches?
    A. Any degree of vertebral body comminution
    B. Vertebral body comminution with displacement of fracture fragments
    C. Posterior elements involvement with ligament injury
    D. Kyphotic deformity less than 30°

    Correct Answer: B

    Explanation:

    The Load Sharing Classification (LSC), developed in 1994 by McCormack and Gaine, is a system used to assess thoracolumbar burst fractures, guiding the surgical approach. The system is based on:

    1. **Degree of vertebral body comminution**: Extent of fragmentation of the vertebral body
    2. **Displacement of fracture fragments**: Movement of bone fragments into the spinal canal

3. **Degree of kyphosis**: Angular deformity resulting from the fracture

   Each factor is scored from 1 to 3, with higher scores indicating more severe injury. The total LSC score ranges from 3 to 9. A higher score suggests increased spinal instability and a greater likelihood of implant failure if only a posterior approach is used.

   Scores ≤6: Generally managed with posterior instrumentation alone.

   Scores >6: Indicates Severely comminuted fractures with significant instability, often necessitating combined anterior (e.g., corpectomy) and posterior surgical approaches to achieve adequate stabilization.

   [48]

12. All of the following are causes of delayed deterioration following spinal cord injuries, EXCEPT:
    A. Posttraumatic syringomyelia
    B. Arachnoiditis
    C. Apoptosis of neurons
    D. Tethered spinal cord

    Correct Answer: B

    Explanation:

    Several conditions can occur as delayed neurological deterioration after spinal cord injuries, usually occur months to years post-injury. Common causes include **posttraumatic syringomyelia**, with symptom onset ranging from 3 months to 34 years, and **subacute progressive ascending myelopathy**, which manifests within 4–86 days, often involving signal changes extending ≥4 levels above the initial injury. Other contributors are **unrecognized spinal instability**, typically diagnosed after an average of 20 days, and **tethered spinal cord**, caused by scar tissue at the injury site. Additionally, **delayed spinal epidural hematomas** (SEH) often occur within 72 h of surgery but may present later. The mechanism of the delayed injuries includes **apoptosis** of neurons and glial cells, and **glial scar formation**, which causes mass effect and releases neurotoxic factors. Therefore, patients with spinal cord injuries require frequent monitoring and follow-up to assess these delayed complications. Arachnoiditisis not a recognized delayed spinal cord condition.

    (GB, p. 1221)

13. A 35-year-old male is brought to the emergency department after a motor vehicle accident. Imaging reveals a burst fracture at L2 involving the vertebral body with retropulsion of bony fragments into the spinal canal. There is also disruption of the posterior longitudinal ligament and ligamentum flavum. Neurologically, the patient has bilateral lower limb weakness and loss of sensation below L2. According to Denis' three-column concept, which of the following statements best describes the significance of this injury?
    A. The involvement of the anterior column alone indicates a stable fracture.
    B. Disruption of the middle column is critical in determining fracture stability.
    C. The posterior column is the primary determinant of mechanical instability.
    D. Injury to the middle and anterior columns typically does not compromise spinal stability.

    Correct Answer: B

Explanation:

Denis' three-column model of the spine is a widely used framework to evaluate the stability of thoracolumbar spine fractures based on CT and anatomical findings. It divides the spine into three columns:

Anterior Column: Includes the anterior half of the vertebral body, anterior annulus fibrosus (AF), and the anterior longitudinal ligament (ALL).

Middle Column: Includes the posterior half of the vertebral body, the posterior AF, and the posterior longitudinal ligament (PLL). This column is crucial in determining spinal stability.

Posterior Column: Includes posterior bony elements (posterior arch) and the posterior ligamentous complex, including the supraspinous and interspinous ligaments, facet joints and their capsules, and the ligamentum flavum (Fig. 7.4).

[50]

14. According to Denis' Three-Column Theory, which of the following is true regarding spinal stability?
    A. Disruption of the anterior column alone causes instability.
    B. Disruption of two columns is sufficient to deem a spinal injury mechanically unstable.
    C. Posterior column disruption is unrelated to spinal stability.
    D. Neurological deficits are unrelated to mechanical instability.

Correct Answer: B

Explanation:

Denis' theory posits that failure of two out of three columns (anterior, middle, or posterior) results in mechanical instability. Neurological deficits, however, add an element of neurological instability.

[50]

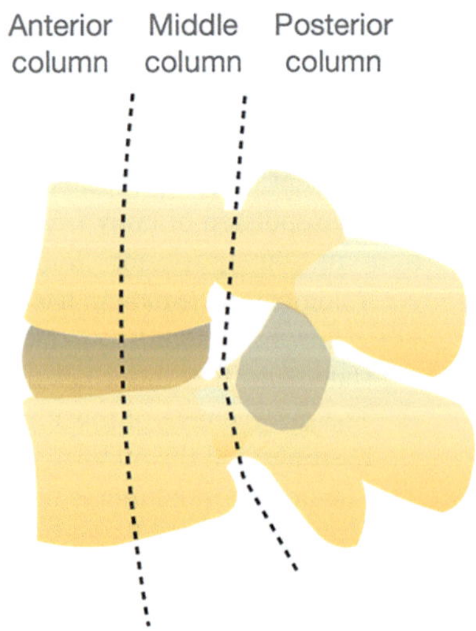

Fig. 7.4 Denis three-column model of the spine

15. A patient suffers a fracture-dislocation at T12–L1 resulting in conus medullaris syndrome. Which of the following clinical features is most characteristic of this condition?
    A. Flaccid paralysis of lower limbs without sensory loss
    B. Mixed upper and lower motor neuron signs with early bladder and bowel dysfunction
    C. Pure upper motor neuron signs in lower limbs
    D. Preservation of reflexes with loss of voluntary movement

    Correct Answer: B

    Explanation:

    Conus medullaris syndrome maybe caused by Injury to the T12–L2 vertebrae, affecting the sacral segments of the spinal cord within the conus medullaris, commonly leads to saddle anesthesia, sensory loss in the lower extremities, incomplete paraplegia and **mixed upper and lower motor neuron signs with early bladder and bowel dysfunction**.

    (SS, p. 520)
16. In evaluating a patient with a suspected spinal fracture, which of the following findings on a lateral thoracolumbar radiograph suggests instability?
    A. Anterior vertebral body compression of 20%
    B. Kyphotic angulation of 5°
    C. Loss of disc height at the injured level
    D. Translation of one vertebral body over another by more than 5 mm

    Correct Answer: D

    Explanation:

    Determining stability in the spine is not straightforward and different models and radiographic features have been developed to assess instability; however, none is solely conclusive. The widely accepted criteria for diagnosing spinal instability, as proposed by Panjabi and White, include sagittal plane translation thresholds of 4 mm anteriorly (5 and more is considered unstable) or 2 mm posteriorly for translational instability. For rotational instability, thresholds are set at >15° for L1–L4, >20° for L4–L5, and >25° for L5–S1. Additionally, sagittal plane angulation exceeding 9° is broadly recognized as indicative of instability.

    [49]
17. Which of the following most accurately reflects White and Panjabi's definition of clinical spinal instability?
    A. The inability of the spine to maintain proper alignment during pathological loads, resulting in severe neurological impairment
    B. Loss of capacity of the spine, under physiological loads, to preserve vertebral relationships, leading to potential nerve damage, deformity, or incapacitating pain
    C. A measurable displacement of vertebral bodies exceeding 3 mm in flexion-extension radiographs
    D. Structural damage to the anterior column leading to immediate mechanical instability and cord compression

    Correct Answer: B

Explanation:

White and Panjabi's definition of clinical instability is "the loss of the capacity of the spine, under physiological loads, to maintain relationships between vertebrae so that no spinal cord or nerve root damage occurs and no incapacitating deformity or pain develops."

(BS, p. 294)

18. A 45-year-old patient presents after a high-impact fall. Radiographic evaluation reveals loss of posterior vertebral body height and retropulsion of bony fragments into the spinal canal. Which of the following most accurately describes this spinal injury?
    A. Compression fracture
    B. Flexion-distraction injury
    C. Burst fracture
    D. Chance fracture

    Correct Answer: C

    Explanation:

    A burst fracture involves the failure of the middle column, typically identified (By Denis) by:
    1. Fracture of the posterior wall cortex of the vertebral body.
    2. Loss of posterior vertebral body height.
    3. Retropulsion of bone fragments into the spinal canal.

    The hallmark of a burst fracture is **middle column involvement with posterior cortex disruption,** often identified on CT.

    This distinguishes it from compression fractures, which do not involve the posterior wall cortex, and from flexion-distraction or chance fractures, which involve tensile forces rather than compression.

    [49]

19. A 62-year-old male presents with a T12 compression fracture following a fall from standing height. Imaging reveals 25% anterior vertebral body height loss without posterior wall involvement. He has back pain but mobilizing. What is the next step in management?
    A. Vertebroplasty
    B. Anterior corpectomy
    C. Thoracolumbar orthosis for 6–12 weeks
    D. Posterior instrumentation

    Correct Answer: C

    Explanation:

    Stable compression fractures without posterior wall involvement or significant neurological deficits are managed conservatively with bracing and activity modification in patient with controlled pain and who is mobile without significant pain. If his pain is not controlled, vertebral augmentation with vertebroplasty or kyphoplasty would be a good option.

    (RS, p. 1339)

20. A 72-year-old postmenopausal woman presents with acute back pain after a minor fall. Radiographs reveal a vertebral body compression fracture. Which of the following factors is **least likely** to contribute to her condition?
    A. Chronic heparin use

B. Low body weight (<58 kg)
C. Family history of vertebral fractures
D. Vitamin C supplementation

Correct Answer: D

Explanation:

Risk factors for osteoporotic fractures include low body weight, smoking, certain medications (e.g., steroids, anticoagulants), postmenopausal status, androgen deprivation therapy, physical inactivity, and low calcium or vitamin D levels. Protective factors include impact exercise and higher body fat. (GB, p. 1209)

21. A 68-year-old male with prostate cancer undergoing androgen deprivation therapy presents with back pain and imaging shows a vertebral compression fracture. Which mechanism is most closely associated with his increased fracture risk?
A. Chronic inflammation leading to microarchitectural bone loss
B. Reduced osteoclast activity due to decreased androgens
C. Enhanced bone resorption relative to deposition
D. Accumulation of microfractures due to physical inactivity

Correct Answer: C

Explanation:

The hallmark of osteoporosis is a decrease in bone mass and quality, which results in a reduction in bone strength. The mineralization of the bones is normal. Cortical and trabecular bone thinning results from an imbalance in bone remodeling where resorption outpaces formation. Because of increased osteoclast activity and decreased bone density in trabecular-rich sites like vertebral bodies, estrogen deficiency, especially after menopause, causes increased bone loss. Cortical bone loss is further exacerbated by aging, which also affects vitamin D metabolism, reduces calcium absorption, and increases parathyroid hormone levels. It makes people more prone to fractures, especially older adults and postmenopausal women. Hip fractures are more common later in life as a result of cumulative bone loss, and vertebral compression fractures are common early in life. Important roles in its development are also played by lifestyle, diet, and genetic factors.

In summary, osteoporosis results from an imbalance in bone remodeling, with resorption outpacing deposition. Androgen deprivation therapy reduces bone density through this mechanism.

(GB, pp. 1208–1209)

22. A 68-year-old woman with a history of postmenopausal osteoporosis presents with a T-score of −2.8 and a history of a recent vertebral compression fracture. She is started on teriparatide therapy. Which of the following is the most accurate description of its mechanism of action?
A. Inhibits osteoclast-mediated bone resorption by targeting RANKL.
B. Increases bone formation by stimulating intermittent osteoblast activity.
C. Prevents bone resorption by inhibiting DNA synthesis in osteoclasts.
D. Enhances bone density through selective estrogen receptor modulation.

Correct Answer: B

Explanation:

Teriparatide, a recombinant PTH (1–34), works by intermittently stimulating osteoblast activity, leading to anabolic bone formation. Unlike bisphosphonates or denosumab, it does not primarily act on osteoclasts or through estrogen receptor modulation.

Other pharmacological treatment of osteoporosis:

The goal of pharmacological management of osteoporosis is to lower the risk of fracture and increase bone mineral density (BMD). Bisphosphonates (such as alendronate, risedronate, and zoledronic acid) and denosumab, which prevent bone resorption, are examples of first-line treatments. Ibandronate and selective estrogen receptor modulators (SERMs), such as raloxifene, are second-line treatments. Calcitonin is an ineffective last-resort treatment. Due to its risks, hormone replacement therapy is no longer as common as it once was. New therapies with promises include sclerostin inhibitors (romosozumab). Vitamin D and calcium supplementation and weight-bearing exercises remain essential for all patients.

(RS, p. 1598)

23. A 75-year-old woman with osteoporosis presents with acute severe back pain following a minor fall. Imaging confirms an osteoporotic vertebral compression fracture (VCF). Based on current evidence, which statement most accurately reflects the role of vertebroplasty or kyphoplasty in her management?
    A. Vertebroplasty consistently demonstrates superior pain relief compared to sham procedures in randomized controlled trials (RCTs).
    B. The American Academy of Orthopedic Surgeons (AAOS) strongly recommends vertebroplasty for acute painful VCFs.
    C. Vertebroplasty is associated with improved physical function and quality of life compared to nonsurgical care in select patients.
    D. Meta-analyses show vertebroplasty provides no significant benefits in pain relief or functional outcomes compared to conservative care.

Correct Answer: C

Explanation:

Evidence regarding vertebroplasty and kyphoplasty for osteoporotic vertebral compression fractures (VCFs) is conflicting. In 2009, the American Academy of Orthopedic Surgeons (AAOS) strongly advised against vertebroplasty and weakly recommended kyphoplasty for pain relief in osteoporotic VCFs, based on randomized controlled trials (RCTs) by Buchbinder and Kallmes, which showed no significant benefit of vertebroplasty over sham procedures. However, methodological flaws, including inconsistent inclusion criteria and patient selection bias, were noted. Subsequent RCTs and meta-analyses provided mixed results. A Cochrane review by Buchbinder showed no difference in pain or quality of life with vertebroplasty compared to sham or conservative care.

While **cement augmentation may benefit select patients, the ideal indications remain undefined.**

(RS, p. 1613)

24. The following levels represent thoracolumbar junction?
    A. T11–T12–L1
    B. T12–L1
    C. T12–L1–L2
    D. T11 till L2

    Correct Answer: A

    Explanation:

    The thoracolumbar junction (T12–L1) is a transitional zone between the stiff, kyphotic thoracic spine and the more mobile, lordotic lumbar spine. Its sagittal alignment is relatively neutral, making it biomechanically susceptible to fractures due to the abrupt change in motion and load distribution. The thoracic spine, supported by the rib cage, provides rigidity, while the lumbar spine permits significant flexion-extension. The lower thoracic vertebrae (T11 and 12) articulate with floating ribs (ribs do not articulate with any bone anteriorly). This also contribute to the vulnerability of the thoracolumbar junction to fractures.

    (SS, p. 95)
25. A 45-year-old male has a fall from a height. CT scan shows a transverse process fracture of L1–L5 in the right side. Which of the following is the most appropriate next step in evaluating for associated injuries?
    A. AP and lateral X-ray of the lumbar spine
    B. MRI to evaluate for ligamentous injury
    C. Extend the CT imaging to include the pelvis
    D. Dynamic flexion-extension radiographs to assess alignment

    Correct Answer: C

    Explanation:

    Lumbar transverse process fractures can be associated with **vertical-shear sacral fractures due to the mechanism of injury specifically** if associated with significant trauma (fall from height in this case). The use of **extended CT imaging** through the pelvis helps in detecting associated pelvic injuries.

    Although lateral radiographs or MRI may be useful, the main objective in this case would be to rule out pelvic fractures that are caused by the transverse process. Without clinical suspicion of instability, flexible-extension radiographs are not needed at this point.

    (RN, p. 1339)
26. Traumatic disc herniations differ from atraumatic herniations primarily due to:
    A. The classification of protrusion and extrusion cannot be used.
    B. The association with high-energy trauma mechanisms
    C. The prevalence of more extra-foraminal disc. The absence of neurologic symptoms in most cases

    Correct Answer: B

    Explanation:

    The hallmarks of traumatic disc herniations include their tendency to develop after high-energy trauma, like road traffic crash, and the challenge of distinguishing them from preexisting herniations in the absence of preinjury imaging.

Both traumatic and atraumatic causes of herniations can be classified into protrusion, or extrusion.

(RN, p. 1339)

27. A patient with a stable compression fracture at T7 is fitted with a brace. When should radiographic and clinical evaluations typically occur to monitor fracture healing and brace effectiveness?
    A. Every week
    B. At 2 weeks and 6 weeks, then every 6–8 weeks
    C. Every 3 months until healed
    D. Only at the end of the treatment period

    Correct Answer: B

    Explanation:

    Bracing is frequently used to treat stable thoracic and lumbar fractures in patients without neurological deficit and no deformity. It provides relative immobilization above and below the injury and prevents unwanted movement such as bending and twisting. Thoracolumbar orthoses are used for upper lumbar and mid-to-low thoracic fractures. For sagittal-plane injuries a hyperextension braces (e.g., Jewett) is used and custom-molded braces for coronal or rotational injuries. Lower lumbar fractures require thoracolumbosacral orthoses, that include a thigh for stabilization. Fractures above T6 may need cervicothoracic orthoses. Upright radiographs are obtained after brace fitting to ensure stability. Follow-up evaluations at 2 and 6 weeks post-injury, and every 6–8 weeks thereafter, ensure proper brace use and fracture stability. Brace weaning begins after clinical and radiographic healing, followed by gradual return to activities once motion and strength are restored.

    (RS, p. 1343)

28. A patient with a flexion-distraction injury of the thoracolumbar spine is at risk of which associated visceral injury?
    A. Bladder rupture
    B. Small bowel perforation
    C. Splenic laceration
    D. Aortic transection

    Correct Answer: B

    Explanation:

    Flexion-distraction (Chance) injuries of the thoracolumbar spine are commonly associated with small bowel perforation, especially in lap belt–only motor vehicle accidents, due to shearing forces on the bowel.

29. In spinal cord injury patients, which of the following is a characteristic feature of neurogenic shock?
    A. Hypertension with bradycardia
    B. Hypotension with bradycardia
    C. Hyperthermia due to loss of thermoregulation
    D. Peripheral vasoconstriction with cool extremities

    Correct Answer: B

Explanation:

Neurogenic shock, typically seen in spinal cord injuries above T6, is characterized by hypotension and bradycardia due to the loss of sympathetic tone and unopposed parasympathetic (vagal) activity. This leads to vasodilation (causing hypotension) and slowed heart rate (bradycardia), distinguishing it from other types of shock, which usually present with tachycardia and peripheral vasoconstriction. Unlike hypovolemic shock, the skin is often warm and dry, not cool and clammy.

30. Which of the following best describes the Frankel grading system used in spinal cord injury assessment?
    A. Classification based on radiographic findings
    B. Scale to grade neurological impairment
    C. System to evaluate pain levels in spinal injury
    D. Tool for predicting long-term functional outcomes

    Correct Answer: B

    Explanation:

    The Frankel grading system is a neurological classification used to assess the degree of spinal cord injury, ranging from Grade A (complete injury with no motor or sensory function) to Grade E (normal motor and sensory function). It evaluates motor and sensory preservation below the level of injury and is primarily used to document the severity of impairment and track neurological recovery over time. It is not based on radiographic findings or pain levels, and while it may correlate with outcomes, its main purpose is not prognostication.

31. Which of the following spinal cord tracts is most susceptible to ischemia following anterior spinal artery injury?
    A. Dorsal columns
    B. Anterior corticospinal tract
    C. Spinocerebellar tract
    D. Lateral corticospinal tract

    Correct Answer: B

    Explanation:

    The lateral corticospinal tract, which carries motor signals from the brain to the limbs, is highly susceptible to ischemia in anterior spinal artery syndrome because it lies within the anterior two-thirds of the spinal cord, the territory supplied by the ASA. Damage to this tract results in motor weakness or paralysis below the level of the lesion.

32. A 40-year-old man with a sacral fracture exhibits weakness in hip extension and knee flexion and diminished sensation at posterior thigh and the knee. Which sacral nerve root is most likely affected?
    A. S1
    B. S2
    C. S3
    D. S4

    Correct Answer: A

Explanation:

The S2 nerve root contributes significantly to the sciatic nerve, which innervates the posterior thigh muscles responsible for hip extension (gluteus maximus) and knee flexion (hamstrings). Sensory fibers from S2 also supply the posterior thigh and upper leg, matching the patient's described sensory loss.

33. Which of the following statements regarding the epidemiology of spinal cord injuries is correct?
    A. The most common cause is penetrating trauma.
    B. Incidence is higher in females than males.
    C. Motor vehicle accidents are the leading cause in young adults.
    D. Most injuries occur in individuals over 65 years old.

    Correct Answer: C

    Explanation:

    Among the various causes of spinal cord injury (SCI), motor vehicle accidents remain the most common cause in young adults, particularly males in their 20s and 30s. These injuries often result from high-velocity trauma involving the cervical or thoracic spine. While falls are more frequent in the elderly, and violence (including penetrating trauma) can cause SCI, they are less common overall. The incidence is also significantly higher in males, not females, likely due to greater exposure to high-risk activities and trauma.
34. A patient with an L5 burst fracture without neurological deficits is being considered for nonoperative management. Which of the following is a contraindication to conservative treatment?
    A. 40% vertebral body height loss
    B. Progressive kyphosis on serial imaging
    C. Associated fracture of the lamina
    D. Absence of canal compromise

    Correct Answer: B

    Explanation:

    While many L5 burst fractures without neurological deficits can be managed nonoperatively, one of the key factors that would shift the decision toward surgery is progressive kyphotic deformity seen on follow-up imaging. This indicates spinal instability, which can eventually lead to mechanical pain, deformity, or even delayed neurological compromise.

    A (40% height loss) may still be acceptable for conservative treatment if the spine remains stable and alignment is preserved.

    C (lamina fracture) is not an absolute contraindication unless it's causing canal compromise or instability.

    D (absence of canal compromise) is actually a favorable sign for nonoperative management.
35. The following levels represent cervicothoracic junction?
    A. C6–C7–T1
    B. C7–T1
    C. C7–T1–T2
    D. C6–T2

    Correct Answer: B

Explanation:

The cervicothoracic junction spans from C7 to T1, marking the transition from the mobile cervical spine to the rigid thoracic spine. This region is clinically significant due to changes in biomechanics and surgical access challenges.

36. One of the following approache(s) are used to do T1 corpectomy:
    A. Thoracotomy
    B. Trans-sternal manubriotomy
    C. Posterior laminectomy of C7–L2
    D. All of the above

    Correct Answer: B

    Explanation:

    T1 corpectomy is anatomically challenging due to its location at the cervicothoracic junction, deep behind the sternum and great vessels. The trans-sternal manubriotomy approach provides direct anterior access to the T1 vertebral body, making it the preferred method in many cases.

37. A 55-year-old woman with ankylosing spondylitis suffers a low-energy fall and presents with severe back pain. Imaging reveals a transverse fracture through the ossified anterior and posterior spinal elements at T11–T12. Which of the following best describes the fracture pattern?
    A. Compression fracture
    B. Chance fracture
    C. Extension-type fracture through a rigid spine
    D. Burst fracture

    Correct Answer: C

    Explanation:

    In patients with ankylosing spondylitis, even low-energy trauma can result in unstable spinal fractures due to the spine's rigidity and loss of normal flexibility. The described transverse fracture through both anterior and posterior elements at T11–T12 is characteristic of an extension-type fracture in a rigid, ankylosed spine.

38. In patients with complete spinal cord injury, which of the following factors is associated with a better prognosis for recovery?
    A. Female patient
    B. Presence of concomitant brain injury
    C. Early initiation of rehabilitation programs
    D. Early high-dose steroids administration

    Correct Answer: C

    Explanation:

    Among patients with complete spinal cord injury, the factor most consistently associated with better functional outcomes is the early initiation of comprehensive rehabilitation. Rehab helps prevent complications like contractures and pressure sores and promotes neuroplasticity, mobility, and independence.

39. Which of the following interventions has been shown to reduce the incidence of heterotopic ossification in spinal cord injury patients?
    A. High-dose steroids
    B. Administration of nonsteroidal anti-inflammatory drugs (NSAIDs)

C. Early surgical excision of ossifications
D. Prolonged immobilization

Correct Answer: B

Explanation:

NSAIDs, particularly indomethacin, have been shown to reduce the risk of heterotopic ossification in patients with spinal cord injuries by inhibiting prostaglandin-mediated bone formation in soft tissues.

40. A patient with a T6 burst fracture exhibits autonomic dysreflexia. Which of the following symptoms is characteristic of this condition?
A. Hypotension and tachycardia
B. Severe hypertension with bradycardia
C. Hyperthermia
D. Diaphoresis below the level of injury

Correct Answer: B

Explanation:

Autonomic dysreflexia is a potentially life-threatening condition seen in patients with spinal cord injuries at or above T6. It results from an exaggerated autonomic response to stimuli (like bladder distention or pain) below the level of injury. This leads to uncontrolled sympathetic discharge, causing severe hypertension, while the intact vagus nerve triggers a reflex bradycardia.

41. One of the following represents MOST challenges to approach upper thoracic spine surgically:
A. Shoulder and scapular musculature
B. Unique type of fractures
C. Smaller and narrow pedicle
D. All of the above

Correct Answer: A

Explanation:

Among the various challenges in approaching the upper thoracic spine, one of the most significant is the presence of the shoulder girdle and scapular musculature, which obstructs both posterior and lateral surgical exposure. These structures limit access, especially in open procedures targeting T1–T4, making positioning and retraction more complex. While smaller pedicles and certain fracture types also pose difficulties, the bulk and anatomical position of the shoulder and scapula are often the primary limiting factors for exposure in this region.

42. In spinal cord injury patients, the development of spasticity is primarily due to which of the following mechanisms?
A. Peripheral nerve demyelination
B. Lower motor neuron damage
C. Loss of inhibitory upper motor neuron control
D. Neurotransmitter depletion

Correct Answer: C

Explanation:

Spasticity following spinal cord injury is primarily caused by the loss of inhibitory signals from upper motor neurons that normally regulate spinal reflexes. When these descending pathways are disrupted, especially in injuries above the level of the reflex arc, the spinal cord becomes hyperexcitable, leading to increased muscle tone, exaggerated reflexes, and spasms.

43. Which of the following is the most appropriate initial imaging modality for a hemodynamically unstable patient with suspected thoracolumbar spine injury?
    A. MRI of the spine
    B. Focused assessment with sonography for trauma (FAST) and lateral spine radiograph
    C. CT scan of the spine
    D. Flexion-extension radiographs

    Correct Answer: B

    Explanation:

    In a hemodynamically unstable patient, the priority is rapid assessment to rule out life-threatening injuries. A FAST exam quickly evaluates for internal bleeding, while a lateral spine radiograph can provide basic but immediate information about potential thoracolumbar spine fractures.

    CT scans (C) offer excellent detail but may not be feasible in unstable patients due to time, positioning, and transport risks.

    MRI (A) is not appropriate as an initial test in trauma, especially in unstable patients.

    Flexion-extension radiographs (D) are contraindicated in acute trauma due to the risk of worsening an unstable injury.

44. The most common location for penetrating injury of the spine is:
    A. Cervical
    B. Thoracic
    C. Lumbar
    D. Sacral

    Correct Answer: B

    Explanation:

    The thoracic spine is the most commonly affected region in penetrating spinal injuries, particularly from gunshot wounds, due to its larger surface area and proximity to vital structures within the thoracic cavity. Although the cervical spine is more exposed anatomically, the thoracic region tends to be involved more frequently in high-velocity trauma, especially in urban settings where firearm-related injuries are more prevalent. (GB, p. 1220)

45. The following is NOT surgical indications for gunshot wound injury to the spine:
    A. CSF leak
    B. Copper jacketed bullet
    C. Compression of a nerve root
    D. Use of high injury missile

    Correct Answer: D

    Explanation:

    The use of a high-velocity missile alone is not an automatic indication for surgery in spinal gunshot injuries. While high-energy projectiles can cause extensive damage, surgical intervention is generally reserved for specific indications such as CSF leaks (A), nerve root or spinal cord compression (C), or persistent neurologic deterioration. The presence of a copper-jacketed bullet (B) is also not an absolute indication unless it causes local toxicity or mechanical issues. Many gunshot injuries to the spine, even from high-energy missiles, can be managed nonoperatively if there is no evidence of instability, compression, or infection.

46. A 30-year-old man presents with back pain after a fall from height. CT scan reveals a vertical sacral fracture extending from S1 to S3, involving the neural foramina. According to Denis classification, which zone is affected?
    A. Zone I
    B. Zone II
    C. Zone III
    D. Zone IV

    Correct Answer: B

    Explanation:

    See question 4 explanation.

47. A high thoracic spinal cord injury (SCI) refers to injury to the spinal cord in the following levels:
    A. T1–T2
    B. T1–T4
    C. T1–T6
    D. T1–T7

    Correct Answer: C

    Explanation:

    A high thoracic spinal cord injury typically refers to injuries occurring between T1 and T6. This region is clinically significant because it includes spinal levels that contribute to sympathetic outflow, and injuries here can lead to complications such as autonomic dysreflexia and impaired cardiovascular regulation.

48. Which of the following is a potential complication of high thoracic spinal cord injury affecting cardiovascular function?
    A. Tachyarrhythmias due to sympathetic overactivity
    B. Neurogenic shock with bradycardia and hypotension
    C. Hypertensive crisis due to catecholamine surge
    D. Cardiac tamponade

    Correct Answer: B

    Explanation:

    High thoracic spinal cord injuries (especially above T6) can disrupt sympathetic outflow, leading to neurogenic shock — a condition marked by bradycardia and hypotension due to unopposed parasympathetic (vagal) activity and loss of vascular tone. This is a well-recognized cardiovascular complication in the acute phase of spinal cord injury.

49. In patients with incomplete spinal cord injury, which of the following findings suggests a favorable prognosis for motor recovery?
    A. Absence of sacral sparing
    B. Presence of pinprick sensation in the lower extremities

C. Loss of motor function below the lesion
D. Age between 40 and 55

Correct Answer: B

Explanation:

In incomplete spinal cord injuries, the presence of pinprick sensation, particularly in the lower extremities and sacral segments, is a strong predictor of favorable motor recovery. This indicates that some spinothalamic and corticospinal tract integrity is preserved, increasing the chances for functional improvement.

50. Which of the following statements about methylprednisolone use in acute spinal cord injury is correct?
A. It is recommended for all patients regardless of time since injury
B. Its use is controversial due to potential complications
C. High-dose steroids are proven to improve neurological recovery
D. It should be administered within 24 h for optimal effect

Correct Answer: B

Explanation:

The use of high-dose methylprednisolone in acute spinal cord injury has been controversial for years. While early studies like the NASCIS trials suggested some potential benefit if given within 8 hours, later analyses questioned the clinical significance of those findings and raised concerns about serious side effects, including infections, GI bleeding, and delayed wound healing. As a result, many guidelines now state that steroid use is optional and not routinely recommended.

51. Which of the following best describes the mechanism of injury in a burst fracture?
A. Flexion-distraction forces
B. Axial compression with or without flexion
C. Hyperextension
D. Shear forces

Correct Answer: B

Explanation:

A burst fracture occurs due to a high-energy axial compression force, often from a fall from height landing on the feet or buttocks. This force causes the vertebral body to fracture and burst outward, extending the fracture line to the posterior cortex of the vertebral body.

Spine Tumors and Vascular Pathology

8

1. What is the most common location for spinal ependymoma?
   A. Cervical spine
   B. Thoracic spine
   C. Lumbar spine
   D. Sacral spine
   Correct Answer: A
   Explanation:
   Spinal ependymomas are the most common intramedullary tumors in adults, accounting for 60% of all glial spinal cord tumors. In children, they are the second most common intramedullary neoplasms, making up 30% of pediatric cases. The peak incidence occurs in the fourth decade of life, with a mean presentation age of 39 years, and they are more prevalent in males than females.
   These tumors are associated with an increased incidence in patients with neurofibromatosis type 2. While ependymomas can develop anywhere along the spinal cord, the **cervical cord is the most frequent location** (44%). Another 23% occur in the cervical cord with extension into the upper thoracic region, and 26% are found exclusively in the thoracic cord.

(RP)

2. Which is the most commonly found tumor in the conus medullaris?
   A. Myxopapillary ependymoma
   B. Schwannoma
   C. Astrocytoma
   D. Hemangioblastoma
   Correct Answer: A
   Explanation:
   Myxopapillary ependymomas are slow-growing gliomas originating from the ependymal cells of the filum terminale. They are the most common tumor of the **conus medullaris, cauda equina, and filum terminale**, comprising 27–30% of all ependymomas and 90% of filum terminale tumors. These tumors typically appear as well-circumscribed, ovoid masses spanning 2–4 vertebral

K. F. AlAli, H. T. Hashim, *Spine Surgery and Peripheral Nerve Surgery*,
https://doi.org/10.1007/978-3-031-98543-0_8

segments, with frequent hemorrhagic features on imaging. MRI is the preferred diagnostic tool, showing hyperintensity on T2-weighted images and strong contrast enhancement on T1-weighted imaging. Symptoms include back pain, radiculopathy, paraparesis, and bladder or bowel dysfunction. It is most common in patients aged 30–40 years, with a male predominance (2:1). Surgical resection offers excellent prognosis, with gross total removal associated with a low recurrence rate (~10%). Subtotal resection or violation of the tumor capsule increases the risk of local recurrence and cerebrospinal fluid (CSF) dissemination. Radiation therapy is an option for incomplete resection or recurrent tumors.

(DI, pp. 811–812)

3. All of the following are features of Myxopapillary ependymoma, EXCEPT:
   A. Glioma with papillary structures and perivascular myxoid change
   B. It has MYCN amplification
   C. Usually located in the filum terminale or conus medullaris
   D. Prognosis is relatively favorable

   Correct Answer: B

   Explanation:

   Myxopapillary ependymoma is a type of glioma characterized by papillary structures and perivascular myxoid changes or, at minimum, focal myxoid microcysts. It demonstrates immunoreactivity for Glial Fibrillary Acidic Protein (GFAP), and for unresolved lesions, a DNA methylation profile aligned with myxopapillary ependymoma can confirm the diagnosis. Histologically, it is desirable to observe papillary arrangements of tumor cells surrounding vascularized fibromyxoid cores. These tumors are typically located in the filum terminale or conus medullaris, consistent with their origin.

   The pathology in the spine associated with MYCN amplification is spinal ependymoma, MYCN-amplified. This is a rare variant of spinal ependymoma with a poor prognosis. It is characterized by small uniform cells forming pseudorosettes or ependymal rosettes in a fibrillary matrix.

   (GB, p. 735)

4. The following tumor represents 50% of the tumors affecting the sacrum?
   A. Osteosarcoma
   B. Chordoma
   C. Ewing's sarcoma
   D. Multiple myeloma

   Correct Answer: B

   Explanation:

   Spinal chordomas are rare malignant tumors originating from remnants of the notochord, most commonly occurring in the sacrococcygeal region. They account for over **50% of primary sacral bone tumors** and are locally aggressive, slow-growing, and osseodestructive. Symptoms often include pain, sphincter disturbances, and nerve root compression, with palpable masses occasionally present on rectal examination. Imaging reveals characteristic features such as centrally located sacral destruction and anterior soft-tissue masses, best visualized with CT and MRI. Diagnosis is confirmed via open or CT-guided posterior biopsy, while transrectal biopsy is avoided to prevent tumor spread.

The preferred treatment is wide en bloc excision combined with postoperative radiation therapy, as piecemeal removal increases the risk of metastasis and recurrence. Radiation options include high-dose external beam radiation therapy (XRT) and intensity-modulated radiation therapy (IMRT), or proton beam therapy. Adverse effects, such as impaired bladder and bowel function, depend on the level of nerve root involvement during sacrectomy. Prognosis varies, with conventional chordomas having a median survival of 6.3 years, while poorly differentiated variants have significantly worse outcomes. (GB, p. 827)

5. A 38-year-old patient presents with low back pain. CT of the lumbar spine reveals a lesion at the L3 vertebra (Fig. 8.1). All of the following are in the deferential diagnosis of such a lesion, EXCEPT:
   A. Giant cell tumor
   B. Eosinophilic granuloma
   C. Osteosarcoma
   D. Osteosclerosis myeloma

   Correct Answer: D

   Explanation:

   This CT shows a lytic expansile vertebral body lesion. All or the options are differential diagnosis of spinal lytic lesion except osteosclerosis myeloma. Multiple myeloma usually presents as lytic and destructive vertebral body lesion. Osteosclerosis myeloma subtype is a rare (3%) subtype that present as sclerotic lesion.

   (DI, p. 749)
6. The presence of which genetic mutation is associated with a better prognosis in spinal oligodendrogliomas?
   A. TP53
   B. EGFR

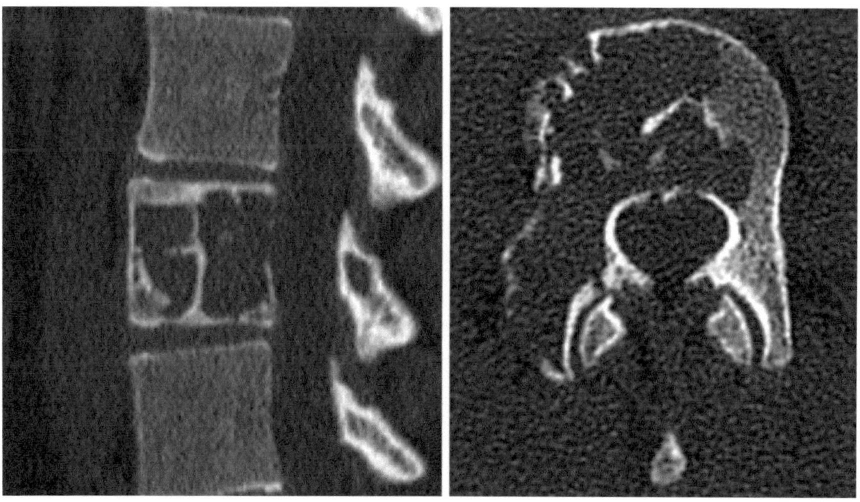

Fig. 8.1 Case 5 CT scan of the lumbar spine reveals a lesion at the L3 vertebra

C. 1p/19q co-deletion
D. BRAF V600E
Correct Answer: C
Explanation:
The presence of a 1p/19q co-deletion is a hallmark genetic mutation in oligodendrogliomas and is associated with a better prognosis. It correlates with improved survival rates and a better response to both chemotherapy and radiation therapy. Other genetic mutations such as **TP53** and **EGFR** are more commonly associated with other glioma subtypes and do not indicate a favorable prognosis in spinal oligodendrogliomas. The **BRAF V600E** mutation is linked with certain low-grade gliomas and other tumor types but is not a typical feature of oligodendrogliomas.
(GB, p. 662)

7. A 32-year-old patient presents with progressive low back pain and weakness in the legs. An MRI is shown below (Fig. 8.2). Which of the following is the most likely diagnosis?
A. Paragangliomas
B. Meningioma
C. Schwannoma
D. Metastasis
Correct Answer: C

Fig. 8.2 Case 7 MRI

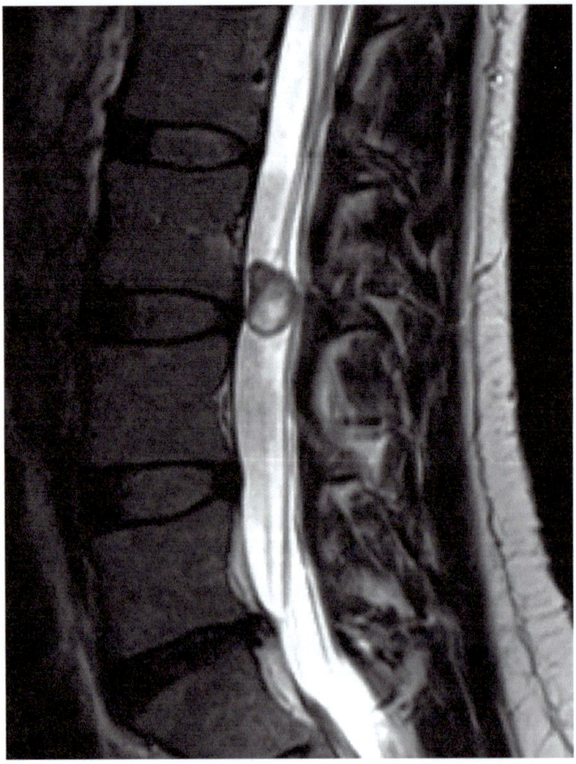

Explanation:

The MRI shows cauda equina mass. The most common tumor in this region is myxopapillary ependymoma, which is not mentioned in the options. **The second most common cauda equina tumors is schwannoma.** Most schwannomas are solitary and sporadic, though they are associated with neurofibromatosis type 2. Small schwannomas can be differentiated from myxopapillary ependymomas by their origin from nerve roots, whereas myxopapillary ependymomas arise from the filum terminale. These tumors almost always enhance on imaging, and hemorrhage, though possible, is less common than in myxopapillary ependymomas. They may also exhibit intrinsic vascular changes such as thrombosis or sinusoidal dilatation, along with cyst formation and fatty degeneration.

Spinal paragangliomas are rare, accounting for only 3.5–3.8% of cauda equina neoplasms, where they almost exclusively occur. Intradural metastases are often multiple and may present as "sugar coating" over the spinal cord and nerve roots.

(RP)

8. What is the most common site for spinal metastasis?
   A. Cervical spine
   B. Thoracic spine
   C. Lumbar spine
   D. Sacral spine

   Correct Answer: B

   Explanation:

   The most common site for spinal metastasis is the thoracic spine, accounting for approximately 70% of cases, followed by the lumbosacral spine (16–22%) and cervical spine (8–15%). The cervical and sacral regions are less commonly involved.

   (RS, p. 1515)

9. A 55-year-old male with a history of lung cancer presents with progressive back pain. Imaging reveals lytic lesions in the thoracic spine. Which pathway is most likely responsible for the spinal metastasis?
   A. Lymphatic spread
   B. Batson's venous plexus
   C. Segmental arteries
   D. Direct invasion

   Correct Answer: C

   Explanation:

   Lung tumors typically spread to the vertebral column via hematogenous dissemination through the segmental arteries. In contrast, breast, gastrointestinal, and prostate tumors spread via Batson's venous plexus.

   (RS, pp. 1515–1516)

10. A 62-year-old woman with breast cancer develops lower back pain. MRI shows multiple osteoblastic lesions in the lumbar spine. What mechanism best explains the tumor's preference for this site?
    A. Increased neoangiogenesis in the vertebral column
    B. Direct invasion from adjacent organs

C. Retrograde spread through Batson's venous plexus
D. Stimulation of osteoblast activity by tumor-secreted factors

Correct Answer: C

Explanation:

Breast cancer often metastasizes to the spine via retrograde venous flow through Batson's venous plexus, facilitated by the valveless nature of this system. This mechanism, combined with osteoblast stimulation by tumor-secreted factors, accounts for osteoblastic lesions.

(RS, pp. 1515–1516)

11. What is the most common primary tumor to metastasize to the spine?
    A. Prostate
    B. Breast
    C. Lung
    D. Kidney

    Correct Answer: C

    Explanation:

    Lung cancer is one of the most common primary malignancies with a high propensity to metastasize to the spine due to its aggressive nature and vascular spread through Batson's venous plexus. It accounts for approximately 17% of spinal metastases in reported series. Other frequent contributors to spinal metastases include lung (16%), prostate, kidney, and thyroid cancers.

    (GB, p. 921)

12. Which of the following is a poor prognostic factor in spinal cord astrocytomas?
    A. Young age at diagnosis
    B. Presence of syrinx
    C. High-grade histology
    D. Cervical location

    Correct Answer: C

    Explanation:

    The histologic subtype of astrocytoma plays a critical role in determining outcomes, as the WHO grade reflects tumor aggressiveness and the likelihood of identifying a dissection plane. Low-grade tumors have a 5-year survival rate exceeding 70%, while high-grade tumors are associated with a significantly lower 5-year survival rate of 18.7%.

    (SSW, p. 2017)

13. What is the most common symptom of spinal metastasis?
    A. Radiculopathy
    B. Myelopathy
    C. Localized back pain
    D. Cauda equina syndrome

    Correct Answer: C

    Explanation:

    Pain is the most common initial symptom of spinal metastases, occurring in up to 95% of patients. It can manifest in three forms: local pain, radicular pain, and mechanical pain. Local pain is typically aching and localized to the affected level, often worsening at night or when lying down. Radicular pain is sharp and shooting, radiating along the dermatome of the involved nerve root, and is frequently bilateral in the thoracic region. Mechanical pain, on the other hand, is usually aggravated by movement.

(GB, p. 922)

14. Which of the following is NOT a component of the Tokuhashi score for predicting survival in patients with spinal metastases?
    A. Severity of the neurological deficit
    B. Number of spinal metastases
    C. Primary tumor site
    D. Pathological fracture from the metastasis

    Correct Answer: D

    Explanation:

    The Tokuhashi score is a prognostic scoring system used to estimate survival in patients with spinal metastases and guide treatment decisions. It assesses six parameters: general condition, number of extraspinal bone metastases, number of spinal metastases, presence of visceral metastases, severity of neurological deficit, and the primary tumor site. Pathological fracture is not a direct component of the Tokuhashi score (Table 8.1).

    Scoring Interpretation:

    - **0–8 points:** Predicted survival <6 months. Palliative care recommended
    - **9–11 points:** Predicted survival ~6–12 months. Palliative surgery may be considered
    - **12–15 points:** Predicted survival >1 year. Aggressive surgical intervention may be considered.

    (SS, p. 625)

15. A 65-year-old woman with metastatic breast cancer presents with worsening back pain and mild lower extremity weakness. Imaging reveals a spinal lesion with soft tissue compression of the spinal canal, but no evidence of bone instability. She is not a surgical candidate due to significant comorbidities. What is the most appropriate management?
    A. Surgical decompression and stabilization
    B. Radiation therapy alone

Table 8.1 Tokuhashi score

Parameter	Scoring criteria	Points
General condition	Poor (bedridden)/moderate (ambulating with assistance)/good (ambulating independently)	0 / 1 / 2
Number of extraspinal bone metastases	≥3/1–2/none	0 / 1 / 2
Number of spinal metastases	≥3/2/1	0 / 1 / 2
Visceral metastases	Non-treatable/Treatable/None	0 / 1 / 2
Severity of neurological deficit	Complete/Moderate/None	0 / 1 / 2
Primary tumor site	Lung, stomach, pancreas/kidney, liver, uterus/thyroid, breast, prostate, rectum, others	0 / 1 / 2

C. Chemotherapy alone
D. Observation with pain management

Correct Answer: B

Explanation:

Radiation therapy is the preferred treatment for radiosensitive tumors, such as breast cancer, in patients with soft tissue compression of the spinal canal and no evidence of spinal instability. It reduces tumor burden, promotes vertebral reossification, and alleviates pain. Radiation therapy is not considered an appropriate initial treatment for spinal canal compromise caused by osseous lesions or for structural instability resulting from metastatic spinal involvement. In cases of metastatic disease with epidural compression, patients treated with spinal cord decompression and reconstruction followed by radiation therapy have shown better outcomes.

Other radiosensitive tumors are prostate and ovarian cancer, lymphoma, myeloma, seminoma, and neuroendocrine carcinoma.

(SS, p. 627)

16. A 59-year-old man with metastatic renal cell carcinoma presents with back pain without neurological deficit. Imaging reveals a large spinal lesion without spinal canal compromise and without instability. What is the most appropriate treatment approach?
    A. Radiation therapy alone
    B. Surgical resection followed by radiation therapy
    C. Chemotherapy alone
    D. Observation with pain management

    Correct Answer: B

    Explanation:

    Renal cell carcinoma is radioresistant, making surgery the preferred initial approach. Other radiosensitive tumors include gastrointestinal adenocarcinoma, metastatic melanoma, thyroid carcinoma, hepatocellular carcinoma, non-small-cell lung carcinoma, and sarcoma.

    (SS, p. 627)

17. Which of the following is NOT a component of the Spine Instability Neoplastic Score (SINS)?
    A. Pain
    B. Tumor location
    C. Neurological deficit severity
    D. Posterior spinal element involvement

    Correct Answer: C

    Explanation:

    The SINS evaluates spinal instability due to neoplastic disease using six components: tumor location, pain, bone lesion quality (lytic, blastic, or mixed), spinal alignment, vertebral body collapse, and posterior spinal element involvement. Neurological deficit severity is not part of the SINS; it is evaluated separately to guide neurological management.

    (SS, p. 627), [36]

18. Which of the following is NOT a typical feature of spinal schwannomas?
    A. Commonly found in thoracic spine
    B. Dumbbell-shaped growth pattern
    C. Intradural extramedullary location
    D. Infiltration of the spinal cord parenchyma

    Correct Answer: D

    Explanation:

    Schwannomas, type of nerve sheath tumors, are slow-growing neoplasms arising from Schwann cells, often seen in the spine. They are commonly **intradural and extramedullary** (70–75%) but may occasionally be extradural or extend through the neural foramen as **dumbbell-shaped** tumors. **Thoracic** localization is most frequent, followed by cervical and lumbar regions. Imaging typically shows well-circumscribed, enhancing masses that are iso-/hypointense on T1-weighted MRI and hyperintense on T2-weighted MRI, with cystic or hemorrhagic changes in some cases. Schwannomas are sporadic in most cases but may be associated with neurofibromatosis type 2 (NF2), characterized by multiple schwannomas, meningiomas, and ependymomas. Gross pathology reveals encapsulated, ovoid lesions with occasional cysts and minimal necrosis. Symptoms often include pain, weakness, and paresthesias, typically in patients aged 30–60 years. Surgical resection is the treatment of choice, and recurrence is rare for solitary lesions. However, patients with NF2 may develop multiple new tumors over time.

    (DI, pp. 769–770)

19. A 48-year-old man with a history of neurofibromatosis type 2 presents with progressive sensory loss and gait instability. MRI shows multiple thoracic intradural extramedullary masses, one at T6 with a dural tail sign, and another at T8 with a cystic component. Histopathological examination of the T6 lesion reveals psammomatous calcifications, while the T8 lesion shows Antoni A and Antoni B areas. Which of the following statements is most accurate?
    A. Both lesions are meningiomas; surgical resection of both is recommended.
    B. The T6 lesion is a meningioma; the T8 lesion is a schwannoma, and resection is curative.
    C. Both lesions are schwannomas; surgical resection is the preferred treatment.
    D. The T6 lesion is a schwannoma; the T8 lesion is a neurofibroma, requiring subtotal resection.

    Correct Answer: B

    Explanation:

    The T6 lesion has classic meningioma features, including a dural tail and psammomatous calcifications, while the T8 lesion demonstrates characteristics of schwannomas, such as Antoni A and Antoni B areas. Both lesions can be surgically resected for symptomatic relief. Neurofibromas and schwannomas are challenging to differentiate on imaging but lack the dural tail seen in meningiomas. Radiation therapy is not the first-line treatment for these surgically accessible lesions.

    (DI, p. 777)

20. Which of the following is NOT a typical feature of primary spinal cord lymphoma?
    A. Association with immunodeficiency states
    B. Typically presents as a leptomeningeal disease
    C. Enhancement on MRI with gadolinium
    D. Predilection for the thoracic spine

    Correct Answer: D

    Explanation:

    Spinal lymphoma includes various lymphoreticular neoplasms that can involve the spine in epidural, osseous, leptomeningeal, or intramedullary locations. It is more commonly secondary to systemic lymphoma but may also present as primary osseous lymphoma, which accounts for 3–4% of malignant bone tumors. Epidural spinal lymphoma is the most frequent form, often in the **thoracic spine**, presenting as an enhancing mass with or without bone involvement.

    (DI, p. 740)
21. Which of the following is NOT a common feature of primary spinal lymphoma?
    A. Epidural location
    B. B cell phenotype
    C. Association with immunodeficiency
    D. Osteoblastic lesions on imaging

    Correct Answer: D

    Explanation:

    Spinal lymphoma includes various lymphoreticular neoplasms that can involve the spine in epidural, osseous, leptomeningeal, or intramedullary locations. It is more commonly secondary to systemic lymphoma but may also present as primary osseous lymphoma, which accounts for 3–4% of malignant bone tumors. Epidural spinal lymphoma is the most frequent form, often in the thoracic spine, presenting as an enhancing mass with or without bone involvement. Imaging may show **lytic bone destruction (not osteoblastic)**, rarely "ivory" vertebrae, and sometimes vertebra plana. Leptomeningeal lymphoma manifests with smooth or nodular pial enhancement, while intramedullary lesions appear as poorly defined masses with surrounding edema.

    Spinal lymphoma predominantly affects adults in their fourth to seventh decades, with a slight male predominance, and is most often of B-cell lineage. Risk factors include immunodeficiency (e.g., AIDS, transplant patients) and Epstein-Barr virus infection. The primary symptom is back pain, with myelopathy in cases of intramedullary involvement. Prognosis varies; primary osseous lymphoma has a favorable outcome with 5-/10-year survival rates of 91% and 87%, respectively. Treatment typically involves chemotherapy and radiation, as spinal lymphoma is highly sensitive to these modalities. Surgical intervention is rarely needed unless for diagnostic or decompressive purposes.

    (DI, p. 740)
22. Which genetic mutation is most commonly associated with the development of intramedullary spinal cord ependymomas?
    A. TP53
    B. NF2

C. IDH1
D. H3 K27M
Correct Answer: B
Explanation:
The **NF2 (neurofibromatosis type 2)** gene mutation is most commonly associated with the development of intramedullary spinal cord ependymomas. NF2 encodes the tumor suppressor protein merlin (schwannomin), and its inactivation is strongly linked to the formation of spinal ependymomas, especially in individuals with neurofibromatosis type 2. These tumors are frequently seen in the cervical spine and are often multiple in patients with NF2. Other mutations, such as **H3 K27M**, are associated with diffuse midline gliomas, while **IDH1** mutations are common in intracranial gliomas, and **TP53** mutations are linked to various malignancies but not specifically ependymomas.
(DI, p. 808)

23. In the context of spinal metastasis, the term "epidural spinal cord compression (ESCC)" is graded using which scale?
A. Frankl scale
B. Bilsky scale
C. McCormick scale
D. Tokuhashi scale
Correct Answer: B
Explanation:
The **Bilsky scale** is specifically designed to assess **epidural spinal cord compression (ESCC)** in the context of spinal metastases. It grades the degree of spinal cord compression based on imaging, particularly MRI, as follows:
- **Grade 0:** No epidural impingement
- **Grade 1:** Epidural impingement without deformation of the spinal cord
- **Grade 2:** Deformation of the spinal cord without signal change
- **Grade 3:** Spinal cord deformation with signal change on T2-weighted imaging

This scale helps guide treatment decisions and predict outcomes. The other options, such as the **Frankl scale**, measure neurological function; the **McCormick scale** assesses disability in intramedullary spinal tumors; and the **Tokuhashi scale** evaluates prognosis in spinal metastases.
(DI, p. 684)

24. Which of the following is a poor prognostic factor for spinal metastasis?
A. Single-level involvement
B. Presence of visceral metastasis
C. Breast cancer primary
D. Response to steroids
Correct Answer: B
Explanation:
The presence of **visceral metastasis** is a poor prognostic factor for spinal metastasis, as it indicates advanced disease and systemic spread, reducing the likelihood of prolonged survival. Prognostic scoring systems like the Tokuhashi score assign lower points to patients with visceral metastases.

- **Single-level involvement** is associated with better outcomes due to localized disease.
- **Breast cancer primary** is often considered a favorable factor because breast cancer responds well to systemic therapies, including radiation and chemotherapy.
- **Response to steroids** can indicate a reversible component of neurologic symptoms, which generally suggests a better prognosis.

  (SS, p. 625)

25. Why is vertebroplasty considered a viable treatment option for patients with spinal metastases?
    A. It reduces the size of the metastatic tumor through chemical ablation.
    B. It provides minimally invasive pain relief and stabilizes the spine with lower morbidity compared to open surgery.
    C. It is more effective than radiation therapy for long-term tumor control.
    D. It is the only treatment option for patients with vertebral body collapse.

    Correct Answer: B

    Explanation:

    The study by Weill et al. evaluated the efficacy and risks of percutaneous injection of acrylic surgical cement (vertebroplasty) for spinal metastases, focusing on pain palliation and stabilization. Among 37 patients undergoing 40 procedures, significant pain relief (≥50% reduction in analgesic use) was observed in 23 cases, with improvement noted within 24 h in most. Vertebroplasty also provided stabilization, with no new instability reported at follow-ups. Cement leakage occurred in 20 cases, with 5 symptomatic complications, including radicular pain and dysphagia, which were generally manageable. Limitations included the absence of a control group, high dropout rates, and heterogeneous treatments. Despite its flaws, the study demonstrated vertebroplasty as a minimally invasive alternative to open surgery, offering **rapid pain relief and partial stabilization for spinal metastases.**

    [37]

26. A 62-year-old patient is diagnosed with a malignant tumor involving multiple levels (L2–L4) with evidence of soft tissue extension (WBB zones 5–9) and infiltration of adjacent structures. The tumor is classified as Stage IIB. What surgical strategy would be recommended based on the WBB (Weinstein, Boriani, Biagini) staging system?
    A. Intralesional curettage with embolization
    B. Radical resection with complete tumor removal
    C. Wide en bloc resection with adjuvant therapy
    D. Palliative decompression and stabilization only

    Correct Answer: C

    Explanation:

    The WBB (Weinstein, Boriani, Biagini) surgical staging system for spinal tumors combines oncologic surgical principles with the spine's unique anatomy to guide treatment planning. It divides the vertebra into 12 zones in a clockwise fashion, with zones 4 and 9 representing the left and right pedicles, respectively.

Additionally, the spine is stratified into five tissue layers extending from the paravertebral extraosseous area to the dura: (A) extraosseous soft tissue, (B) intraosseous superficial, (C) intraosseous deep, (D) extraosseous extradural, and (E) extraosseous intradural. In the cervical spine, a sixth layer, "F," is added to account for vertebral artery or intervertebral foramen involvement. The system also defines various en bloc tumor excision techniques, including posterior arch resection, vertebrectomy, and sagittal resection, performed through a range of surgical approaches.

Lower-grade malignancies (Stage IA and IB) are managed with either marginal resection combined with adjuvant therapy or wide en-bloc excision. In contrast, higher-grade malignancies (Stage IIA and IIB) **necessitate wide resection along with adjuvant therapy**.

[38]

27. A 48-year-old patient with thyroid cancer presents with a moderate-growth spinal tumor, treatable visceral metastases, and isolated spinal involvement. Imaging confirms the lesion is in the lumbar spine. The patient's Tomita score is 5. What treatment strategy is most appropriate according to the Tomita system?
   A. Wide en bloc excision
   B. Intralesional excision with or without marginal excision
   C. Nonoperative palliative care
   D. Supportive care with radiation only

   Correct Answer: B

   Explanation:

   The study by Tomita et al. (2001) proposed a prognosis-based scoring system to guide surgical management for spinal metastases, focusing on survival prediction and treatment stratification. The system evaluates three factors: (1) malignant grade of the primary tumor (slow, moderate, or rapid growth), (2) presence and treatability of visceral metastases, and (3) localization of bone metastases (isolated to the spine or not). Patients are assigned scores from 2 to 10, which guide treatment: lower scores favor aggressive surgery (e.g., en bloc resection), mid-range scores suggest intralesional excision or stabilization, and high scores recommend nonoperative palliative care. In phase 1, retrospective analysis demonstrated strong correlation between survival and total prognostic scores, while phase 2 prospectively validated the scoring system's application. Patients with lower scores showed longer survival and better local tumor control with more aggressive surgeries. Limitations include lack of data on comorbidities and adjunct therapies (e.g., radiotherapy), and some deviations from recommended treatments. Despite these drawbacks, the Tomita scoring system has become a widely used tool for decision-making in metastatic spinal disease (Table 8.2).

   [39]

28. A 62-year-old patient with metastatic prostate cancer presents with severe back pain and no neurological deficits. Imaging reveals a low-grade epidural disease without significant spinal cord compression. The patient has not undergone

Table 8.2 The Tomita scoring system summary table

Factor	Scoring criteria	Score
Malignant grade of tumor	Slow growth	1
	Moderate growth	2
	Rapid growth	3
Visceral metastases	None	1
	Present but treatable	2
	Present and untreatable	3
Bone metastases	Isolated to the spine	1
	Not isolated to the spine	2
Total score	**Treatment recommendation**	
2–3	Wide or marginal en bloc excision	
4–5	Intralesional excision ± marginal excision	
6–7	Palliative decompression and stabilization	
8–10	Nonoperative palliative care	

prior radiation therapy. Which treatment approach is most appropriate based on the Spine Oncology Study Group (SOSG) recommendations?

A. Surgical decompression and stabilization
B. Conventional radiotherapy
C. Stereotactic body radiosurgery
D. Nonoperative palliative care

Correct Answer: B

Explanation:

SOSG guidelines recommend conventional radiotherapy for spinal metastases in cases without instability, prior radiation, or high-grade epidural compression. Prostate cancer is a favorable histology for conventional radiotherapy, and the patient's lack of significant compression makes conventional radiotherapy an effective option to control pain and maintain functionality. Stereotactic body radiosurgery is not prioritized in this situation as conventional radiotherapy is sufficient.

The Spine Oncology Study Group highlights conventional radiotherapy (CRT) as a standard for spinal metastases, achieving 60–80% ambulation and 50–70% pain relief. Stereotactic body radiosurgery (SBRS) shows superior pain relief (85–100%), and effectiveness in radio-resistant tumors. CRT offers variable dosing with longer courses improving motor outcomes, while SBRS ensures excellent local control (~90%) and serves as a primary, adjunct, or re-irradiation option. Rarely, disease progression occurs at adjacent levels or in the epidural space.

The Spine Oncology Study Group (SOSG) recommends CRT for non-unstable metastases without prior radiation or high-grade cord compression and SBRS for radio-resistant tumors. Limitations of the study include heterogeneity in patient populations, inconsistent outcome measures, and reliance on mostly retrospective studies. SBRS is gaining prominence as a first-line treatment for select cases, reducing the need for invasive surgeries. However, vertebral compression fractures (VCFs) are a notable complication (11–39%), with risk factors including lytic lesions and high-dose fractions. Pre-SBRS cement augmentation may reduce VCF risk in susceptible patients.

[40]

29. A multidisciplinary tumor board reviews a case of a 60-year-old patient with a large, localized primary spinal tumor. Based on Enneking and WBB staging systems, en bloc resection is deemed feasible. What is the most critical factor in determining the success of this procedure?
    A. The patient's age and overall health status
    B. The use of advanced reconstructive techniques
    C. Achieving negative surgical margins
    D. Minimizing operative time to reduce complications

    Correct Answer: C

    Explanation:

    Achieving negative surgical margins is the most critical factor for the success of en bloc resection, as it directly impacts the likelihood of long-term disease-free survival and reduces the risk of local recurrence.

    A systematic review evaluated the outcomes of en bloc resection versus intralesional resection for primary spine tumors. En bloc resection, where the tumor is removed intact with adequate margins, offers the best long-term disease-free survival, especially for low-grade malignant tumors such as chordomas and chondrosarcomas. However, it is technically challenging, resource-intensive, and associated with high morbidity, including nerve root sacrifice, hemorrhage, and infections. Open biopsies and prior intralesional resections reduce the likelihood of achieving appropriate margins and disease-free survival, emphasizing the importance of preoperative CT-guided biopsies. Enneking and Weinstein-Boriani-Biagini (WBB) staging systems help determine feasibility. While en bloc resection improves oncologic outcomes, its high complication rate necessitates treatment at specialized centers with multidisciplinary teams. Study limitations of the study include low patient numbers, lack of randomized controlled trials, and insufficient evaluation of quality of life and adjunctive therapies. Despite these challenges, **en bloc resection remains the gold standard for maximizing disease-free survival when feasible**.

    [41]

30. A 45-year-old female is incidentally found to have a hyperintense lesion on T1 and T2 imaging at the L3 vertebra during evaluation for nonspecific back pain. The lesion exhibits a "polka-dot" appearance on axial CT. What is the most appropriate management?
    A. Observation with serial imaging
    B. Radiation therapy
    C. Vertebroplasty
    D. Surgical excision

    Correct Answer: A

    Explanation:

    Spinal hemangiomas are often asymptomatic and discovered incidentally. The "polka dot" sign, also referred to as the salt and pepper sign, occurs in vertebral intraosseous hemangiomas due to the replacement of normal cancellous bone with thickened vertical trabeculae surrounded by fatty marrow or vascular spaces. **Observation** is appropriate unless the lesion causes pain or neurological symptoms, in which case vertebroplasty or surgery may be considered.

(DI, pp. 520–522)

31. Spinal hemangioblastomas are most commonly associated with which genetic syndrome?
    A. Neurofibromatosis type 1
    B. Von Hippel-Lindau disease
    C. Tuberous sclerosis
    D. Li-Fraumeni syndrome

    Correct Answer: B

    Explanation:

    Spinal hemangioblastomas are highly associated with Von Hippel-Lindau (VHL) disease, an autosomal dominant genetic condition. VHL is characterized by the development of multiple hemangioblastomas in the central nervous system (CNS), including the spinal cord, cerebellum, and retina, as well as other tumors like renal cell carcinoma and pheochromocytomas. Neurofibromatosis type 1, tuberous sclerosis, and Li-Fraumeni syndrome are not commonly linked to spinal hemangioblastomas.

    (GB, p. 646)

32. The etiology of von Hippel-Lindau disease is:
    A. Mutations in the VHL tumor suppressor gene located on chromosome 3
    B. Absence of the VHL tumor suppressor gene located on chromosome 3
    C. Mutations in the VHL tumor suppressor gene located on chromosome 13
    D. Absence of the VHL tumor suppressor gene located on chromosome 13

    Correct Answer: A

    Explanation:

    The **VHL gene**, a tumor suppressor located on **chromosome 3p25.3**, encodes the VHL protein, which is part of the VCB-CUL2 protein complex. Most cases are inherited as an autosomal dominant mutation with ~95% penetrance by age 60, but ~20% arise from spontaneous mutations during early development. The second mutation in susceptible organs (e.g., brain, kidney, and retina) leads to loss of functional VHL protein, enabling cyst or tumor formation. About 4% of carriers with the mutant gene remain asymptomatic.

    (GB, p. 646)

33. A 50-year-old healthy male with severe back pain, weight loss, and a noticeable decrease in appetite. Plain radiographs of the spine show a "winking owl sign." CT scan showed T9 body lesion. CT chest, abdomen, and pelvis were unremarkable.

    What is the most appropriate next step in management?
    A. CT-guided biopsy of the spine
    B. Radiation therapy

C. Pain therapy
D. Surgical decompression

Correct Answer: A

Explanation:

Bone metastases of unknown primary tumors are a significant clinical challenge, particularly when presenting as spinal metastases. They are characterized by the absence of identifiable primary malignancy despite thorough investigation. The spine is the most common site for skeletal metastases, especially in the thoracic region. Autopsy studies reveal that the primary site is identified in approximately 70% of cases, but only 25–30% are diagnosed during life. Lung, gastrointestinal, and renal cancers are among the most common occult primary sites, with adenocarcinomas comprising the majority of these cases.

Biopsy is crucial in these cases and first step in diagnosis, with a diagnostic success rate of 80–90% when combined with advanced immunohistochemical and molecular studies. Core needle biopsy under CT guidance is preferred for its high yield and low complication rate. Despite these diagnostic efforts, the prognosis for the spinal metastases without known origin remains poor, with median survival ranging from 6 to 12 months.

[42]

34. A 35-year-old woman presents with slowly progressive numbness and weakness in both legs, worsening over the past year. MRI shows an intramedullary lesion at the thoracic level, hypointense on T1, hyperintense on T2, with a cystic component.

What is the most likely diagnosis?

A. Schwannoma
B. Ependymoma
C. Astrocytoma
D. Hemangioblastoma

Correct Answer: C

Explanation:

Astrocytomas are the **most common intramedullary spinal cord tumors in younger adults**, particularly in the thoracic region. The lesion's MRI characteristics—T1 hypointensity, T2 hyperintensity, and the presence of a cystic component—are typical of astrocytomas. These tumors often present with slowly progressive neurological deficits, such as numbness and weakness.

- **Schwannoma (A)**: Typically, an extramedullary lesion, not intramedullary, and arises from nerve roots.
- **Ependymoma (B)**: More common in older adults; often shows a more well-defined mass with associated hemosiderin cap on imaging.
- **Hemangioblastoma (D)**: May have cystic components but is more often associated with Von Hippel-Lindau disease and a vascular mural nodule.

(DI, p. 804)

35. The most common type of spinal lymphoma is:
    A. Primary spinal epidural non-Hodgkin's lymphoma
    B. Primary spinal epidural Hodgkin's lymphoma
    C. Spinal intramedullary lymphoma
    D. Metastatic or secondary lymphoma
    Correct Answer: D
    Explanation:
    The most common type of spinal lymphoma is **primary spinal epidural non-Hodgkin's lymphoma**. It usually originates in the epidural space and can cause spinal cord compression, presenting with back pain, weakness, or sensory changes.
    Primary spinal epidural Hodgkin's lymphoma is extremely rare, as Hodgkin's lymphoma more commonly affects lymph nodes.
    Spinal intramedullary lymphoma is rare and occurs within the spinal cord parenchyma.
    Metastatic or secondary lymphoma to the spine is less frequent than primary epidural lymphoma, although it can occur in the context of systemic lymphoma.
    (GB, p. 979)
36. The spinal meningiomas predominately affects female; however, in the following region the male to female ratio is 1:1:
    A. Cervical
    B. Thoracic
    C. Lumbar
    D. Sacral
    Correct Answer: C
    Explanation:
    Spinal meningiomas predominantly affect females due to the influence of hormonal factors, particularly in the thoracic and cervical regions. However, in the **lumbar region**, the male-to-female ratio is approximately 1:1. Lumbar meningiomas are relatively rare compared to those in the thoracic spine, where they are most common and have a strong female predominance.
    Cervical and Thoracic regions show a marked female predominance.
    Sacral meningiomas are uncommon and also exhibit female predominance.
    The unique ratio in the lumbar region may reflect anatomical or hormonal differences affecting tumor incidence in this area.
    (GB, p. 981)
37. 67-year-old female presents with progressive lower extremity weakness and bowel incontinence. MRI reveals an intradural, extramedullary lesion at T8 with homogeneous contrast enhancement and a dural tail. Histopathology shows spindle-shaped cells arranged in a whorled pattern with psammoma bodies. What genetic mutation is most commonly associated with this tumor?
    A. NF1 gene mutation
    B. NF2 gene mutation
    C. TP53 mutation
    D. VHL gene mutation
    Correct Answer: B

Explanation:

Spinal meningiomas are intradural, extramedullary tumors commonly associated with NF2 mutations, especially in multiple meningiomas or in younger patients. They have a characteristic dural tail sign on MRI. The other mutations are associated with different tumors: NF1 with neurofibromas, TP53 with various cancers, and VHL with hemangioblastomas.

(GB, p. 981)

38. According to Asazuma classification system for dumbbell spinal schwannomas, Type IIIa is:
    A. Intradural and extradural and are restricted to the spinal canal
    B. Intradural and extradural foraminal
    C. Intradural and extradural paravertebral
    D. Extradural and intravertebral

    Correct Answer: B

    Explanation:

    The **Asazuma classification system** categorizes dumbbell spinal schwannomas based on their anatomical extent:

    Type I: Intradural and extradural, confined to the spinal canal with constriction at the dura

    Type II: Entirely extradural, with subtypes:

    IIa: Confined to the neural foramen

    IIb: Spanning the spinal canal and paravertebral space

    IIc: Extending into both foraminal and paravertebral regions

    Type III: Combined intradural and extradural:

    IIIa: Foraminal involvement

    IIIb: Paravertebral involvement

    Type IV: Extradural with intravertebral extension

    Type V: Extradural with extralaminar and laminar invasion

    Type VI: Multidirectional bone erosion

    Craniocaudal spread is designated as **IF** (intervertebral foramina) and **TF** (transverse foramina), indicating the number of levels involved (e.g., IF stage 2 = two foramina affected).

    (GB, p. 982)

39. The following type of spinal tumors has the most motor deficit when resected surgically:
    A. Cervical schwannomas
    B. Thoracic schwannomas
    C. Lumbar neurofibromas
    D. Lumbar schwannomas with extradural extension

    Correct Answer: A

    Explanation:

    During nerve sheath tumors resection, it is often possible to preserve some fascicles of the affected nerve root, complete resection of the nerve root may sometimes be necessary. New deficits may not develop, particularly in cases with large tumors, as the affected fascicles are frequently nonfunctional, and adjacent nerve roots may compensate. The risk of motor deficits is greater with

schwannomas compared to neurofibromas, higher in **cervical** tumors than lumbar ones, and increases with cervical tumors that have extradural extension.
(GB, p. 982)

40. What is the current WHO grade classification for Myxopapillary ependymoma as of the 2021 update?
    A. Grade I
    B. Grade II
    C. Grade III
    D. Grade IV

    Correct Answer: B
    Explanation:
    As of the fifth edition, 2021 WHO Classification of Tumors of the Central Nervous System, **myxopapillary ependymomas** have been upgraded to **Grade II**. Previously classified as Grade I, this change reflects their potential for local recurrence and dissemination, particularly within the cerebrospinal fluid.
    (RP)

41. In the context of Myxopapillary ependymoma, which histological feature is most characteristic?
    A. Rosenthal fibers
    B. Perivascular pseudorosettes
    C. Homer Wright rosettes
    D. Verocay bodies

    Correct Answer: B
    Explanation:
    Perivascular pseudorosettes are a hallmark histological feature of ependymomas, including myxopapillary ependymomas. These structures consist of tumor cells arranged radially around blood vessels with an intervening zone of fibrillary processes, creating a characteristic appearance.
    Rosenthal fibers: Seen in pilocytic astrocytomas, not ependymomas.
    Homer Wright rosettes: Associated with medulloblastomas and neuroblastomas.
    Verocay bodies: Characteristic of schwannomas, not ependymomas.
    This feature, along with the myxoid background and papillary architecture, helps distinguish myxopapillary ependymomas histologically.
    (RP)

42. Which of the following immunohistochemical markers is commonly positive in myxopapillary ependymomas?
    A. Synaptophysin
    B. AE1/AE3
    C. EMA (Epithelial Membrane Antigen)
    D. Desmin

    Correct Answer: B
    Explanation:
    Myxopapillary ependymomas are immunohistochemically positive for GFAP, S100, vimentin, CD99, **AE1/AE3**, and NCAM1.

Synaptophysin: Associated with neuronal tumors, not ependymomas.

EMA: Occasionally positive in ependymomas but not characteristic of myxopapillary subtype.

Desmin: Marker for muscle tumors, not ependymomas.

AE1/AE3 positivity is a significant feature of myxopapillary ependymomas, alongside other markers like GFAP and S100.

(RP)

43. During the surgical resection of a solid spinal hemangioblastoma, the surgeon encounters significant bleeding. Which of the following intraoperative techniques is most likely to control the bleeding effectively?
   A. Use of bipolar cautery
   B. Application of hemostatic agents
   C. Preoperative embolization
   D. Intraoperative radiation therapy

   Correct Answer: C

   Explanation:

   Solid hemangioblastomas are more challenging to remove and should be approached similar to arteriovenous malformations (AVMs). Piecemeal removal is avoided; instead, surgery focuses on working along the tumor's margin and devascularizing its blood supply. A useful technique involves shrinking the tumor by placing bipolar forceps along its surface and applying coagulation. Preoperative embolization can also be beneficial in reducing the tumor's vascularity.

   (GP, p. 825)

44. Patient with nocturnal back pain has lumbar puncture that showed clotted and xanthochromia of CSF. This condition is called:
   A. Froin's syndrome
   B. Queckenstedt's test
   C. Clotted CSF syndrome
   D. Xantho CSF test

   Correct Answer: A

   Explanation:

   Froin's Syndrome is a clinical condition characterized by **xanthochromia** and **hypercoagulability** of cerebrospinal fluid (CSF) caused by **blockage of CSF flow** due to spinal cord or cauda equina lesions. This syndrome is typically associated with:

   Stasis of CSF: Caused by complete or near-complete obstruction of CSF flow at a specific level of the spinal cord (spinal cord tumors, stenosis)

   High protein content: Due to local inflammation or tumor breakdown products, leading to xanthochromia.

   Hypercoagulability: Resulting from fibrinogen and protein accumulation in the CSF.

   (GB, p. 987)

45. A 55-year-old female undergoes surgery for an intramedullary spinal cord tumor. During the procedure, the surgeon uses somatosensory evoked potentials (SSEPs) and motor evoked potentials (MEPs) for intraoperative monitoring. Suddenly, there is a significant drop in MEP amplitude. What is the most appropriate immediate action?
    A. Increase the depth of anesthesia
    B. Check for technical issues with the monitoring equipment
    C. Proceed with tumor resection
    D. Administer a muscle relaxant

    Correct Answer: B

    Explanation:

    A sudden drop in **motor evoked potential (MEP)** amplitude during surgery is a critical finding that may indicate compromised spinal cord or nerve root function. The immediate priority is to rule out technical issues with the monitoring equipment, **as false alarms** can occur due to poor electrode contact, disconnection, or other technical factors.

    Increase the depth of anesthesia: Deeper anesthesia can suppress MEPs and may worsen the issue if it is not the underlying cause.

    Proceed with tumor resection: Continuing surgery without identifying the cause of the MEP drop could result in permanent neurological deficits.

    Administer a muscle relaxant: Muscle relaxants interfere with MEP signals and are contraindicated when monitoring is required.

    If no technical issues are found, the surgeon must promptly assess and address potential surgical or vascular causes (e.g., traction on neural tissue or ischemia).

46. During the resection of an intramedullary spinal cord tumor, the intraoperative neurophysiological monitoring team reports a loss of D-wave signals. What does this finding most likely indicate?
    A. Technical malfunction of the monitoring equipment
    B. Potential irreversible damage to the corticospinal tract
    C. Temporary ischemia of the spinal cord
    D. Normal variation in monitoring signals

    Correct Answer: B

    Explanation:

    The D-wave is a direct electrophysiological recording of corticospinal tract function. Loss of D-wave signals during intraoperative neurophysiological monitoring is a serious finding and most commonly indicates potential irreversible damage to the corticospinal tract. Technical malfunction of the monitoring equipment: While technical issues can cause signal loss, this is less likely with D-waves, as they are highly stable and less affected by anesthesia or physiological changes compared to other signals like MEPs. Temporary ischemia of the spinal cord: While ischemia may transiently affect MEPs, the loss of D-wave signals suggests more severe and potentially permanent corticospinal injury. Normal variation in monitoring signals: D-wave loss is not considered a normal variation; it is a significant warning requiring immediate action to prevent permanent neurological deficits. Preservation of D-wave signals during surgery correlates with better long-term motor outcomes, even if MEPs are temporarily lost.

(GB. p. 989)

47. The preferred initial treatment for small a symptomatic spinal cord hemangioblastoma is:
   A. Stereotactic radiosurgery
   B. Chemotherapy
   C. Observation
   D. Surgical resection

   Correct Answer: D

   Explanation:

   Even if small, a symptomatic spinal cord hemangioblastoma requires surgical resection as the preferred initial treatment. These tumors are highly vascular but often well-circumscribed, and early removal can prevent progressive neurological deterioration due to compression or cyst formation. Microsurgical techniques allow for safe and effective resection in most cases.

   (GB, p. 825)

48. The presence of a "drop metastasis" in the spinal canal is most commonly associated with which primary brain tumor?
   A. Glioblastoma multiforme
   B. Medulloblastoma
   C. Meningioma
   D. Craniopharyngioma

   Correct Answer: B

   Explanation:

   "Drop metastasis" refers to the dissemination of tumor cells through the cerebrospinal fluid (CSF), leading to metastatic deposits along the spinal canal. This phenomenon is most commonly associated with **medulloblastoma**, a primary brain tumor that typically arises in the posterior fossa. Medulloblastomas are known for their propensity to spread via the CSF to the spinal cord, creating nodular deposits along the leptomeninges.

   (GB, p. 744)

49. The most common histological subtype of spinal cord astrocytoma in adults is:
   A. Pilocytic astrocytoma
   B. Anaplastic astrocytoma
   C. Glioblastoma
   D. Fibrillary astrocytoma

   Correct Answer: D

   Explanation:

   Fibrillary astrocytoma is the most common histological subtype of spinal cord astrocytoma in adults. These tumors are diffusely infiltrative and typically present as low-grade (WHO Grade II) but may progress to higher grades (anaplastic astrocytoma or glioblastoma) over time. They commonly occur in the thoracic spinal cord.

   (DI, p. 804)

50. A 17-year-old male presents with localized thoracic pain, worse at night, and partially relieved by NSAIDs. CT shows a well-defined lytic lesion with central mineralization in the posterior elements of the T8 vertebra. What histological feature is most likely to confirm the diagnosis?
    A. Presence of physaliphorous cells
    B. Interlacing trabeculae of woven bone surrounded by osteoblasts
    C. Small, round blue cells with a Homer-Wright rosette pattern
    D. Spindle cells with nuclear pleomorphism and mitotic figures

    Correct Answer: B

    Explanation:

    Osteoblastoma is a benign bone tumor (>1.5 cm) commonly found in the posterior spinal elements, especially the cervical spine. It appears as a well-circumscribed, expansile lesion on CT and may cause significant peritumoral edema visible on MRI, sometimes mimicking malignancy. It often presents in males aged 10–30 with dull pain, scoliosis, or neurological symptoms from nerve compression. They are highly vascular with **osteoblast-lined trabeculae and variable woven bone**. Peritumoral edema results from prostaglandin release. Aggressive osteoblastoma may exhibit nuclear pleomorphism and cortical breakthrough.

    Differential diagnoses include osteoid osteoma, aneurysmal bone cysts (often co-existing with osteoblastoma), metastases, and osteogenic sarcoma. Treatment involves surgical curettage with bone grafting, sometimes preceded by embolization for vascular tumors. Osteoblastomas have a slow growth pattern, with recurrence rates of 10–15% (higher in aggressive forms).

    The other options describe features of chordoma, Ewing sarcoma, and osteosarcoma, respectively.

    (DI, pp. 705–706)

51. The primary mechanism of action of bisphosphonates in the treatment of spinal metastases is:
    A. Inhibition of osteoclast-mediated bone resorption
    B. Direct cytotoxic effect on tumor cells
    C. Inhibition of angiogenesis
    D. Activation of osteoblasts

    Correct Answer: A

    Explanation:

    Bisphosphonates are primarily used in the treatment of spinal metastases to reduce bone loss, pain, and associated complications. They achieve this by **inhibiting osteoclast-mediated bone resorption**. Bisphosphonates bind to hydroxyapatite in bone, and when osteoclasts attempt to resorb bone, the drugs are internalized, leading to decreased osteoclast activity, induction of apoptosis, and reduction in bone destruction.

    (GB, p. 1211)

52. In the management of metastatic epidural spinal cord compression, which of the following factors is NOT typically considered in the decision-making process?
    A. Presence of systemic metastases
    B. Primary tumor histology
    C. Patient's life expectancy
    D. None of the above

    Correct Answer: D

    Explanation:

    All the listed factors: **Presence of systemic metastases**, **primary tumor histology**, and **patient's life expectancy**—are integral to the decision-making process in managing metastatic epidural spinal cord compression.

    Systemic metastases: The extent of disease affects the feasibility and goals of treatment (e.g., palliation vs prolongation of survival).

    Primary tumor histology: Tumor type influences response to treatments such as radiation or chemotherapy (e.g., radiosensitive tumors like lymphoma respond well to radiation).

    Life expectancy: Guides the intensity of intervention, with more aggressive treatments reserved for patients with longer anticipated survival.

    (RS, pp. 1547–1548)

53. The most common non-neoplastic lesion that can mimic a spinal epidural metastasis on imaging is:
    A. Disc herniation
    B. Epidural abscess
    C. Hematoma
    D. Arachnoid cyst

    Correct Answer: B

    Explanation:

    Spinal epidural abscess is the most common non-neoplastic lesion mimicking spinal epidural metastasis on imaging due to its mass effect.

    Spinal epidural metastasis typically appears as a well-circumscribed, extraosseous soft tissue mass that is hypointense on T1, hyperintense on T2, with diffuse enhancement. It often involves contiguous vertebral lesions, causing posterior vertebra or pedicle destruction without affecting intervertebral discs, and may present with craniocaudal elongation, paravertebral extension, and compression fractures. In contrast, a spinal epidural abscess is often associated with spondylodiscitis or instrumentation, spans multiple segments, and shows peripherally enhancing necrotic abscesses or homogeneously enhancing phlegmon on contrast imaging. MRI findings include iso-to-hypointensity on T1, hyperintensity on T2 and Short-Tau Inversion Recovery (STIR), and hyperintensity on Diffusion-Weighted Imaging (DWI) with Apparent Diffusion Coefficient (ADC) hypointensity. It may cause dural enhancement, anterior epidural venous enhancement, and spinal cord signal changes due to compression, ischemia, or direct infection. These imaging differences help differentiate between infectious and neoplastic epidural lesions.

    (DI, p. 594)

54. Which of the following best describes the NOMS framework for decision-making in metastatic spine tumors?
    A. Neurological and oncological factors exclusively guide treatment.
    B. It incorporates neurological, oncological, mechanical, and systemic considerations.
    C. It relies solely on tumor histology and radiosensitivity.
    D. It excludes systemic disease burden as a factor.

    Correct Answer: B

    Explanation:

    The NOMS (Neurologic, Oncologic, Mechanical, and Systemic) framework comprehensively incorporates neurological, oncological, mechanical, and systemic considerations to guide treatment. It accounts for factors such as myelopathy, tumor radiosensitivity, spinal instability, and the patient's overall health to tailor interventions.

    (BS, pp. 1325–1342)

55. In the randomized trial by Patchell et al., comparing surgery plus radiotherapy (RT) to RT alone for metastatic spinal cord compression, which of the following outcomes showed significant improvement in the surgical group?
    A. Pain relief and overall survival
    B. Recovery of ambulation and bowel/bladder continence
    C. Reduction in tumor size and prevention of recurrence
    D. Radiographic tumor control and shorter hospital stays

    Correct Answer: B

    Explanation:

    The study demonstrated that patients undergoing surgery followed by RT had significantly better recovery of ambulation (62% vs 19%) and maintained bowel/bladder continence for a longer duration (155 days vs 17 days) compared to RT alone.

    [31]

56. A 55-year-old male presents with localized lower back pain and a kyphotic deformity. Imaging reveals a solitary, expansile lesion in the L2 vertebra with cortical destruction but no soft tissue mass. Serum protein electrophoresis shows a monoclonal spike. What is the best definitive treatment?
    A. High-dose corticosteroids
    B. Surgical stabilization and local radiation therapy
    C. Chemotherapy with bortezomib
    D. Observation with periodic imaging

    Correct Answer: B

    Explanation:

    Plasmacytoma is a neoplasm originating from a single clone of plasma cells, similar to multiple myeloma, but it is diagnosed based on the following criteria:

    - Absence of additional lesions on a complete skeletal survey (excluding bone scans)
    - No evidence of myeloma on bone marrow aspirate
    - Serum and urine electrophoresis showing no detectable monoclonal immunoglobulin protein

Solitary plasmacytomas is treated with **local radiotherapy** (40–60 Gy), with or without autologous stem cell transplantation, is standard. **Surgical intervention** is preferred for neurologic involvement, spinal deformity or instability. Gross total tumor resection or total spondylectomy with adjuvant radiotherapy reduces local recurrence and progression to multiple myeloma. Long-term bisphosphonate therapy (~2 years) effectively prevents osteolysis and bone loss.

Systemic chemotherapy is reserved for multiple myeloma. Observation is not appropriate due to risk of progression to myeloma.

(GB, pp. 930–931)

57. A 14-year-old male presents with severe back pain, fever, and weight loss. Imaging shows a lytic lesion in the T10 vertebral body with a large paraspinal soft tissue mass. Biopsy demonstrates small, round blue cells with CD99 positivity. What is the recommended initial treatment?
    A. En bloc surgical resection
    B. Radiation therapy alone
    C. Chemotherapy followed by local control
    D. Observation with serial imaging

    Correct Answer: C

    Explanation:

    Ewing sarcoma is an aggressive childhood cancer that includes the Ewing sarcoma family of tumors (ESFT), such as Askin tumor and peripheral primitive neuroectodermal tumor (PNET). It commonly affects the sacrum or vertebral body and appears as a permeative lytic lesion with a "moth-eaten" bone pattern and wide zone of transition on imaging. MRI best identifies tumor extent, often showing soft tissue masses with central necrosis and heterogeneous enhancement. Differential diagnoses include lymphoma, leukemia, osteosarcoma, osteomyelitis, and metastatic neuroblastoma. Histologically, it consists of small round cells with high mitotic activity, often linked to EWSR1 genetic translocations. Most cases occur before age 20, with a male predominance. Metastases to the lungs, lymph nodes, and bones occur in 30% of cases. Treatment involves a multimodal approach with **chemotherapy** and radiation therapy. En bloc excision is considered when feasible, particularly in cases of neurological deficits or spinal instability. Long-term survival can be achieved in over 50% of localized cases, although complications like recurrence or secondary malignancies are common.

    (DI, pp. 735–736)

58. A 50-year-old male presents with chronic, progressive lower back pain. Imaging reveals an expansile, destructive lesion in the L5 vertebral body with calcifications. Biopsy demonstrates lobules of hyaline cartilage with atypical chondrocytes in a myxoid stroma. Which radiological feature is most characteristic of this tumor?
    A. Osteoblastic activity on bone scan
    B. Hypointense signal on T2-weighted MRI

C. Mineralized rings and arcs pattern on CT
D. Soap-bubble appearance on plain radiographs

Correct Answer: C

Explanation:

Chondrosarcomas are malignant cartilage-producing tumors, and the mineralized rings and arcs pattern on CT is characteristic of hyaline cartilage. They often present as expansile lesions with cortical destruction and calcifications. Soap-bubble appearance is typical of benign giant cell tumors.

(RP)

59. A 58-year-old female presents with generalized weakness and bone pain. Serum protein electrophoresisreveals a significant M-spike, and 24-h urine analysis detects Bence-Jones protein. A technetium-99m bone scan is negative, but X-rays show generalized osteoporosis with no specific sclerotic lesions. Bone marrow biopsy reveals 12% myeloma cells. Which additional finding would confirm the diagnosis of multiple myeloma?
A. Positive antinuclear antibody (ANA) test
B. Low serum calcium levels
C. Normal serum immunoglobulin levels
D. Osteolytic lesions on X-ray or CT

Correct Answer: D

Explanation:

The diagnosis of multiple myeloma is based on cytologic, clinical, and laboratory criteria. Cytologic evidence includes ≥10% plasma or myeloma cells in the bone marrow or a biopsy-proven plasmacytoma. Clinical criteria include the presence of an M-protein (monoclonal component) in the serum (>3 g/dL) or urine, **osteolytic lesions on imaging** or generalized osteoporosis with >30% plasma cells in the marrow, and detection of myeloma cells in ≥2 peripheral blood smears. Key diagnostic tests include 24-h urine analysis for Bence-Jones protein (monoclonal kappa or lambda light chains present in 75–80% of cases) and blood tests such as serum protein electrophoresis with immunofixation and free light chain assay to detect monoclonal proteins. Complete blood count (CBC) often reveals anemia due to marrow infiltration, and serum creatinine levels are assessed for prognosis. Imaging, particularly skeletal surveys, reveals characteristic "punched-out" lytic lesions or osteoporosis, while technetium-99m bone scans are typically negative in untreated multiple myeloma. Bone marrow biopsy, demonstrating ≥10% myeloma cells, is essential for confirmation. Diagnosis requires a combination of cytologic and clinical/laboratory findings for specificity.

(GB, p. 930)

60. A 16-year-old female presents with localized back pain and swelling over the thoracolumbar region. Imaging shows an expansile lesion with a fluid-fluid level in the posterior elements of T10. Histology reveals blood-filled spaces lined by fibroblasts and osteoclast-like giant cells. What is the most appropriate initial treatment?
A. En bloc resection
B. Curettage with bone grafting

C. Radiotherapy
D. Chemotherapy

Correct Answer: B

Explanation:

Aneurysmal bone cysts (ABCs) have a characteristics imaging of expansile lesion with a fluid-fluid level in the posterior vertebral elements and typical histology of blood-filled spaces lined by fibroblasts and osteoclast-like giant cells. It is an expansile, tumor-like osteolytic lesion characterized by a highly vascular honeycomb structure of blood-filled cavities separated by connective tissue septa, surrounded by a thin cortical bone shell that may expand. Accounting for 15% of spine tumors, ABCs peak in incidence during the second decade of life. The etiology is debated and may involve preexisting tumors (e.g., osteoblastoma, giant cell tumor, fibrous dysplasia, or chondrosarcoma) or acute fractures. Treatment typically involves **intralesional curettage**, but incomplete excision carries a high recurrence rate of 25–50%.

(GB, p. 979)

61. A 30-year-old male with a history of a giant cell tumor in the vertebral column underwent intratumoral curettage six months ago. He now presents with recurrent localized pain. Imaging shows residual tumor without evidence of metastasis. What is the most appropriate management?
A. Revision surgery for resection
B. Start bisphosphonate therapy
C. Initiate radiotherapy
D. Observe with periodic imaging

Correct Answer: A.

Explanation:

Giant cell tumors (GCTs) of bone, also known as osteoclastomas, are benign but locally aggressive lesions arising from osteoclasts, often categorized alongside aneurysmal bone cysts. These tumors typically occur in adolescence and are most common in the knees and wrists, but neurosurgical cases usually involve the skull (particularly the sphenoid bone) or the vertebral column, with about 4% occurring in the sacrum. GCTs are lytic, causing bony collapse, and can exhibit pseudomalignant behavior, including recurrence and occasional pulmonary metastases. Evaluation includes MRI for soft tissue assessment, CT for bony destruction and surgical planning, and chest CT to check for metastases. Treatment involves intratumoral curettage, often preceded by embolization, with a recurrence rate of ~20%. **Recurrence requires revision surgery for resection of if surgery is feasible.** Radiotherapy is reserved for unresectable recurrences due to risks of malignant transformation. Osteoclast-inhibiting drugs like bisphosphonates or RANKL inhibitors (e.g., denosumab) have shown success after subtotal resection. Cryosurgery is rarely used in spinal cases because of risks to neural structures. Close follow-up with MRI or CT every 3 months is essential to monitor for recurrence.

(GB, pp. 995–996)

62. A 28-year-old male presents with chronic radicular pain and difficulty walking. MRI reveals an intradural, extramedullary lesion at the lumbar level with a hypointense rim on T1 and hyperintensity on T2-weighted imaging. Histology shows keratinized squamous epithelium and cholesterol clefts. What is the most likely cause of this lesion?
    A. Trauma-induced epidermal implantation
    B. Congenital inclusion
    C. Malignant transformation of dermoid cyst
    D. Secondary to chronic infection

    Correct Answer: B

    Explanation:

    Epidermoid cyst, also known as an epidermoid tumor, is a benign, non-neoplastic spinal mass arising from epidermal elements. It is commonly located in the cauda equina or lumbosacral region, with imaging typically showing a CSF-isointense mass on T1 and mildly hyperintense on T2, with restricted diffusion on DWI to distinguish it from arachnoid cysts. Most cases are from **congenital inclusion**, while acquired forms are linked to lumbar punctures or surgery. Symptoms are often asymptomatic or progress slowly, causing compressive radiculopathy or myelopathy. Diagnosis involves MRI, particularly DWI, for its ability to detect mass effects. Microscopically, epidermoid cysts have an outer connective tissue capsule lined with **stratified squamous epithelium**. The central contents consist of desquamated epithelial keratin and **cholesterol crystals**, which stain positively for EMA and cytokeratin.

    Treatment is complete surgical excision, which offers the best neurological outcome, though recurrence is common with incomplete removal. Malignant transformation is exceedingly rare.

    (DI, p. 100)

63. A 47-year-old male presents with lower back pain, radicular symptoms, and occasional headaches. MRI shows a hyperintense intradural lesion at L2 on T2-weighted imaging, with marked enhancement post-contrast. The lesion is highly vascular on angiography. Histology reveals cells with salt-and-pepper chromatin in a Zellballen pattern. What is the most specific immunohistochemical marker for this tumor?
    A. GFAP
    B. S100
    C. Synaptophysin
    D. CD34

    Correct Answer: C

    Explanation:

    A paraganglioma, also known as a glomus tumor or extra-adrenal pheochromocytoma, is a WHO grade 1 rare benign spinal tumor most commonly found in the cauda equina or filum terminale as an intradural, extramedullary mass. It appears hypervascular on imaging, with intense contrast enhancement and prominent flow voids on MRI, while CT may show vertebral scalloping and foraminal enlargement due to bony remodeling. MRI is the preferred diagnostic tool, though distinguishing paraganglioma from ependymoma and schwannoma and require histopathological confirmation.

Histopathologically, it is well-differentiated, featuring zellballen architecture with compact nests of chief (type I) cells surrounded by sustentacular (type II) cells, sinusoidal blood vessels, and chromogranin- and **synaptophysin-positive** staining. Electron microscopy reveals dense core neurosecretory granules. Symptoms include chronic back pain, radiculopathy, sensory or motor deficits, and, rarely, secretory activity (e.g., hypertension, palpitations). These tumors are slow-growing, with recurrence rates of <5% following gross total resection. Treatment involves surgical excision, which is usually curative, and preoperative embolization may be performed to minimize intraoperative hemorrhage.

(DI, pp. 799–800)

64. A 35-year-old female with a history of neurofibromatosis type 1 (NF1) presents with unilateral radicular pain and paresthesia. MRI reveals an intradural, extramedullary lesion at the C7-T1 level that is hypointense on T1, hyperintense on T2, and enhances homogeneously with contrast. What is the most likely finding on histopathology?
   A. Antoni A and Antoni B areas
   B. Spindle cells with wavy nuclei in mucoid matrix
   C. Rosenthal fibers and eosinophilic granular bodies
   D. Small, round blue cells

   Correct Answer: B

   Explanation:

   Neurofibromas are non-encapsulated tumors that infiltrate between nerve fascicles, complicating resection. They typically affect superficial cutaneous nerves but may involve larger, deep-seated nerves. Microscopically, they consist of Schwann cells and fibroblasts (**Spindle cells with wavy nuclei**) embedded in a rich **mucoid collagen matrix**. Immunohistochemically, Schwann cells are S100-positive, while the stromal component expresses CD34.

   In contrast, Antoni A/B areas are seen in schwannomas, Rosenthal fibers in pilocytic astrocytomas, and small round blue cells in malignant small round cell tumors like Ewing sarcoma.

   (RP)

65. What is the most common location for spinal cavernous malformations?
   A. Cervical spine
   B. Thoracic spine
   C. Lumbar spine
   D. Sacral spine

   Correct Answer: B

   Explanation:

   Spinal cavernous malformations most often occur in the thoracic spine, then in the cervical and lumbar regions. They make up 5% of all spinal vascular lesions and are more common in females (2:1).

   (HS, p. 278)

66. What is the estimated annual hemorrhage rate for spinal cavernous malformations?
    A. 0.5–1%
    B. 1.4–4.5%
    C. 10–20%
    D. 50–66%

    Correct Answer: B

    Explanation:

    The hemorrhage rate for spinal cavernous malformations is 1.4–4.5% per patient-year. However, the chance of repeat hemorrhage can reach 66% per year.

    (HS, p. 278)
67. Which MRI sequence is best for diagnosing spinal cavernous malformations?
    A. T1 MRI
    B. T2 MRI
    C. Flair sequence
    D. Gradient recalled echo (GRE) sequence

    Correct Answer: D

    Explanation:

    MRI with gradient-recalled echo (GRE) sequences is the best imaging method. Cavernous malformations appear as "popcorn-like" lesions with hemosiderin-stained rims and no flow voids.

    (HS, p. 278)
68. At what age do symptomatic hemorrhages from spinal cavernous malformations most commonly occur?
    A. Second decade (10–20 years)
    B. Third decade (20–30 years)
    C. Fourth decade (30–40 years)
    D. Fifth decade (40–50 years)

    Correct Answer: C

    (HS, p. 278)
69. What is the most effective treatment for symptomatic spinal cavernous malformations with recurrent hemorrhage?
    A. Radiation therapy
    B. Conservative management with steroids
    C. Gross total excision
    D. Endovascular embolization

    Correct Answer: C

    Explanation:

    For symptomatic cavernous malformations with recurrent hemorrhage, gross total excision is the best treatment. Surgery prevents future bleeds and stabilizes neurological function.

70. Which type of spinal arteriovenous fistula (AVF) is the most common?
    A. Intradural-dorsal AVF
    B. Intradural-ventral AVF
    C. Extradural AVM
    D. Intramedullary AVM

    Correct Answer: A

    Explanation:

    Intradural-dorsal AVF accounts for 60–80% of all spinal vascular lesions. It occurs due to venous outflow dysfunction and mainly affects middle-aged men in the thoracolumbar spine.

    (HS, p. 280)
71. What is the most common symptom of an intradural-dorsal AVF?
    A. Sudden paralysis
    B. Severe radicular pain without weakness
    C. Progressive myelopathy with gait and sphincter dysfunction
    D. Acute meningeal signs

    Correct Answer: C

    Explanation:

    Intradural-dorsal AVFs cause progressive myelopathy, leading to gait instability and bladder dysfunction. Symptoms result from venous congestion rather than hemorrhage.

    (HS, p. 280)
72. Where do intramedullary spinal AVMs most commonly occur?
    A. Cervical spine
    B. Thoracic spine
    C. Lumbar spine
    D. Sacral spine

    Correct Answer: A

    (HS, p. 280)
73. What is a classic angiographic finding in intradural-ventral AVFs?
    A. Sluggish venous outflow with delayed emptying
    B. Direct shunting between the anterior spinal artery (ASA) and a vein
    C. Multiple fistulous points at different spinal levels
    D. Normal arterial and venous anatomy with only mild congestion

    Correct Answer: B

    Explanation:

    Intradural-ventral AVFs show direct arteriovenous shunting between the ASA and a ventral vein. The ASA often forms a "hairpin loop" and may be displaced from the midline.

    (HS, p. 280)

74. What is the preferred treatment for extradural spinal AVMs?
    A. Endovascular embolization
    B. Surgical resection
    C. Radiation therapy
    D. Conservative management

Correct Answer: A

Explanation:

Extradural AVMs are **high-flow lesions** best treated with **endovascular embolization**. Surgery is reserved for cases with persistent compression or hemorrhage.

(HS, p. 280)

75. What is the best treatment for intradural-dorsal arteriovenous fistulas (AVFs)?
    A. Endovascular embolization with coils
    B. Microsurgical clip occlusion
    C. Radiation therapy
    D. Conservative management with anticoagulation

Correct Answer: B

Explanation:

The gold standard for intradural-dorsal AVFs is microsurgical clip occlusion at the fistulous point. Endovascular embolization is an alternative but has a higher risk of recurrence.

(HS, p. 280)

9 Spine Infections

1. Which imaging feature is the most characteristic of early vertebral osteomyelitis on MRI?
   A. Hypointense vertebral marrow on T1WI with endplate erosion
   B. Hyperintense vertebral marrow on T2WI without endplate changes
   C. Increased bone density on plain radiographs
   D. Preserved disc space with hypointense signal on T2WI
   Correct Answer: A
   Explanation:
   Early vertebral osteomyelitis often manifests on MRI as hypointense vertebral marrow on T1-weighted imaging accompanied by endplate erosion. These changes represent inflammation and early bone destruction. T2-weighted imaging typically shows hyperintense signals in the disc and vertebral marrow due to edema. Radiographic findings lag behind and are often negative for up to 2–8 weeks after symptom onset. Disc space preservation is less likely in active osteomyelitis.
   (DI, p. 562)
2. Which organism is the most common cause of vertebral osteomyelitis?
   A. *Escherichia coli*
   B. *Salmonella*
   C. *Staphylococcus aureus*
   D. *Pseudomonas aeruginosa*
   Correct Answer: C
   Explanation:
   Staphylococcus aureus is the most common organism in vertebral osteomyelitis. It is frequently associated with hematogenous spread from bacteremia. *Escherichia coli* is more common among gram-negative infections, while *Salmonella* is seen in sickle cell patients. *Pseudomonas aeruginosa* is typically associated with intravenous drug use or postoperative infections.
   (DI, p. 562)

K. F. AlAli, H. T. Hashim, *Spine Surgery and Peripheral Nerve Surgery*,
https://doi.org/10.1007/978-3-031-98543-0_9

3. A 65-year-old diabetic patient presents with lumbar spine pain and fever. Blood cultures are positive for Staphylococcus aureus. What is the next best step in management?
   A. Immediate surgical debridement
   B. Empirical antitubercular therapy
   C. Initiation of IV antibiotics and MRI of the spine
   D. Percutaneous biopsy of the affected vertebrae
      Correct Answer: C
      Explanation:
      The patient has a typical risk factor for vertebral osteomyelitis or discitis: Diabetes. The history is also suggestive of an infectious spine condition: Fever and positive blood culture. Therefore, MRI of the spine, which is usually diagnostic for vertebral osteomyelitis or discitis, is indicated.
      (DI, p. 562)
4. A 52-year-old with a history of chronic kidney disease. He has back pain and rapidly progressive onset of paraparesis. T1 contrast MRI is shown (Fig. 9.1). Which one of the following is most likely?
   A. Spinal brucellosis
   B. Spinal lipomatosis

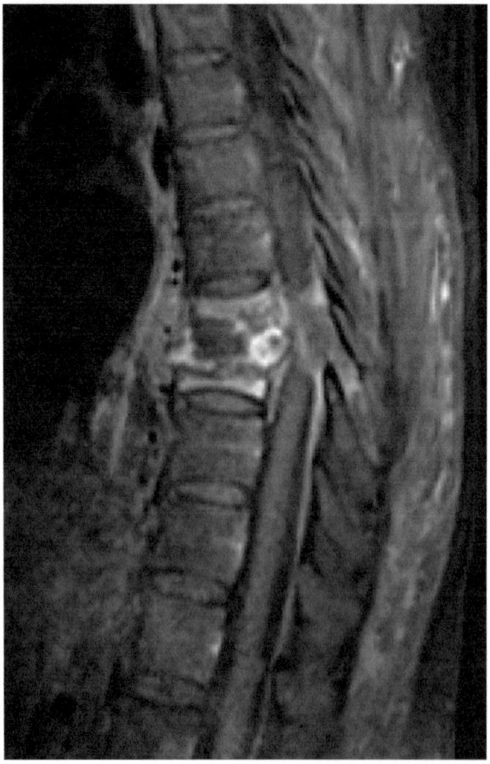

Fig. 9.1 Case 4 T1 contrast MRI

C. Spinal metastasis
D. Discitis with epidural abscess

Correct Answer: D

Explanation:

The patient immunocompromised (chronic kidney disease), which is a risk factor for discitis. The MRI showed destruction at a mid-thoracic level disc space with enhancement involving the two vertebrae and enhancing epidural collection suggestive of discitis with epidural abscess.

(DI, p. 562)

5. What is the most recommended empirical antibiotic regimen for suspected postoperative discitis?
A. Metronidazole and amoxicillin
B. Vancomycin and ceftriaxone
C. Clindamycin and gentamicin
D. Rifampin and isoniazid

Correct Answer: B

Explanation:

The combination of vancomycin (for gram-positive coverage, including methicillin-resistant Staphylococcus aureus [MRSA]) and ceftriaxone (for gram-negative coverage) is a standard empirical regimen for postoperative spine infections pending culture results.

(RS, p. 1816)

6. A patient with a history of sickle cell disease presents with back pain and fever. An MRI shows spinal osteomyelitis and discitis. Which organism is most likely responsible?
A. *Pseudomonas aeruginosa*
B. *Salmonella species*
C. *Mycobacterium tuberculosis*
D. *Candida albicans*

Correct Answer: B

Explanation:

In patients with sickle cell disease and spinal osteomyelitis, *Salmonella* is the more common organism.

(DI, p. 362)

7. Regarding spinal infection mechanism of spread:

7a. All of the following are spreading pathways for spinal infections, EXCEPT:
A. Direct extension
B. Lymphatic channels
C. Hematogenous dissemination
D. Neural pathway

7b. What is the most common mechanism for hematogenous spread of infection to the spine?
A. Arterial dissemination
B. Batson's plexus
C. Direct lymphatic spread
D. Contagious spread from skin infections

Correct Answers: 7a: D, 7b: B

Explanation:

Spinal infections can spread by different routes: Direct extension, lymphatic channels, hematogenous dissemination, and cerebrospinal fluid pathways. Hematogenous dissemination is considered the primary mechanism for spinal infection spreading. It can be via arterial or venous routes. The arterial supply to the vertebral bodies includes end-arteriole networks that lack anastomoses, making these regions particularly susceptible to bacterial seeding. Segmental arteries supply two adjacent vertebral bodies and the intervening disc, leading to typical patterns of disc space infection. Venous spread occurs via Batson's plexus (**the most common hematogenous route**), a valveless venous network running parallel to the spine, interconnected with the vena cava, portal system, azygos, intercostal, pulmonary, and renal veins. Blood flow in this plexus is pressure-dependent, influenced by thoracoabdominal pressure fluctuations.

(RN, p. 1527)

8. Regarding tuberculous spondylitis:

8a. Which of the following findings on histopathological examination is most indicative of tuberculous spondylitis?

A. Noncaseating granulomas
B. Neutrophilic infiltrate
C. Caseating granulomas
D. Eosinophilic infiltrate

8b. It commonly affects:

A. Cervical
B. Thoracic
C. Lumber
D. Sacral

8c. The primary site of infection is usually:

A. Anterior vertebral body
B. Posterior vertebral body
C. Paraspinal muscles
D. Posterior spine elements

8d. The usual route of spreading is:

A. Direct extension
B. Cerebrospinal fluid pathways
C. Hematogenous dissemination
D. Neural pathway

Correct Answers: 8a: C, 8b: B, 8c: A, 8d: C

Explanation:

Tuberculous spondylitis (TS) is a granulomatous infection of the spine and adjacent soft tissue caused by *Mycobacterium tuberculosis*. It commonly affects the **mid-thoracic or thoracolumbar spine**, with the **anterior vertebral body** as the primary site of infection. Key imaging findings include vertebral collapse, gibbus deformity, sparing of intervertebral discs, large paraspinal abscesses, and epidural soft tissue masses, which may cause spinal cord compression. Spread occurs **hematogenously** or through lymphatics, and the infection may extend beneath the longitudinal ligaments or involve posterior elements. Clinically, TS presents with chronic back pain, focal tenderness, and neurologic deficits like paraparesis and kyphosis, while fever is less common. Diagnosis is supported by MRI (most sensitive), elevated erythrocyte sedimentation rate (ESR), and QuantiFERON assays. Microscopic histopathological features are **caseating granulomas** and nonspecific inflammatory reactions.

Treatment includes prolonged antituberculous therapy (≥1 year), with surgery reserved for cases involving neurologic deficits (cord compression) or severe spinal deformity or instability. Early diagnosis and intervention significantly improve outcomes, reducing the risk of permanent deficits or death.

(DI, p. 570)

9. A 58-year-old male patient presents with low back pain and imaging suspected of a spinal infection. He has a positive ESR and C-reactive protein (CRP), but multiple blood cultures are negative. What is the next best step for identifying the pathogen?
   A. Repeat blood cultures
   B. CT-guided biopsy
   C. Start empirical broad-spectrum antibiotics
   D. Lumbar puncture

   Correct Answer: B

   Explanation:

   When suspecting spinal infections and blood cultures are negative, CT-guided biopsy is indicated and the gold standard. A systematic review and meta-analysis [25] found the diagnostic yield of image-guided biopsy to be 48% versus 76% achieved by open surgical biopsy. Factors that reduced diagnostic yield were prior antibiotic exposure, but not statistically significant. Fluoroscopy-guided biopsy showed a slightly higher yield (55%) than CT-guided biopsy (44%), though this was also statistically insignificant.

   [25]

10. Regarding spinal brucellosis:

    10a. Which of the following is NOT a typical feature of spinal brucellosis?
    A. Sacroiliitis
    B. Epidural abscess formation
    C. Skip lesions
    D. Involvement of the posterior elements of the spine

    10b. Spinal brucellosis commonly affects which level:
    A. Cervical
    B. Thoracic
    C. Lumber
    D. Sacral

10c. One of the following is a distinctive imaging feature of spinal brucellosis:
A. Posterior endplate involvement
B. Preservation of posterior elements.
C. Large paraspinal collection
D. All of the above

10d. Brucellosis infection is:
A. Granulomatous infection
B. Suppurative infection
C. Necrotizing infection
D. Viral infection

10e. The recommended antibiotic regimen for spine brucellosis is:
A. Amoxicillin and metronidazole for at least 6 weeks
B. Ciprofloxacin and ceftriaxone for at least 4 weeks
C. C. Doxycycline and rifampin for at least 6 weeks
D. Azithromycin and rifampin for at least 2 weeks

Correct Answers: 10a: D, 10b: C, 10c: B, 10d: A, 10e: C

Explanation:

Spinal brucellosis (Brucellar Spondylitis) is a granulomatous infection caused by *Brucella* species, primarily affecting the **lower lumbar spine** (L4) and sacroiliac joints. It spreads hematogenously or via direct extension, producing localized vertebral osteomyelitis and discitis. Drinking unpasteurised camel milk is a known mechanism for brucellosis acquisition. The infection commonly involves the anterior endplate and vertebral body with **preservation of posterior elements**. Imaging features include endplate irregularity, vertebral sclerosis, and disc destruction, with minimal paraspinal tissue involvement and absence of significant spinal deformity. MRI is the diagnostic modality of choice, revealing hypointense T1 and hyperintense T2 changes, along with epidural or paraspinal abscesses that may cause cord compression. Chronic back pain, fever, and neurologic deficits are typical clinical presentations. Diagnosis is aided by serological testing, with a *Brucella* titer ≥1:160 or rising titers, and blood cultures which are positive in up to 70% of acute cases. Treatment involves prolonged antibiotic therapy with doxycycline and rifampin for at least 6 weeks, often extending to 3 months in spondylitis cases. Surgical intervention is rarely needed unless neural compression or severe abscesses are present. Early diagnosis and treatment generally lead to favorable outcomes.

(RS, p. 1559; DI, p. 583)

11. All of the following are standard antibiotic treatments for methicillin-resistant Staphylococcus aureus (MRSA) spinal infections, EXCEPT:
A. Vancomycin
B. Linezolid
C. Cefazolin
D. Daptomycin

Correct Answer: C

Explanation:

Standard treatments for MRSA spinal infections are Vancomycin, Linezolid, and Daptomycin. Cefazolin is a first-generation cephalosporin and not effective for treating methicillin-resistant *Staphylococcus aureus* (MRSA).

(GB, p. 343) [26]

12. Regarding spinal epidural abscess:

12a. What is the most common location?

A. Cervical spine
B. Thoracic spine
C. Lumbar spine
D. Sacral spine

12b. All of the following are risk factors for spinal epidural abscess, EXCEPT:

A. Diabetes
B. IV drug use
C. Recent spinal surgery
D. Recent trauma

12c. What is the second most common causative organism?

A. *Staphylococcus aureus*
B. *Escherichia coli*
C. *Streptococci species*
D. *Pseudomonas aeruginosa*

12d. The most critical factor in prognosis is:

A. Timing of surgical intervention
B. Patient age and comorbidities
C. The specific organism causing the infection
D. The type of initial antibiotic therapy

Correct Answers: 12a: B, 12b: D, 12c: B

Explanation:

Spinal epidural abscess (SEA) is a potentially devastating condition, causing spinal cord compression. Risk factors include diabetes, IV drug use, and recent spinal surgery. SEA typically presents with severe localized back pain, fever, and neurological deficits, although systemic signs may sometimes be absent. Most SEAs are posterior to the cord, with **thoracic** levels being the most frequent site (followed by lumbar, then cervical spine). Hematogenous spread, primarily from skin infections, IV injections, or other systemic infections like UTIs or respiratory infections, is the most common route of origin. *Staphylococcus aureus* is the predominant causative organism, followed by gram-negative bacteria (*Escherichia coli*) and then streptococci. MRI is the diagnostic modality of choice. Management includes early surgical intervention, particularly in cases with neurological deterioration, combined with targeted antibiotic therapy for at least 6 weeks. Prognosis depends on prompt treatment, with delayed intervention leading to irreversible neurological damage and higher mortality rates.

(GB, p. 381)

13. In vertebral osteomyelitis, which imaging finding is most suggestive of a vascular etiology such as septic emboli?
    A. Involvement of the anterior vertebral body
    B. Involvement of multiple, non-contiguous vertebral levels
    C. Predominant involvement of the posterior elements
    D. Isolated disc space infection without vertebral involvement

    Correct Answer: B

    Explanation: Vertebral osteomyelitis resulting from hematogenous dissemination of septic emboli can exhibit various imaging patterns and may manifest as either solitary or multiple intraosseous lesions.

    [27]
14. Which of the following is the most common fungal pathogen associated with spinal intradural infections in both immunocompetent and immunocompromised patients?
    A. *Candida albicans*
    B. *Exserohilum rostratum*
    C. *Aspergillus* spp.
    D. *Cryptococcus neoformans*

    Correct Answer: C

    Explanation:

    Aspergillus spp. is the most common pathogen causing spinal intradural fungal infections, regardless of immune status.

    (RS, pp. 1650–1651)
15. All of the following are the findings during cerebrospinal fluid (CSF) analysis in spinal intradural fungal infections, EXCEPT:
    A. Mild leukocytosis
    B. Elevated protein levels
    C. Decreased glucose levels
    D. Negative fungal cultures

    Correct Answer: C

    Explanation:

    CSF analysis in spinal intradural fungal infections typically shows mild to moderate leukocytosis, increased protein levels, and normal glucose levels. Fungal cultures are often negative, positive in only 10%–30% of cases. Decreased glucose levels are more characteristic of bacterial or tuberculous meningitis rather than fungal infections.

    (RS, pp. 1650–1651)
16. What is the recommended treatment strategy for spinal intradural fungal infections with positive culture?
    A. Short-duration antifungal therapy only
    B. Long-duration antifungal therapy
    C. Short-duration antifungal therapy with high-dose corticosteroids
    D. Long-duration antifungal therapy with broad-spectrum antibiotics

    Correct Answer: B

Explanation:

The recommended treatment for spinal intradural fungal infections involves long-duration antifungal therapy, with voriconazole or amphotericin B. Corticosteroids and antibiotics are not standard treatments for fungal infections and may worsen the condition.

(RS, pp. 1650–1651)

17. Which of the following is a characteristic feature of spinal infection caused by *Pseudomonas aeruginosa*?
    A. Commonly occurs at the lumbar spine
    B. Rapidly progressive neurologic deficits
    C. Involvement of the intervertebral disc only
    D. Usually found in heroin IV users

    Correct Answer: D

    Explanation:

    Spinal *Pseudomonas aeruginosa* infection is usually seen in heroin IV users. These patients also have a high risk for *Staphylococcus aureus* infections or multiple organisms.

    (RN, pp. 1526)

18. What is the best suitable initial empirical antibiotic treatment for a patient with probable spinal tuberculosis?
    A. Isoniazid, rifampicin, vancomycin, and meropenem
    B. Isoniazid, rifampicin, pyrazinamide
    C. Isoniazid, rifampicin, pyrazinamide, and ethambutol
    D. Isoniazid, rifampicin, and metronidazole

    Correct Answer: C

    Explanation:

    The Centers for Disease Control and Prevention (CDC), the Infectious Diseases Society of America (IDSA), and the American Thoracic Society (ATS) recommend a four-drug regimen as the standard empirical treatment for spinal tuberculosis (Pott's disease) until the susceptibility pattern of the specific strain is established. The initial phase is often for 2 months, followed by 4–7 months of therapy with isoniazid and rifampin.

    (GB, p. 358 and p. 389)

19. In the context of spinal infection, which laboratory test exhibits the best specificity for infection?
    A. Leukocyte count
    B. Erythrocyte sedimentation rate
    C. C-reactive protein
    D. Procalcitonin

    Correct Answer: D

    Explanation:

    Procalcitonin is a biomarker that is especially indicative of bacterial infections.

    It increases markedly in reaction to bacterial endotoxins and pro-inflammatory cytokines and stays diminished in viral or non-infectious inflammatory situations.

Its specificity makes it a valuable indicator for distinguishing bacterial spinal infections from other causes of increased inflammatory markers.

[28]

20. What is a potential concern following surgical debridement or decompression for spinal tuberculosis?
    A. Recurrence of infection
    B. Postoperative wound dehiscence
    C. Development of a postoperative epidural abscess
    D. Progressive spinal deformity

    Correct Answer: D

    Explanation:

    Progressive collapse can lead to vertebra plana and the development of acute kyphotic or gibbus deformity. This angular deformity, combined with epidural granulation tissue and bony fragments, may result in spinal cord compression. It results mainly from the collapse of the anterior column.

    (RP/tuberculous spondylitis)

21. Which of the following is a characteristic feature of actinomycotic infection of the spine?
    A. Rapidly progressing infection
    B. Primarily caused by *Actinomyces israelii*
    C. Affects a single vertebra without adjacent tissue involvement.
    D. Occurs without any prior mucosal injury.

    Correct Answer: B

    Explanation:

    Actinomycotic spinal infections are rare and mostly induced by *Actinomyces israelii*. It is marked by abscess development, tissue fibrosis, and sinus tracts that expel sulfur granules, which are indicative of actinomycosis.

    (SSW, p. 1501)

22. Regarding spinal infections among children under 20 years of age:

    22a. Which of the following is the most commonly involved region?
    A. Cervical spine
    B. Thoracic spine
    C. Lumbar spine
    D. Sacral spine

    22b. One of the following is a frequent pathogen in this age group:
    A. *Haemophilus influenzae*
    B. *Clostridium difficile*
    C. *Pseudomonas aeruginosa*
    D. *Treponema pallidum*

    Correct Answers: 22a: C, 22b: A

    Explanation:

    Spinal infections in children, particularly under the age of 20 and with a peak incidence between 2 and 3 years, are likely due to residual feeding arteries in the nucleus pulposus that involute by 20–30 years of age. The **lumbar spine** is most commonly affected. Symptoms vary by age, with younger children refusing to walk or sit, while older children (>9 years) often experience back pain. Low-grade fever is common, while WBC may sometimes be elevated. ***Haemophilus influenzae*** is a frequent pathogen in this group. Most cases resolve within 9–22 weeks with proper management, including antibiotics. Surgery is rare and reserved for cases with spinal instability, poor response to antibiotics, or recurrence.

(GB, p. 390)

23. Regarding spinal hydatid disease:

23a. Which of the following is a characteristic feature?

A. Multiloculated osteolytic cystic lesions
B. Vividly enhancing cystic lesions
C. Skip lesions with cervical region
D. Lytic lesions with a periosteal reaction

23b. The causative organism is:

A. *Taenia solium*
B. *Schistosoma mansoni*
C. *Toxoplasma gondii*
D. *Echinococcus species*

23c. The ideal regime of oral treatment for a hydatid cyst is:

A. Albendazole for 1–3 months
B. Albendazole and praziquantel combination for 6 months
C. Mebendazole for 2 weeks
D. Albendazole and ivermectin

Correct Answers: 23a: A, 23b: D, 23c: A

Explanation:

Spinal hydatid cysts are a rare echinococcal infection caused by the tapeworm ***Echinococcus species.*** They typically involve the thoracic, lumbar, or sacral spine. MRI and CT are diagnostic and biopsy is required to confirm. These cysts are **multiloculated** and T2 hyperintense in MRI with minimal or no enhancement. Vertebrae are the most commonly affected bony site. Disc spaces are generally spared. The recommended treatment is oral anti-parasitic drugs like albendazole for 1–3 months. Surgical decompression is reserved for cases with neural element compression. Without treatment, the disease progresses indolently but can lead to severe complications like fractures and anaphylaxis if cysts rupture.

(DI, p. 623)

24. Which species of Schistosoma is most commonly linked to the spinal cord in neuroschistosomiasis?

A. *Schistosoma haematobium*
B. *Schistosoma intercalatum*
C. *Schistosoma mansoni*
D. *Schistosoma japonicum*

Correct Answer: C

Explanation:

Neuroschistosomiasis, or bilharziasis, is caused by the Schistosoma parasite, predominantly the *Schistosoma mansoni* species in the spine.

(DI, p. 626)

25. What is the recommended timing for the administration of prophylactic antibiotics in spinal surgery to ensure optimal efficacy?
    A. At the time of skin closure
    B. 1–2 h before the surgical incision
    C. 30 min to 1 h before the surgical incision
    D. Immediately after the procedure

    Correct Answer: C

    Explanation:

    Prophylactic antibiotics, like cefazolin, should be administered 30 min to 1 h before surgery to achieve adequate tissue levels at incision and may be redosed for prolonged procedures.

    (RS, p. 1814)

26. A 51-year-old patient with a history of intravenous drug use presents with low back pain. MRI confirmed spondylodiscitis features. Blood cultures were negative. Which of the following is the most likely pathogen?
    A. *Candida albicans*
    B. *Mycobacterium tuberculosis*
    C. *Bartonella henselae*
    D. *Staphylococcus epidermidis*

    Correct Answer: A

    Explanation:

    Spinal *Candida albicans* is a fungal infection and usually associated with immunocompromised patients, intravenous drug use, and prolonged urinary catheters.

    Treatment involves antifungal medications such as amphotericin B or voriconazole, sometimes. Delayed management or intramedullary extension often results in poor prognosis, with high mortality rates.

    (RS, p. 1650)

27. A 1-year-old child is diagnosed with an intramedullary abscess secondary to an infected dermoid cyst. Which MRI finding is most characteristic?
    A. Non-enhancing cystic lesions with surrounding edema
    B. Septated cystic cavities with rim enhancement
    C. Diffuse T2 hyperintensity without enhancement
    D. Linear enhancement of nerve roots

    Correct Answer: B

    Explanation:

    Intramedullary abscesses often show septated, cystic, rim-enhancing lesions on MRI. Children with midline congenital dermal sinuses have high risk for spinal infections.

    [30]

28. Which of the following MRI findings is most characteristic of viral myelitis in children?
    A. Ring-enhancing lesions in the spinal cord
    B. Diffuse T2 hyperintensity in the spinal cord without significant expansion
    C. Enhancement limited to nerve roots with normal spinal cord signal
    D. T2 hypointensity with adjacent bone marrow edema

    Correct Answer: B

    Explanation:

    Viral myelitis typically presents as non-specific, diffuse T2 hyperintensity in the spinal cord without significant expansion or mass effect.

    [30]

29. A child with herpes zoster presents with segmental weakness. MRI shows focal enhancement near the dorsal nerve roots. Which of the following findings would support a diagnosis of varicella-zoster virus myelopathy?
    A. Diffuse T1 hypointensity with rim enhancement
    B. Necrosis or hemorrhage within the spinal cord
    C. Peripheral calcification within abscesses
    D. Thickening and nodular enhancement of nerve roots

    Correct Answer: B

    Explanation:

    Varicella-zoster virus myelopathy may involve direct invasion of the spinal cord, manifesting as necrosis or hemorrhage, along with enhancement near the dorsal nerve roots.

    [30]

Spine Deformity, Scoliosis, and Biomechanics

10

Check spine measurements GP 1312

1. All of the following are risk factors for developing proximal Junctional Kyphosis (PKJ), EXCEPT:
   A. Smoking
   B. Osteoporosis
   C. Parkinson's disease
   D. Short segment fusion
      Correct Answer: D
      Explanation:
      Long segment fusion is a known risk factor for PJK.
      (RSS, p. 117)
2. Smith-Petersen osteotomy (SPO) can achieve, approximately:
   A. 5 degrees of kyphotic correction per vertebral level
   B. 10 degrees of kyphotic correction per vertebral level
   C. 15 degrees of kyphotic correction per vertebral level
   D. 20 degrees of kyphotic correction per vertebral level
      Correct Answer: B
      Explanation:
      SPO is a posterior column shortening procedure used to correct spinal deformities. It can achieve 10 degrees of kyphotic correction per vertebral level.
      (RSS, p. 123)
3. Pedicle subtraction osteotomy (PSO) can achieve, approximately:
   A. 10–15 degrees of correction in lumbar lordosis
   B. 15–20 degrees of correction in lumbar lordosis
   C. 20–25 degrees of correction in lumbar lordosis
   D. 30–35 degrees of correction in lumbar lordosis
      Correct Answer: D
      (RSS, p. 127)

K. F. AlAli, H. T. Hashim, *Spine Surgery and Peripheral Nerve Surgery*,
https://doi.org/10.1007/978-3-031-98543-0_10

4. 56-year-old patient who had long segment thoracolumbar fusion developed pseudoarthrosis with sagittal imbalance, one of the following regarding the indicated pedicle subtraction osteotomy (PSO) is true:
   A. Interbody fusion above and below PSO is the most predictable way to achieve fusion
   B. Postrio-lateral fusion above and below PSO is the most predictable way to achieve fusion
   C. In-line connectors should be avoided
   D. All of the above
   Correct Answer: A
   Explanation:
   The best approach for achieving fusion in pedicle subtraction osteotomy (PSO) involves multiple techniques. **Interbody fusion above and below PSO** provides strong anterior column support, improving fusion rates.
   (RSS, p. 128)
5. Lumbar lordosis is typically measured from:
   A. Superior end plate of L1 to superior end plate of L5
   B. Superior end plate of L1 to inferior end plate of L5
   C. Superior end plate of L1 to superior end plate of S1
   D. Superior end plate of L1 to inferior end plate of S1
   Correct Answer: C
   (RSS, p. 128)
6. The most common genetic mutation associated with congenital scoliosis is:
   A. FGFR3
   B. PAX1
   C. TBX6
   D. GDF6
   Correct Answer: C
   Explanation:
   Congenital scoliosis is due to vertebral segmentation or formation failure. The most common genetic mutation occurs at TBX6 gene.
   (70)
7. Which factor is most associated with curve progression in adult scoliosis?
   A. Osteophyte formation
   B. Single-level rotatory subluxation
   C. Thoracic curves <30°
   D. Curve magnitude >30°
   Correct Answer: D
   Explanation:
   Curve progression is common in adult scoliosis, especially in degenerative scoliosis. Progression rates range from 1° to 6° per year, averaging 3° per year. Key risk factors include multiple rotatory subluxations, curves >30°, and minimal osteophyte formation. In adult idiopathic scoliosis, curves >50° progress at <1° per year, while thoracic curves <30° rarely progress. Since curve magnitude >30° is a major predictor of progression, it is the correct answer.

8. What is the optimal sagittal balance parameter for adult spinal deformity surgery?
   A. SVA (Sagittal vertical axis) < 2 cm
   B. SVA < 5 cm
   C. SVA < 7 cm
   D. SVA < 10 cm
   Correct Answer: B
   Explanation:
   Sagittal vertical axis (SVA), also called the plumb line, is the horizontal distance between the C7 plumb line and the posterior superior corner of the S1 vertebral body. Below 5 cm is considered normal and called positive sagittal vertical axis (Fig. 10.1).
9. Which of the following statements best describes the biomechanics of the cervical spine following a multilevel anterior cervical corpectomy and fusion with plating?
   A. The construct is primarily loaded in compression with minimal shear forces
   B. The anterior plate prevents extension but allows flexion at the operated levels
   C. The construct has increased risk of screw pullout due to cantilever bending forces

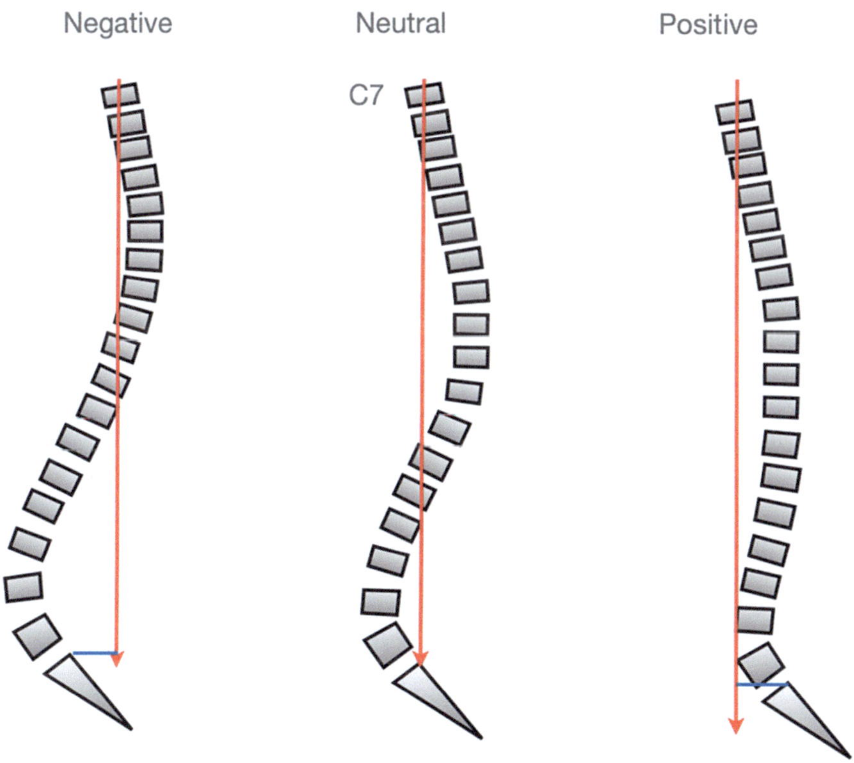

Fig. 10.1 Plumb line or sagittal vertical axis measurement

D. The anterior plate provides sufficient stability to allow immediate full range of motion

Correct Answer: C

Explanation:

Multilevel anterior cervical corpectomy with plating is subject to cantilever bending forces, which increase the risk of **screw pullout** due to the mechanical stress. This is a known complication of anterior cervical constructs, particularly in cases involving long constructs.

(SSW, p. 1626)

10. A posterior column osteotomy (PCO) is planned to increase flexibility at the apex of a rigid thoracic scoliosis curve. Which of the following steps is critical to avoid neural injury during this procedure?
    A. Perform the osteotomy with the screws already in place to stabilize the segment.
    B. Ensure that the interspinous ligaments remain intact between the osteotomy levels.
    C. Prepare pedicle screw tracts before performing the osteotomies, then insert the screws after osteotomy completion.
    D. Place cross-links between screws before performing the osteotomy to provide additional stability.

    Correct Answer: C

    Explanation:

    Preparing screw tracts before the osteotomy allows for controlled screw placement without risking displacement into the spinal canal. Performing osteotomies first and then attempting to insert screws increases the risk of neural injury if the canal has been opened.

    (EM, p. 137)

11. In scoliosis surgery, the Ponte osteotomy is performed at the level of:
    A. The apex of the curve
    B. The end vertebrae
    C. The neutral vertebrae
    D. Every level where screws are placed

    Correct Answer: A

    Explanation:

    Ponte osteotomy also known as extension osteotomy is similar to the Smith-Peterson osteotomy. It involves resection of inferior and superior facets, ligamentum flavum, and sometimes the spinous process. It is commonly used in scoliosis and the resection is usually at the apex of the curve.

    (RS, p. 532)

12. Why is sagittal spinal alignment more important than coronal alignment in predicting disability?
    A. It correlates more with pain and function.
    B. Coronal alignment is rarely a cause of pain.
    C. Coronal deformity does not progress over time.
    D. Sagittal alignment does not change with age.

Correct Answer: A

Explanation:

Studies show that sagittal imbalance is more closely linked to pain and disability than coronal deformity. Patients with poor sagittal alignment often struggle with standing and walking, leading to worse quality of life.

(GB, p. 1312)

13. What is the normal range of lumbar lordosis (LL)?
    A. 5–20°
    B. 10–40°
    C. 30–60°
    D. 50–90°

    Correct Answer: B

    Explanation:

    Normal lumbar lordosis (LL) ranges from 10° to 40°. LL should be about 30° greater than thoracic kyphosis to maintain proper spinal balance. Excessive or reduced LL can lead to back pain and postural issues.

    (GB, p. 1313)

14. Which spinopelvic parameter is fixed after skeletal maturity and does not change with posture?
    A. Pelvic incidence (PI)
    B. Pelvic tilt (PT)
    C. Sacral slope (SS)
    D. Sagittal vertical axis (SVA)

    Correct Answer: A

    Explanation:

    Pelvic incidence (PI) is a fixed anatomical parameter that does not change with posture or degeneration. It helps determine how much lumbar lordosis is needed for a balanced spine. PI = SS + PT, meaning pelvic tilt and sacral slope adjust to maintain balance (Fig. 10.2).

    (GB, p. 1313)

15. Where does the **majority of lumbar lordosis (LL) occur** in normal sagittal alignment?
    A. L1–L3
    B. L2–L4
    C. L4–S1
    D. Evenly distributed across all lumbar vertebrae.

    Correct Answer: C

    Explanation:

    Most lumbar lordosis occurs at L4–S1, with 28% at L4–L5 and 39% at L5–S1. The Roussouly classification helps understand how LL varies between individuals and influences spine surgery planning.

    (GB, pp. 1313–1314))

16. Which Cobb angle is required to classify a spinal curve as scoliosis?
    A. 5°
    B. 10°

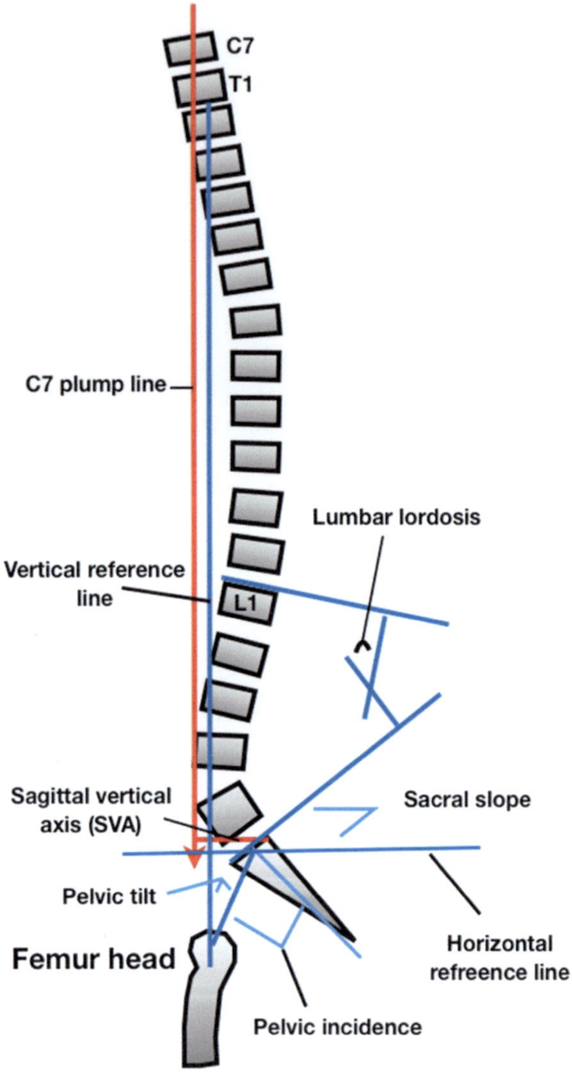

Fig. 10.2 Spine parameters measurements

C. 15°
D. 20°

Correct Answer: B

Explanation:

Scoliosis refers to an abnormal spine curvature in the coronal plane if the Cobb angle is greater than 10 degrees. Anything less than that is usually just spinal asymmetry and not considered real scoliosis.

(GB, p. 1319)

17. Which is the most common type of idiopathic scoliosis?
    A. Infantile (0–3 years)
    B. Juvenile (4–9 years)
    C. Adolescent (10–17 years)
    D. Adult idiopathic scoliosis (≥18 years)
    Correct Answer: C
    Explanation:
    Adolescent idiopathic scoliosis (>18 years) is the most common type of idiopathic scoliosis. It commonly occurs in females. It typically presents as thoracic dextroscoliosis (convex to the right).
    (GB, p. 1319)
18. What is the key predictor of progression of the curve in adolescent idiopathic scoliosis?
    A. Thoracic levoscoliosis
    B. Cobb angle <25°
    C. Presence of back pain
    D. Skeletal maturity
    Correct Answer: D
    Explanation:
    Curve progression is most likely during the growth period. Skeletally immature patients with larger curves are at the highest risk of progression.
    (GB, pp. 1319–1326)
19. Regarding bracing in adolescent idiopathic scoliosis (AIS), which statement is CORRECT?
    A. Bracing reverses scoliosis.
    B. Bracing is only used in skeletally mature patients.
    C. Bracing is recommended for curves >50°.
    D. Bracing prevents curve progression but does not correct scoliosis.
    Correct Answer: D
    Explanation:
    Bracing does not correct scoliosis. It only helps prevent progression in skeletally immature patients with curves of 25–40°. It is ineffective in skeletally mature patients.
    (GB, p. 1324)
20. Which curve magnitude is an indication for surgery in adolescent idiopathic scoliosis?
    A. Thoracic curve >30°
    B. Thoracolumbar/lumbar curve >35°
    C. Main thoracic curve >50°
    D. Lumbar curve >25°
    Correct Answer: C
    Explanation:
    Surgery is indicated for thoracic curve >50° and thoracolumbar or lumbar curve >40–45° as these curves tend to progress despite skeletal maturity.
    (GB, p. 1324)

21. What is the most common curve pattern in adolescent idiopathic scoliosis (AIS)?
    A. Thoracic levoscoliosis
    B. Thoracic dextroscoliosis
    C. Lumbar dextroscoliosis
    D. Double major scoliosis

    Correct Answer: B

    Explanation:

    AIS commonly occurs as thoracic dextroscoliosis (convex to the right). Thoracic levoscoliosis (left curve) is rare and should raise suspicion for an underlying condition such as spinal cord pathology, tumor, or syringomyelia.

    (GB, p. 1324)
22. Which adolescent idiopathic scoliosis (AIS) patient has the highest risk of curve progression?
    A. 16-year-old with a 15° curve
    B. 13-year-old with a 25° curve
    C. 11-year-old with a 35° curve
    D. 10-year-old with a 50° curve

    Correct Answer: D

    Explanation:

    The risk of curve progression depends on age and Cobb angle. Younger patients have more growth remaining. Patients with larger curves (>50°)have higher progression risk. Curves >50° often progress into adulthood, requiring surgery.

    (GB, pp. 1319–1326)
23. When should MRI be considered in adolescent idiopathic scoliosis (AIS)?
    A. In all AIS cases.
    B. Only if the Cobb angle is >50°.
    C. If the patient has thoracic levoscoliosis or neurological symptoms.
    D. Only if surgery is planned.

    Correct Answer: C

    Explanation:

    MRI is not routine for AIS. It is indicated for atypical scoliosis cases (e.g., thoracic levoscoliosis, neurological deficits, or syndromic features). These findings may indicate an underlying spinal pathology like Chiari malformation, syringomyelia, or tumor.

    (GB, pp. 1319–1326)
24. Which method is most commonly used to assess skeletal maturity in adolescent idiopathic scoliosis (AIS)?
    A. Cobb angle
    B. Lenke classification
    C. Leg length measurement
    D. Sander's maturity scale

    Correct Answer: D

Explanation:

The Sander's maturity scale (based on hand X-rays) is the most accurate method to assess growth potential. Risser staging (iliac crest ossification) is less reliable. Skeletal maturity is crucial for bracing and surgery decisions.

(GB, pp. 1319–1326)

25. What is the purpose of the Lenke classification in adolescent idiopathic scoliosis (AIS)?
    A. Determine which curves will progress
    B. Classify AIS based on severity
    C. Identify which curves need fusion in surgery
    D. Measure spinal flexibility

    Correct Answer: C

    Explanation:

    The Lenke classification is the gold standard for classifying AIS before surgery. It determines which curves are structural and need fusion, using curve type, lumbar modifier, and sagittal alignment modifier.

    (GB, pp. 1319–1326)
26. How many curve types are defined in the Lenke classification?
    A. 3
    B. 5
    C. 6
    D. 7

    Correct Answer: C

    Explanation:

    The Lenke classification includes six curve types based on which spinal regions are involved. These types help guide surgical planning by identifying major and minor curves that require fusion.

    (GB, pp. 1319–1326)
27. What defines a major curve in the Lenke classification?
    A. The largest curve present
    B. Any curve with a Cobb angle >25°
    C. The most painful curve
    D. Any curve that is flexible on bending films

    Correct Answer: A

    Explanation:

    The major curve is the largest Cobb angle curve in a patient with multiple spinal curves. It is always structural and is the main focus for surgical correction.

    (GB, pp. 1319–1326)
28. Which of the following indicates that a minor curve is structural in the Lenke classification?
    A. The Cobb angle decreases to <25° on side-bending films
    B. The curve is larger than the major curve
    C. Side-bending films show a residual Cobb angle ≥25°
    D. The patient has back pain in the minor curve area

    Correct Answer: C

Explanation:

A structural curve does not correct to <25° on side-bending X-rays. Structural curves must be included in fusion surgery to prevent future progression.

(GB, pp. 1319–1326)

29. What does the lumbar modifier in the Lenke classification describe?
    A. The severity of thoracic kyphosis
    B. The overall spinal flexibility
    C. The risk of scoliosis progression
    D. The relationship of the central sacral vertical line (CSVL) to the lumbar curve

    Correct Answer: D

    Explanation:

    The lumbar modifier (A, B, or C) classifies how the lumbar curve aligns with the pelvis using the central sacral vertical line (CSVL). It helps determine if the lumbar curve should be included in fusion surgery.

    (GB, pp. 1319–1326)

30. What does the thoracic sagittal modifier in the Lenke classification indicate?
    A. The flexibility of the thoracic curve
    B. The severity of scoliosis progression
    C. The degree of thoracic kyphosis
    D. The likelihood of successful bracing

    Correct Answer: C

    Explanation:

    The thoracic sagittal modifier (–, N, or +) categorizes thoracic kyphosis (T5–T12 Cobb angle):

- "–" if <10° (hypokyphosis)
- "N" if 10–40° (normal)
- "+" if >40° (hyperkyphosis)

This helps guide surgical planning for proper sagittal balance.

(GB, pp. 1319–1326)

Pediatric Spine

11

1. The following cervical conditions are contraindication to participate in contact sports, EXCEPT:
   A. Odontoid abnormalities
   B. Klippel-Feil anomaly
   C. Cervical spinal bifida occulta
   D. Atlantooccipital fusion
   Correct Answer: C
   Explanation:
   This is a mild and typically asymptomatic condition. It is not considered a contraindication for sports participation in most cases. Other options are all contraindication to participate in contact sports.
   (GB, p. 1126)
2. A 9-year-old presents with scoliosis and leg weakness. MRI shows a syrinx extending from T6 to T12 without associated Chiari malformation. What is the most appropriate next step in management?
   A. Observation
   B. Posterior spinal fusion
   C. Syrinx drainage
   D. MRI of the brain and craniocervical junction
   Correct Answer: D
3. A 10-year-old boy presents with progressive neck pain and headaches, worse with coughing or straining. His parents report clumsiness, intermittent arm weakness, and occasional numbness in his hands over the past several months. His MRI is shown (Fig. 11.1). What is the best management for this condition?
   A. Observation with serial imaging
   B. Arachnoid to peritoneal shunt
   C. Suboccipital craniectomy with C1 laminectomy
   D. C1–C2 posterior fusion
   Correct Answer: C

K. F. AlAli, H. T. Hashim, *Spine Surgery and Peripheral Nerve Surgery*,
https://doi.org/10.1007/978-3-031-98543-0_11

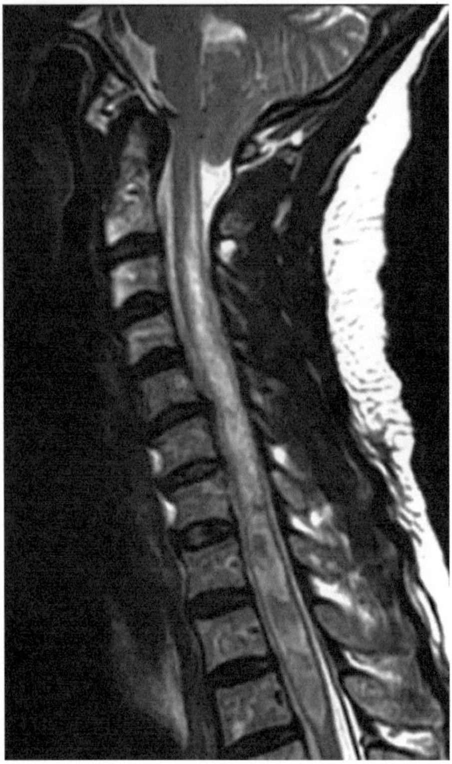

Fig. 11.1 Case 3 MRI

Explanation:

This is a case of Chiari I malformation with syrinx. Patient has typical symptoms of Chiari I malformation, neck pain, and headaches, worse with coughing or straining. Surgical intervention for Chiari I malformation is generally recommended for symptomatic individuals. Syrinx presents in 30–70% of the patients. In most cases syrinx will resolve after suboccipital decompression.

(GB, p. 296)

4. Which of the following statements regarding spinal cord injury without radiographic abnormality (SCIWORA) is true?
   A. It is most commonly seen in elderly patients with spondylosis.
   B. MRI is essential for diagnosis and may reveal ligamentous injury or cord edema.
   C. Prognosis is generally poor.
   D. It is caused by penetrating trauma leading to neural injury.

   Correct Answer: B

   Explanation:

   SCIWORA (spinal cord injury without radiographic abnormality) is a neurological injury with normal plain radiographs and CT scans, primarily affecting children. The pediatric spine's greater elasticity, compared to the less distensible spinal cord, predisposes to stretch injuries despite normal bony imaging. **MRI is the preferred diagnostic modality**. MRI might show intramedullary hemorrhage/edema, ligamentous disruption, disc and herniation. The cervical region and cervicothoracic junction are most commonly involved; thoracolumbar involvement, associated with high-energy trauma, can occur. Due to potential spontaneous reduction of initial displacement, these injuries are treated as potentially unstable. Delayed-onset SCIWORA (up to 96 h post-injury) can occur with ligamentous instability. Management involves 12 weeks of external immobilization. Recurrent neurological deterioration, though rare, can occur post-stabilization, emphasizing the importance of continued immobilization. Laminectomy was proposed in the past; however, it was shown to be ineffective.

(SS, p. 419)

5. One of the following signs is characteristic for Chiari 1 malformation:
   A. Downbeat nystagmus
   B. Dissociated sensory loss
   C. Truncal ataxia
   D. Abnormal gag reflex

   Correct Answer: A

   Explanation:

   Downbeat nystagmus is uncommon but characteristic in Chiari I malformation. It is characterized by involuntary eye movements where the quick component is directed downwards, even when the eyes are looking straight ahead. This type of nystagmus strongly suggests a structural abnormality in the posterior fossa, frequently involving the area where the brainstem meets the spinal cord (cervicomedullary junction).

   (GB, pp. 297 and 586)

6. Chiari I malformation is linked or associated with several conditions. In that context, answer the following:

   6a. Which of the following is NOT typically associated with Chiari I malformation?
   A. Arachnoid cysts in the posterior fossa
   B. Foramen magnum meningioma
   C. Craniosynostosis involving the sagittal suture only
   D. Hypermobility of the craniovertebral junction

   6b. Acquired Chiari I malformation has been linked to:
   A. Congenital heart defects
   B. Lumboperitoneal shunting
   C. Trisomy 21
   D. Maternal exposure to teratogens

   6.c. Which upper cervical spine abnormality is often seen in conjunction with Chiari I malformation?
   A. Cervical spondylosis
   B. Occipitalization of the atlas
   C. Atlantoaxial subluxation due to rheumatoid arthritis
   D. Cervical disc herniation at C5–C6

6d. Which of the following conditions might explain some treatment failures of suboccipital craniectomy in Chiari I patients?

A. Ehlers-Danlos syndrome
B. Klippel-Feil syndrome
C. Retained rhomboid roof
D. Pseudotumor cerebri

Correct Answers: 6a: C, 6b: B, 6c: B, 6d: D

Explanation:

Chiari I malformation frequently presents with concurrent anatomical variations within the posterior cranial fossa. These associations encompass a spectrum of osseous and soft tissue anomalies. Diminutive posterior fossa volume may arise from occipital bone hypoplasia, attributable to aberrant development of occipital somites of para-axial mesodermal origin, or from a low-lying tentorium cerebelli. Paradoxically, instances of osseous hypertrophy or superior displacement of the occipital bone constituting the posterior fossa floor have also been documented. The presence of intracranial space-occupying lesions represents another significant association, encompassing arachnoid cysts (affecting both retrocerebellar and supratentorial compartments), neoplastic processes (including, but not limited to, foramen magnum meningiomas and cerebellar astrocytomas), and augmented dural vascularity. Acquired Chiari I malformation occurs with any process encroaching on intracranial volume, such as chronic subdural hematomas or hydrocephalus, can be implicated. Iatrogenic Chiari I malformation, an acquired form, has been documented following **lumboperitoneal shunting** or multiple lumbar punctures. Moreover, the presence of arachnoid adhesions, cicatricial changes, or fibrotic tissue enveloping the brainstem and cerebellar tonsils in proximity to the foramen magnum constitutes a further recognized association. Concurrent abnormalities of the upper cervical spine are frequently observed, including hypermobility of the craniovertebral junction, Klippel-Feil syndrome, **occipitalization of the atlas**, and anterior indentation of the foramen magnum, as exemplified by basilar invagination and odontoid retroversion. Finally, certain systemic conditions, such as Ehlers-Danlos syndrome, **pseudotumor cerebri** (which may confound surgical outcomes following suboccipital craniectomy in the context of Chiari-pseudotumor cerebri syndrome), craniosynostosis (especially involving multiple or all cranial sutures, termed pansynostosis), and the infrequent persistence of the rhomboid roof, represent additional comorbidities encountered in association with Chiari I malformation.

(GB, p. 296)

7. A 3-month-old infant is diagnosed with lipomyelomeningocele. Questions 7a–c are regarding lipomyelomeningocele:

7a. Which of the following statements regarding the anatomical characteristics of lipomyelomeningocele is INCORRECT?

A. The lipoma is distinct from normal epidural fat, exhibiting a different texture and consistency.
B. The dura is dehiscent at the level of the dorsal myeloschisis.

C. The subarachnoid space typically bulges ipsilateral to the lipoma.
D. The lipoma may extend cephalad under intact arches and potentially into the central canal.

7b. The parents inquire about the likelihood of neurological improvement following surgery. Based on the provided information, which of the following is the MOST accurate response?
A. Complete resolution of all neurological deficits is expected in the majority of cases.
B. Approximately 75% of patients will experience stabilization of their neurological status, with a smaller percentage showing improvement or worsening.
C. Surgical intervention is primarily for cosmetic purposes and has minimal impact on neurological outcomes.
D. Foot deformities associated with lipomyelomeningocele will consistently resolve after surgery.

7c. The patient will have surgical intervention. Which of the following intraoperative findings is MOST crucial for successful untethering of the spinal cord?
A. Identification and sectioning of the fibrovascular band connecting the cephalic lamina to the bifid lamina.
B. Complete resection of the subcutaneous lipoma for cosmetic purposes.
C. Extensive debulking of the lipoma extending into the central canal, regardless of potential neural injury.
D. Primary closure of the dura without addressing the placode.

Correct Answers: 7a: C, 7b: B, 7c: A

Explanation:

Lipomyelomeningocele is a congenital condition characterized by a subcutaneous lipoma extending through a midline defect in the lumbodorsal fascia, vertebral neural arch, and dura, merging with a tethered spinal cord. This fatty tumor, sometimes termed lipoma of the cauda equina, is associated with a dorsally split conus medullaris (myeloschisis), often at the level of the bifid spine. The meningocele sac with the neural tissue is usually constricted by a fibrovascular band connecting the cephalic lamina to the bifid lamina. The lipomatous tissue in lipomyelomeningocele differs significantly from typical epidural adipose tissue, which exhibits a looser, more areolar structure. Characteristically, the subarachnoid space demonstrates a contralateral displacement or bulging relative to the side of the lipoma. Cutaneous stigmata, such as fatty pads, dimples, or port-wine stains, are almost universally present. Neurological findings vary, with sensory loss in sacral dermatomes being the most common abnormality. X-rays usually show spina bifida and MRI demonstrate a low-lying conus, and the lipomatous mass. Surgical intervention, typically initiated around 2 months of age, aims to release the tethered cord, reduce lipoma bulk, with goal to stabilize neurological functions.

(GB, pp. 284–285)

8. Regarding tethered cord syndrome:

8a. A child with a tethered cod and scoliosis, following untethering procedure, what is CORRECT regarding the outcome for the patient's scoliosis?

A. Scoliosis correction is always sufficient after the untethering procedure.
B. Untethering does not affect the progression of scoliosis and a separate scoliosis surgery is needed.
C. Mild Scoliosis (<10°) is usually stabilized after untethering procedure.
D. Scoliosis usually worsens after untethering surgery.

8b. During tethered cord release surgery, the most reliable technique for distinguishing the filum terminale from nerve roots is:

A. Visual inspection of the filum's reddish color compared to the yellowish nerve roots.
B. Filum have cord-consistency compared to the softer nerve roots.
C. The filum is located within the central canal, while nerve roots are located more laterally.
D. Presence of ligamentous-like strands within the filum and with a vessel on its surface.

Correct Answers: 8a: C, 8b: D

Explanation:

Tethered cord syndrome, characterized by a low laying conus medullaris, frequently co-occurs with a thickened, shortened filum terminale or intradural lipoma. Tethering is common in myelomeningocele (MM), clinical evaluation is crucial, given the near-constant radiographic presence of tethering.

The clinical picture varies, may include cutaneous stigmata (e.g., hypertrichosis, subcutaneous lipomata), lower motor function deficit, muscular atrophy, sensory deficit, vesical dysfunction (occasionally presenting in isolation), back pain, and spinal deformities such as scoliosis or kyphosis. In patients with MM, exacerbation of pre-existing scoliosis, spasticity, gait disturbance, or urodynamic abnormalities warrants investigation for tethered cord, following exclusion of cerebrospinal fluid shunt complications and intracranial hypertension. Usually, pain suggests tethering, whereas painless decline raises suspicion of syringomyelia.

Early surgical untethering may ameliorate progressive scoliosis, particularly in cases of minimal curvature (<10°). Because of the possibility of iatrogenic bladder injury, preoperative cystometry is recommended, particularly for continent patients. Vertebral osteotomy is taken into consideration for recurrent occurrences. Surgical techniques range from simple filum sectioning to lipoma removal. Intraoperative filum identification relies on a **characteristic surface vessel**, a pale microscopic appearance, and collagenous fascicles, with intraoperative electrophysiological studies providing definitive confirmation. In myelomeningocele (MM), permanent untethering of the spinal cord is typically not feasible. However, repeated untethering procedures during childhood (2–4 times) may suffice until the child completes growth, after which tethering may no longer pose a problem. Tethering that is addressed early in childhood can recur, particularly during adolescent growth spurts. Postoperative cerebrospinal fluid (CSF) leaks occur in approximately 15% of cases.

Fig. 11.2 Case 9 CT scan

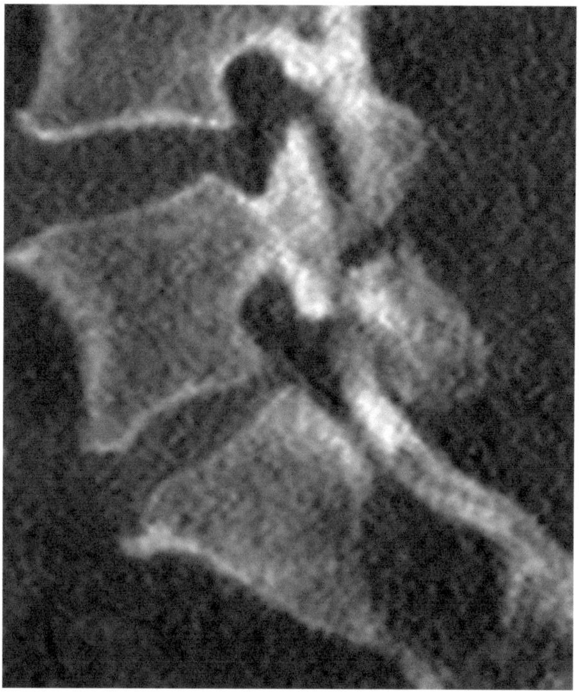

9. A 16-year-old soccer player presents with low back pain that worsens with hyperextension. CT scan is seen below (Fig. 11.2). What is the most likely mechanism of injury?
   A. Axial loading of the spine
   B. Hyperflexion of the spine
   C. Repeated hyperextension and rotation
   D. Sudden impact trauma

   Correct Answer: C

   Explanation:

   Isthmic spondylolysis often results from repetitive spinal hyperextension and rotation, particularly in athletes involved in sports like gymnastics, soccer, diving, dance, and wrestling.

   (SS, p. 345)
10. A 10-year-old boy with legs weakness was found to have a split cord syndrome with two hemicords divided by rigid spectrum and each hemicord covered by a separate dura. Answer the following questions (10a–d):

   10a. Which of the following conditions is most frequently associated with diastematomyelia in pediatric patients?
   A. Tethered cord syndrome
   B. Scoliosis
   C. Syringomyelia
   D. Arnold-Chiari malformation

10b. This type of split cord syndrome will feature the following cutaneous stigmata:

A. Nevi
B. Hypertrichosis
C. Dermal sinuses
D. All of the above

10c. Surgery is planned, the best surgical strategy is:

A. Tethered filum terminally is done initially then resection of the median septum
B. Tethered filum terminale be postponed following the removal of the median septum
C. The resection of the median septum is solely enough
D. All strategies are valid options

10d: The distinctive difference between this type of split cord syndrome and the other type is:

A. This type is also known as diastematomyelia.
B. This type commonly features spinal bifida occulta at the lumbosacral region.
C. The other type does not require untethering.
D. All of the above are correct.

Correct Answers: 10a: A, 10b: D, 10c: B, 10d: A

Explanation:

Split cord malformation (SCM) is a division of the spinal cord into two hemicords in the sagittal plane. It is divided into 2 types (Pang classification):

Type I SCM (described in the question), also known as **diastematomyelia,** is featured by two separate hemicords. Each of the hemicord has central canal covered within separate dural tubes and divided by a rigid osseocartilaginous median septum. Cutaneous stigmata are usually seen such as nevi, hypertrichosis, lipomas, dermal sinuses, or hemangiomas. The treatment is surgery by untethering with osseous septum resection and dural reconstruction into single dural tube. In order to avoid proximal cord retraction against the remaining osseous structure, **it is essential that the division of the tethered filum terminale be postponed following the removal of the median septum**.

Type II SCM, also known as diplomyelia, features two hemicords contained within a single dural sac, separated by a non-rigid fibrous median septum. Usually there is no vertebral anomalies at the level of the split. Spinal bifida occulta is frequently seen in the lumbosacral region. Treatment involves surgical **untethering** at the level of the spina bifida occulta.

(GB, p. 292)

11. Which primary bone tumors are most likely to involve the spine in the pediatric population?

A. Osteoid osteoma and plasmocytoma
B. Osteosarcoma and Ewing sarcoma
C. Chondrosarcoma and giant cell tumor
D. Multiple myeloma and chordoma

Correct Answer: B

Explanation:

Common spine tumor diagnoses vary by age group. In patients aged 10–30 years, common tumors include Langerhans cell histiocytosis, osteoid osteoma, osteoblastoma, osteochondroma, giant cell tumor (GCT), aneurysmal bone cyst (ABC), osteosarcoma, and Ewing sarcoma. Between ages 30 and 50, chordoma, chondrosarcoma, and hemangioma are more prevalent. In patients older than 50, metastatic tumors, myeloma, and lymphoma are the most frequently encountered spinal tumors.

(SS, pp. 347 and 608)

12. A 4-year-old child presents with progressive scoliosis and mild gait disturbance. MRI of the lumbar spine shows a fatty intradural lesion at the filum terminale without spinal cord tethering. What is the most appropriate next step in management?
   A. Surgical excision of the lipoma
   B. Observation with serial MRI
   C. Radiation therapy
   D. Spinal cord detethering

   Correct Answer: B

   Explanation:

   Isolated lipomas of the filum terminale refers to the asymptomatic presence of fat within a normal-appearing filum terminale, with no imaging signs of tethered spinal cord and a normally positioned conus medullaris. On imaging, it is best identified as a linear fat signal on T1-weighted MRI, extending from the conus to the sacrum, with no enhancement or associated dysraphism. CT shows punctate fat attenuation in the dorsal lumbar thecal sac. Differential diagnoses include intraspinal lipoma (thicker filum, low-lying conus), tethered cord, and lipomyelocele. Typically, an incidental finding in 4–6% of autopsies, it is congenital, asymptomatic, and **requires no treatment** unless associated with other pathologies. Symptomatic lesions suggest an intraspinal lipoma rather than a fibrolipoma.

   (DI, p. 42)

13. A 12-year-old male presents with neck pain after a minor fall during sports. Cervical CT is seen below (Fig. 11.3). What is the subtype of the condition seen on the CT scan?
   A. Os odontoideum—dystopic type
   B. Os odontoideum—orthotopic type
   C. Odontoid fracture—type II
   D. Persistent ossiculum terminale

   Correct Answer: A

   Explanation:

   In the orthotopic type, the ossicle is located in the position of the normal dens and moves in conjunction with the C1 arch. In the dystopic type (seen in this case), the ossicle is located adjacent to the clivus and may fuse with the occiput and move in concert with the clivus (SS, p. 353)

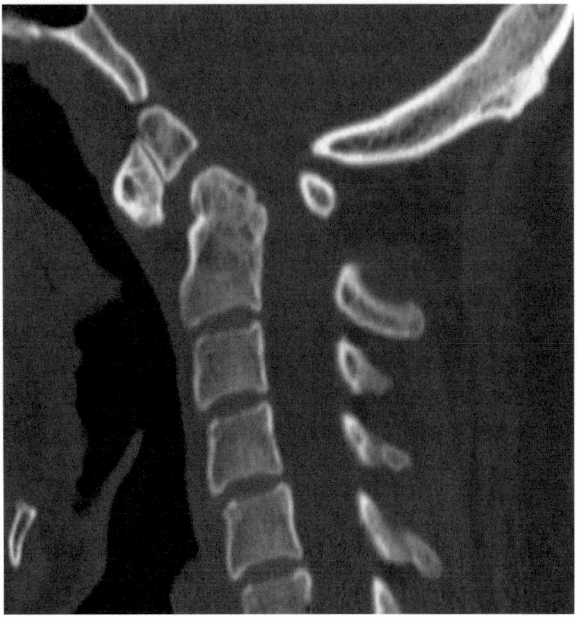

Fig. 11.3 Case 13 cervical CT scan

14. A 10-year-old male presents with neck pain. CT scan shows a single, single lytic lesion in the C4 vertebral body (Fig. 11.4). Biopsy reveals cells with Birbeck granules. What is the most likely clinical course?
    A. Spontaneous regression
    B. Rapid progression with systemic involvement
    C. Recurrence after surgery
    D. High mortality without chemotherapy

    Correct Answer: A

    Explanation:

    Langerhans cell histiocytosis, also known as eosinophilic granuloma, is a disorder characterized by abnormal proliferation of Langerhans cells, resulting in granulomatous skeletal lesions. It usually affects children and young adults. Spinal involvement is common at the thoracic region. Imaging reveals lytic vertebral lesions, often leading to vertebra plana while sparing the intervertebral discs and posterior elements. Clinical presentations vary from asymptomatic to localized pain, swelling, and neurologic deficits. Histopathology showed Langerhans cell histiocytosis shows abnormal granulomatous histiocytes and characteristic **Birbeck granule** inclusions within the cytoplasm.

    Although recurrence is conceivable, most lesions **spontaneously regress** over months to years. The degree of the disease determines the prognosis; single-system diseases frequently regress spontaneously without treatment, whereas multisystem diseases may need immunomodulation or chemotherapy. Usually, bracing, local therapies, or observation are used as forms of treatment. Surgery may be necessary in advanced cases, primarily if instability is present.

    (DI, p. 762)

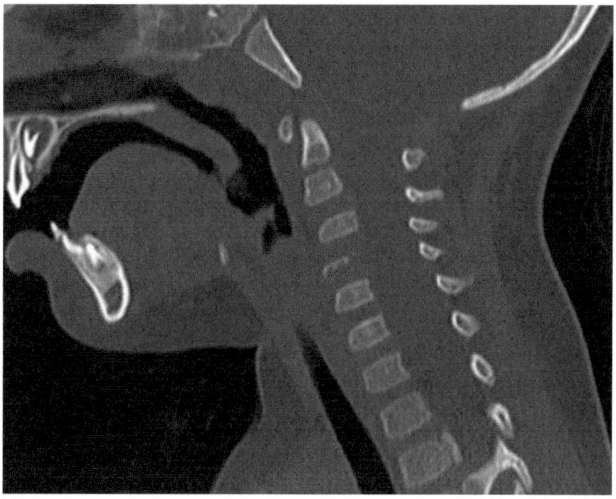

Fig. 11.4 Case 14 CT scan showing a single, single lytic lesion in the C4 vertebral body

15. Which of the following is the most common presenting symptom in pediatric patients with atlantoaxial instability?
    A. Neck pain
    B. Headache
    C. Gait disturbance
    D. Torticollis

    Correct Answer: D

    Explanation:

    In children with atlantoaxial instability, particularly those experiencing atlantoaxial rotatory subluxation, a common form in the pediatric population—the most frequent presenting symptom is torticollis, often described as a painful head tilt or "cock-robin" position.
16. A 7-year-old boy presents with torticollis and neck pain after a minor fall. Radiographs show rotatory subluxation of C1 on C2:

    16a. Based on the Fielding & Hawkins classification, which type involves anterior displacement of C1 with 3.1–5 mm of anterior shift?
    A. Type I
    B. Type II
    C. Type III
    D. Type IV

    16b: In case of a child with respiratory tract infection and rotatory subluxation of C1 and C2, the condition is known as:
    A. Greenberg syndrome
    B. Gabriel syndrome
    C. Grisel syndrome
    D. Gharib-Lennot syndrome

    16c: The patient also presented with lateral head tilt to one side, rotation to the other side, and slight flexion. This head position is called:
    A. Cock robin position
    B. Robin hood position

C. Black robin position
D. Robin nodding position

16d. Which of the following surgical procedures is preferred for the management of a C1–C2 rotatory subluxation that has failed conservative treatment?
A. Anterior cervical discectomy and fusion
B. Occipitocervical fusion
C. Odontoid screw fixation
D. C1–C2 posterior fusion

Correct Answers: 16a: B, 16b: C, 16c: A, 16d: D

Explanation:

Atlanto-axial rotatory fixation can be associated with trauma, rheumatoid arthritis, and respiratory tract infection (Grisel syndrome). Commonly present with torticollis with typical head position of Cock robin position (lateral head tilt to one side, rotation to the other side, and slight flexion). It is categorized into four types according to the Fielding and Hawkins classification:

- Type I: The atlas is rotated on the odontoid without anterior displacement (most common).
- Type II: The atlas is rotated on one lateral articular process with 3–5 mm of anterior displacement, suggesting injury to the transverse ligament.
- Type III: The atlas rotates on both lateral articular processes with anterior displacement over 5 mm, indicating damage to both the transverse and alar ligaments.
- Type IV: Involves rotation with posterior displacement of the atlas

Treatment is case based. For Grisel syndrome, treatment is with proper antibiotic with traction followed by immobilization (collar). In all other cases, treatment is with traction followed with immobilization. If this failed **C1–C2 posterior fusion** is needed.

(GP, p. 1159)

Correct Answer: B

(GP, p. 1159)

17. 11-year-old with trisomy 21:

17a: All of the following are spinal condition associated with this child's condition, EXCEPT:
A. Occipito-cervicial instability
B. C1 hypoplasia
C. Spinal stenosis
D. Spinal lipomatosis

17b: What is the most important radiographic measurement when assessing for atlantoaxial instability in this patient?
A. Atlantodental interval
B. Cervical lordosis
C. Pavlov ratio
D. Degree of basilar invagination

17c: The most possible cause of death in this patient's condition is:
A. Pulmonary hypertension
B. Congenital heart disease
C. Leukemia
D. Hypothyroidism

Correct Answers: 17a: D, 17b: A, 17c: B

Explanation:

Trisomy 21 or Down syndrome is a genetic disorder caused by presence of extra copy of chromosome 2. Clinically, it has variable presentations, commonly varies degree of intellectual disabilities. These patients can have several spinal diseases like occipito-cervical instability, atlanto-axial instability, C1 hypoplasia, occipital condyle hypoplasia, os odontoideum, spinal stenosis, and scoliosis. The incidence of atlantoaxial instability is 20% and usually occur before the age of 10 due to laxity of the transverse atlantal ligament, therefore patients need to be screened by cervical X-ray with measurements of atlanto-dental interval (ADI). For ADI of > 4.5 C1-C2 fusion is recommended in symptomatic patient if cord compression presence is observed in MRI.

Patients with down syndrome can have other non-spinal conditions that affect their life span, such as congenital heart disease (most common cause of mortality), pulmonary hypertension, leukemia, hypothyroidism, repeated respiratory infections, sleep apnea, and Alzheimer's disease.

(GB, p. 1381)

18. A 13-year-old gymnast girl with long lasting low back pain:

18a. One of the following to CORRECT about pediatric lumbar disc herniation:
A. The diagnosis is usually achieved faster in pediatric patients.
B. Cauda equina syndrome is more prevalent in pediatric patients.
C. Reactive scoliosis always presents in pediatric patients with lumbar disc herniation.
D. Pediatric patients tend to have a lower success rate with nonoperative treatment compared to adults.

18b. The distinct feature lumbar disc herniation in pediatric patients in comparison to adult, the pediatric lumbar disc herniation:
A. Occur more at upper lumbar levels
B. Has fewer neurological findings
C. Straight leg raising sign is almost always negative
D. All of the above

18c. Reactive scoliosis presence in pediatric lumbar disc herniation due to:
A. The child avoiding stressing the back in the symptomatic side
B. Back muscle weakness in the symptomatic side
C. A higher water content of the pediatric intervertebral disc
D. A congenital spinal deformity unrelated to nerve compression

18d. Axial Lumbar CT scan is done in this patient and shows a central rim of calcification at the upper level of L4–L5 level. The diagnosis is:
A. Old calcified L4–L5 disc herniation due to repetitive trauma
B. Apophyseal ring fracture

C. Schmorl's node with reactive calcification
D. Juvenile ankylosing spondylitis with disc involvement

Correct Answers: 18a: D, 18b: D, 18c: A, 18d: B

Explanation:

Pediatric lumbar disc herniation is not as common as in adult patients. Most of the cause of low back pain in children is due to muscle strain and usually associated with history of trauma. The diagnosis of lumbar disc herniation in the pediatric patients is usually delayed compared to an adult. Also compared to adult, pediatric lumbar disc herniation occur more at upper lumbar levels, has fewer neurological findings and straight leg raising sign is almost always negative. **Reactive scoliosis may present (not always) due to child avoiding stressing the back in the systematic side. Pediatric patients tend to have a lower success rate with nonoperative treatment compared to adults.** This is due to increased elasticity and higher water content of the immature intervertebral discs and association with apophyseal ring fracture. As in adult, surgery is indicted if symptoms persist and conservative management failed or when neurological deficit is present.

Apophyseal ring fracture is present in 1/3 of the patients. It is a fracture occurring at the junction of the vertebral body and its cartilaginous ring apophysis, typically before the apophysis fully fuses around age 18. It commonly affects the L4–L5 or L5–S1 levels and is prevalent in males engaged in sports involving repetitive flexion and rotation. Surgery often required to remove the fractured bone fragment, associated cartilage, and disc material.

(SS, p. 345)

19. A 12-year-old girl presents with a rapidly progressive thoracic scoliosis. MRI reveals a large intradural mass compressing the spinal cord:

19a. Which of the following is the most likely diagnosis?
A. Ependymoma
B. Astrocytoma
C. Neurofibroma
D. Meningioma

19b. What is the possible etiology of the scoliosis in this patient:
A. Asymmetric destruction of the spinal cord causing multifidus muscle atrophy
B. Idiopathic muscular imbalance unrelated to the spinal cord
C. Primary dysfunction of the erector spinae muscles
D. Bilateral motor neuron paralysis affecting the paraspinal muscles

Answers: 19a: B, 19b: A

Explanation:

Spinal astrocytoma is the most common intradural intramedullary tumor in the pediatric patients. It is occasionally asymmetric and exophytic lesion leading to asymmetrical destruction of the spinal cord casing weakness to the paraspinal muscles specifically multifidus muscle. This cause scoliosis with convexty to atrophied muscles side.

[51]

20. The following statement is FALSE regarding radiographic lines used to assess basilar invagination:
    A. McGregor's line: From the posterior edge of the hard palate to the lowest point of the occiput.
    B. Chamberlain's line considered abnormal if the odontoid tip lies more than 3 mm above it.
    C. McRae's line, drawn across the foramen magnum, is abnormal if the odontoid extends above it.
    D. The Digastric line assesses the relationship between the atlas and axis by measuring the distance between the digastric notches.

    Answer: D (Fig. 11.5)

    Explanation:

    Before the era of CR scan, several lines were described to assess basilar invagination on cervical X-ray:

- **McGregor's Line** is drawn from the posterior edge of the hard palate to the lowest point of the occiput and helps diagnose basilar invagination if the odontoid tip extends above it.
- **Chamberlain's Line** is considered abnormal if the odontoid process extends more than **5 mm** (not 3 mm) above it.
- **McRae's Line** is a line across the foramen magnum. It is abnormal if the odontoid tip extends beyond this line, indicating basilar invagination.
- **The Digastric Line** measures the position of the skull base but does **not** directly assess the relationship between the atlas and axis.

21. A pediatric patient with congenital scoliosis:

    21a. What is the most common cause of congenital scoliosis
    A. Hemivertebra
    B. Neuromuscular disorders
    C. Chromosomal anomalies
    D. Scheuermann's disease

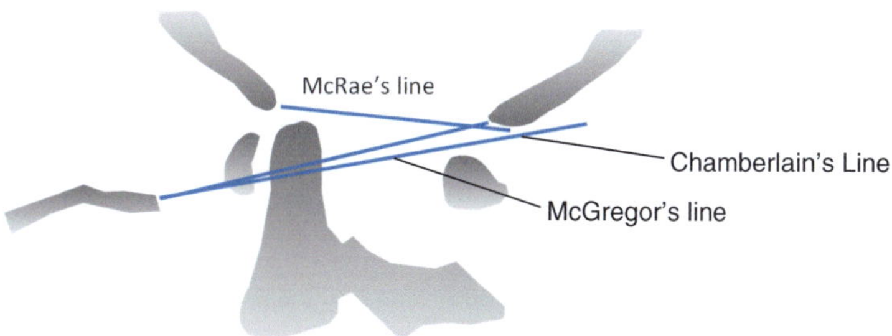

Fig. 11.5 Illustration of occipito-cervical junction showing the line measurements that can be used to assess basilar invagination

21b. The possible etiology of the correct answer in question 21a is:
A. Impairment of neuromuscular junctions
B. Chromosomal deletion syndromes
C. Uneven growth of the vertebral endplates
D. Vertebral segmentation anomalies

Correct Answers: 21a: A, 21b: D

Explanation:

Congenital scoliosis is usually caused by abnormal segmentation (hemivertebra) or formation of the vertebrae. Hemivertebra is caused by segmentation abnormality where chondral center and ossification in one side.

(RP)

22. A term newborn girl is delivered via cesarean section following prenatal ultrasound that revealed a lumbar spine defect (Fig. 11.6).

22a. The embryological base of this condition is:
A. Anterior neuropore closure failure
B. Posterior neuropore closure failure
C. Failure of neural crest cell migration
D. Over proliferation of mesodermal tissues

22b. The following condition is almost always associated with the diagnosis of this child:
A. Chiari II malformation
B. Tethered cord syndrome
C. Hydrocephalus
D. Spina bifida occulta

22c. The appropriate antibiotics regimen for this condition (if ruptured) is:
A. Meningitis dose ceftriaxone
B. Cefazolin and vancomycin
C. Nafcillin and gentamicin
D. All of the above

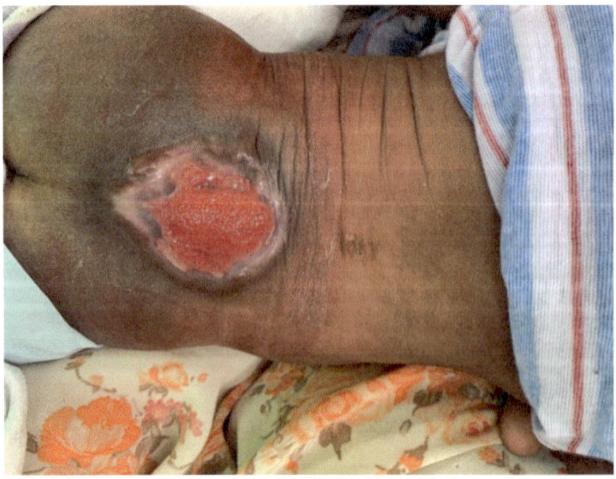

Fig. 11.6 Case 22 lumbar spine defect

22d. In the management of this condition, the timing of surgical closure should ideally be within:
A. 24 h of birth
B. 48 h of birth
C. 72 h of birth
D. 1 week of birth

Correct Answers: 22a: B, 22b: A, 22c: D, 22d: B

Explanation:

The diagnosis is myelomeningoceleis (MMC). Its embryological bases are failure of posterior neuropore closure. Posterior neuropore is a caudal opening of the neural tube during embryonic development. It typically closes by day 28 of gestation. The etiology of MMC is multifactorial with increased risk with material folate deficiency. Hydrocephalus is present in 60–80%. Patient with Chiari 2 malformation almost always have MMC. Infection is a concern in ruptured MMC and all patients should be covered by antibiotics. Recommended regime is Nafcillin and gentamicin.

All MMC need closure surgery, ideally within 48 h of birth. Early closure of myelomeningoceleis does not improve neurological outcome; however, it decreases the infections risk.

(GB, pp. 281–282)

23. A 5-year-old female was found to have incidental L5–S1 spondylolisthesis in an abdominal CT scan. He has no back pain:

23a. What is the nosy likely type of spondylolisthesis in this patient?
A. Developmental
B. Isthmic
C. Traumatic
D. Degenerative

23b. All of the following changes can be seen in the CT of this patient, EXCEPT:
A. Hypoplastic L5 transverse processes
B. Deficient L5 and S1 laminae
C. Elongation of the pars interarticularis
D. L5–S1 facet arthritis

23c. All of the following indicate of progression of the spondylolisthesis in this patient, EXCEPT:
A. Female gender
B. Young age at presentation
C. Degree of spondylolisthesis 25–50%
D. Instability on dynamic radiographs

23d. Based on Spinal Deformity Study Slip Severity Group classification, type 2 of this type of spondylolisthesis is:
A. Slip less than 25% and Pelvic incidence less than 45°
B. Slip between 25–50% and Pelvic incidence less than 45°
C. Slip less than 50% and pelvic incidence between 45° and 60°
D. Slip more than 50% and pelvic incidence between 45° and 60°

Correct Answers: 23a: A, 23b: D, 23C: C, 23d: C

Explanation:

This patient likely has developmental spondylolisthesis. It is usually featured with dysplastic changes at the site of slippage like abnormalities in the lumbosacral facets, underdeveloped L5 and S1 laminae, elongation of the pars interarticularis, rounded sacral dome, sacral endplate irregularities, a trapezoidal L5 vertebra, and hypoplastic L5 transverse processes. It is divided into high- and low-dysplastic types.

The **Spinal Deformity Study Group Classification of Spondylolisthesis** categorizes developmental spondylolisthesis based on slip severity and pelvic incidence (PI). For low-grade slips (<50%), the classification is further divided into three types based on pelvic incidence (PI): Type 1 for PI < 45°, Type 2 for PI between 45° and 60°, and Type 3 for PI > 60°. These types all exhibit sacropelvic balance. Type 4 represents low-grade slips with a balanced sacropelvis and spinopelvis. High-grade slips (≥50%) are classified as Type 5A when there is unbalanced sacropelvic alignment but balanced spinopelvic alignment. Type 5B applies when there is unbalanced sacropelvic alignment with lumbosacral kyphosis (LSK) <80° or a pelvic femoral angle (PFA) ≥10°. Finally, Type 6 denotes high-grade slips with both unbalanced sacropelvic and spinopelvic alignment.

(BS, p. 235; SS, pp. 412–413)

24. A newborn is found to have a cutaneous change in his lumbar region (see Fig. 11.7):

The best next step to approach this child is:

A. Bed side resection of this skin anomaly
B. Reassurance that this will regress and fall within 12 months
C. Full neurological exam of the child
D. Lumbar X-ray to look for skeletal anomalies

Correct Answer: C

Explanation:

Caudal appendages or human tails are rare anatomical anomalies that found in the lumbosacral or coccygeal region, and are classified as true tails or

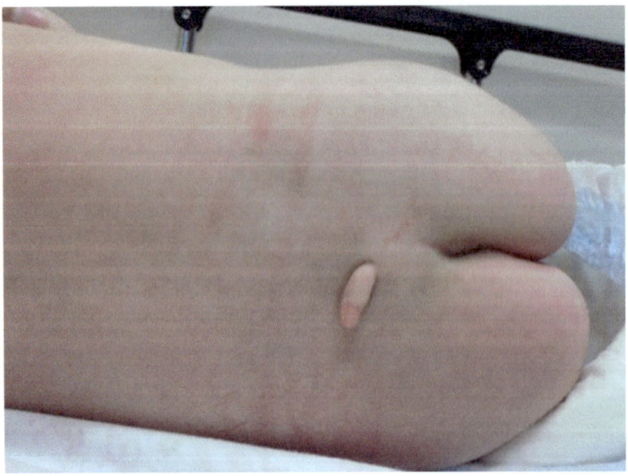

Fig. 11.7 Case 24 cutaneous change in the lumbar region

pseudo-tails. True tails are remnants of the embryonic tail that fail to regress during the fourth to eighth weeks of gestation. They consist of normal tissues such as fat, muscle, and nerves, and are not associated with other anomalies. Pseudo-tails, on the other hand, often result from abnormal tissue growth and are frequently linked to conditions like spinal dysraphism, dermal sinuses, or lipomas. Proper evaluation involves **neurological examinations and imaging studies (Spine MRI)** to exclude underlying abnormalities. Surgical excision is the treatment of choice.

[52]

25. A newborn is found to have a dimple in her lower lumbar region (see Fig. 11.8):

25a. What is the likely embryological explanation of this condition:

A. Incomplete ectoderm and endoderm dysjunction in the fourth week of gestation
B. Failure of primary neurulation during the third week of gestation
C. Persistence of the embryonic tail due to incomplete regression
D. Disrupted somite segmentation leading to vertebral anomalies

25b. The primary clinical potential concern that might lead to mortality in this baby is:

A. Hydrocephalus
B. Severe scoliosis leading to respiratory compromise
C. Meningitis
D. Congenital heart defect

25c. The next appropriate step in the management of this patient is:

A. Immediate surgical excision
B. Lumbosacral MRI
C. Routine observation with follow-up in 6 months
D. Genetic testing to confirm diagnosis

Correct Answers: 25a: A, 25b: C, 25c: B

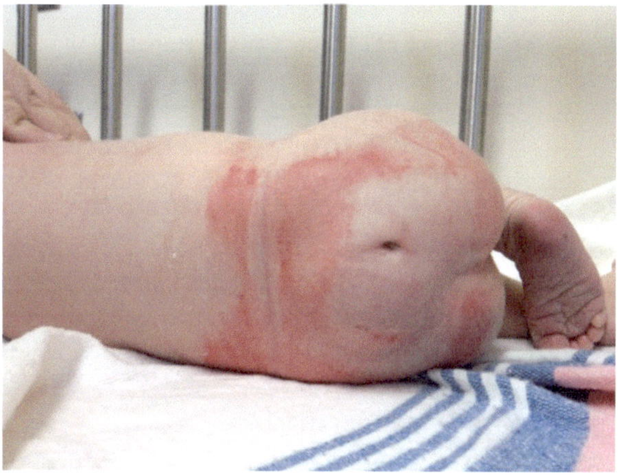

Fig. 11.8 Case 25 picture showing dimple in her lower lumbar region

Explanation:

This showed a dermal sinus tract which is a midline dimple that can occur in any region of the neuroaxis, typically in the lumbosacral area. It is usually due to incomplete ectoderm and endoderm dysjunction in the fourth week of gestation. It can be an isolated findings or can be associated with spinal dysraphism. The tract is usually covered with squamous epithelium. This condition can be associated with tethered cord or dermoid; however, the main concern is recurrent infections with protentional meningitis. MRI of the spine is essential to evaluate if the dermal sinus is connected to any neuro tissue and also to look for other associated anomalies. Treatment is surgical excision by following the tract down to the its origin with removal of epithelial linings and any dermoid or epidermoid lesions and also untethered the cord if needed.

(BS, p. 164)

26. One of the following is CORRECT about neurenteric cysts in pediatric patients:
   A. Primarily composed of neural tissue
   B. Typically located in the anterior mediastinum
   C. Frequently present with isolated symptoms unrelated to the spine
   D. Almost always associated with other spinal abnormalities

   Correct Answer: D

   Explanation:

   Neurenteric cysts is uncommon congenital condition. They result from failure of closure between endoderm and ectoderm. They tend to occur at cervical or thoracic spine. They almost always have associated other spinal anomalies like hemivertebra, spinal bifida, and split cord syndrome.

   (BS, p. 168)

27. A pediatric patient with a fibroblast growth factor receptor (FGFR) 4p mutation. He has increased risk of the following spinal conditions:
   A. Scoliosis
   B. Spinal stenosis
   C. Cervicomedullary compression
   D. All of the above

   Correct Answer: D

   Explanation:

   Mutation of FGFR-4p leads to impairment of endochondral ossification that manifest clinically as Achondroplasia. It is the most common cause of dwarfism. Achondroplasia is associated with several spinal conditions such as scoliosis, thoracolumbar kyphosis, lumbar hyperlordosis, spinal stenosis, and cervicomedullary compression (foramen magnus stenosis or basilar invagination).

   (SS, p. 405)

28. A 11-year-old boy with low laying posterior hair line presents with restricted cervical movement and legs weakness. CT scan is seen (Fig. 11.9):

   28a. The classic triad of this syndrome presents in approximately:
      A. 90% of the patient
      B. 70% of the patients

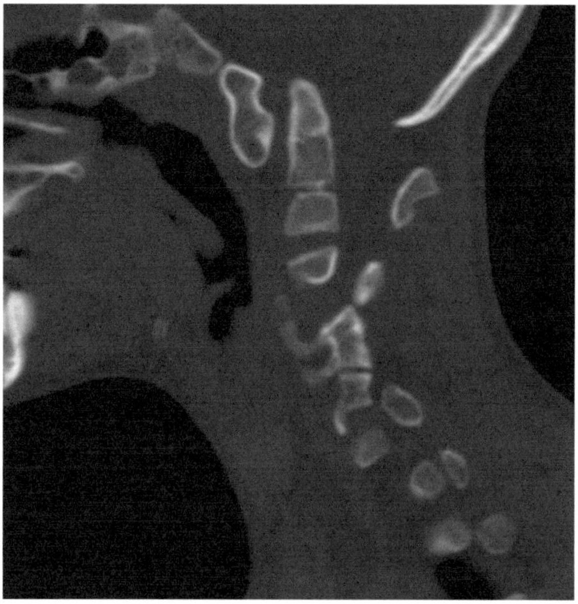

Fig. 11.9 Case 28 CT scan

C. 50% of the patients
D. 10% of the patients

28b. All of the following conditions are associated with the patient's condition, EXCEPT:

A. Sprengel's deformity
B. Synkinesis
C. Clubfoot
D. Cleft palate

28c. The appropriate treatment for this patient is:

A. Conservative with physical therapy
B. Foramen magnum decompression and occipito-cervcial fusion
C. Cervical traction alone for 6 months
D. All are valid options.

Correct Answers: 28a: C, 28b: C, 28c: B

Explanation:

This patient has Klippel-Feil syndrome which is a congenital condition that has triad of, low laying hair line, limited cervical movement and short neck. This triad presents in 50% or less of the patients. Patients usually have multiple fused cervical vertebrae. They also might have basilar invagination (seen in the CT of this patients) with compression to the cervicomedullary junction. Other associated conditions include: sprengel's deformity (raised scapula), synkinesis (mirror involuntary and undesirable hands or facial movements), cleft palate, facial palsy, and ptosis.

This patient has symptomatic basilar invagination with significant compression to the cervicomedullary junction. This needs decompression surgery (like transoral odontoid resection) and occipito-cervical fusion.

(GB, p. 289)

29. A newborn with a large sacrococcygeal teratoma is most at risk for which of the following complications?
    A. Malignant transformation
    B. Tethered cord syndrome
    C. High-output cardiac failure
    D. Urinary incontinence

    Correct Answer: C

    Complication:

    Sacrococcygeal teratoma is germ cell tumor of coccyx that can be benign of malignant. It is a highly vascular a tumor and heart failure of the neonate is a protentional complication.

    (DI, p. 127)

30. A 16-year-old patient with Marfan syndrome presents with a new onset of back pain and lower extremity weakness. The most likely spinal pathology is:
    A. Dural ectasia
    B. Spondylolisthesis
    C. Spinal stenosis
    D. Lumbar scoliosis

    Correct Answer: A

    Explanation:

    Marfan syndrome is an autosomal dominant condition of the connective tissues. Patients can present with low back pain usually due to dural ectasia which is weakness of the dura that leads to ballooning and expansion of the dura. Patients can have low back pain or/and radiculopathy.

    (RP)

31. The pediatric spinal injury tends to affect ligaments more than bones due to:
    A. Ligamentous laxity
    B. High head-to-body weight ratio
    C. Immaturity of paraspinal muscles
    D. All of the above

    Correct Answer: D

    Explanation:

    Pediatric patients tend to have ligamentous more than bony spinal injuries due to ligamentous laxity, high head-to-body weight ratio, immaturity of paraspinal muscles and underdeveloped uncinate processes in the cervical spine.

    (GB, p. 1121)

32. The following can mimic spinal injuries in pediatric patients, EXCEPT:
    A. Pseudospread of the atlas
    B. Synchondroses
    C. Pseudosubluxation
    D. Hemivertebra

Correct Answer: D

Explanation:

Several normal anatomical features in pediatric patients can resemble spinal injuries and fractures. Normal synchondroses may mimic fractures and the knowledge of their anatomical features are essential. Pseudospread of the atlas which is defined as a total overlap of more than 2 mm between the C1 lateral masses and C2 on an AP open-mouth radiograph. This finding can be mistaken for a Jefferson fracture. Normal anterior displacement (pseudosubluxation) may present in children specifically at C2–C3 level.

Hemivertebra is a distinctive congenital condition that the least option to resemble spinal fracture.

(GB, p. 1121)

Revision Spine Surgery

12

1. Which approach has the lowest risk of recurrent disc herniation when treating recurrent lumbar disc herniation?
   A. Redo microdiscectomy
   B. Posterior lateral fusion
   C. TLIF
   D. B and C
   Correct Answer: C
   Explanation:
   Interbody fusion techniques, such as TLIF has the highest chance in preventing further disc herniation by removing the disc entirely and replacing it with an interbody cage when treating recurrent lumbar disc herniation. Posteriolateral fusion involved fusion at the posterior-lateral area and does not involve complete disc removal. It reduces the risk of herniation, but not as effective as interbody fusion.
   Redo microdiscectomy addresses the herniation but does not stabilize the spine, leaving a higher chance of recurrence.
   [18]
2. When performing a revision microdiscectomy for recurrent lumbar disc herniation, which technique reduces the risk of dural tear in the presence of epidural fibrosis?
   A. Sharp dissection of the scar tissue
   B. Use of a microscope and minimal scar manipulation
   C. Laminotomy with extensive scar resection
   D. All of the above
   Correct Answer: B
   [8]

K. F. AlAli, H. T. Hashim, *Spine Surgery and Peripheral Nerve Surgery*,
https://doi.org/10.1007/978-3-031-98543-0_12

3. A 50-year-old with history of lumbar fusion presents with symptomatic adjacent segment disease and sagittal imbalance. What is the most important element in a successful revision surgery?
   A. Use of Iliac crest graft for fusion
   B. Correction of the lordosis
   C. Dynamic lumbar stabilization
   D. Avoiding instrumentation

   Correct Answer: B

   Explanation:

   The key element in a successful revision surgery for adjacent segment disease in a patient with history of lumbar fusion is proper sagittal alignment. If lordosis is not corrected, symptoms frequently persist and functional outcomes are poor. Though they can help with fusion, the use of instruments and bone grafts is secondary to alignment correction and the final result.

   (RSS, p. 205)
4. A 58-year-old female develops persistent neck pain and myelopathy 3 years after C5–C6 ACDF. Imaging shows persistent pseudoarthrosis, adjacent segment degeneration at C6–C7, and kyphotic angulation at the fused level. Which surgical approach is best for this patient?
   A. Posterior cervical fusion with laminectomy at C5–C7
   B. Revision C5–C7 ACDF
   C. Combined anterior and posterior fusion from C5 to C7
   D. Observation with cervical bracing

   Correct Answer: C

   Explanation:

   In cases of pseudarthrosis with kyphotic angulation and adjacent segment degeneration, combined anterior and posterior fusion is often required to achieve stability, correct sagittal alignment, and decompress the neural elements. While a revision ACDF may address pseudarthrosis, the kyphotic deformity and ASD necessitate posterior stabilization to ensure a durable correction and fusion.
5. The overall complication of same level revision ACDF is:
   A. Up to 5%
   B. Up to 25%
   C. Up to 50%
   D. Up to 85%

   Correct answer: B

   Explanation:

   The overall complication rate for revision surgery at the index level of ACDF ranges from 10% to 25%, depending on the approach used—anterior, posterior, or circumferential. Common complications include dysphagia, transient hoarseness, and radiculopathy. Despite these risks, most patients experience significant symptom relief following revision surgery.

   (RSS, p. 43)

6. A 46-year-old male with history of unilateral vocal cord paralysis after C5–C6. He has recurrent disc herniation and revision C5–C6 ACDF is planned. One of the following is appropriate regarding the revision surgery:
   A. Same side revision surgery
   B. Contralateral side revision surgery
   C. Posterior C5–C6 laminectomy and lateral mass fusion
   D. All of the above

   Correct Answer: A

   Explanation:

   In a patient with history of unilateral vocal cord paralysis, the surgical approach for the same level revision surgery should be on the same side to prevent bilateral recurrent laryngeal nerve palsy. Bilateral paralysis can have severe consequences, potentially necessitating permanent tracheostomy placement.

   (RSS, p. 42)
7. One of the following is an indication for converting cervical total disc replacement (artificial disc) to ACDF is:
   A. Loosening of the artificial disc
   B. Heterotopic ossification
   C. Mechanical neck pain
   D. All of the above

   Correct Answer: D

   Explanation:

   Indications for revision surgery of conversion of cervical total disc replacement to ACDF are recurrent neurological issues, severe neck pain, device loosening or causing local pathology (like dysphagia), heterotopic ossification, device failure (like fracture), device ejection, or patient reactions to device components or debris.

   (RSS, p. 52)
8. The following step can help in achieving good fusion in revision C1–C2:
   A. Stripping and packing the C1–C2 joints with bone graft
   B. Avoiding re-do C1–C2 Harms technique and use of laminar wire.
   C. Adding Halifax clamp and leaving the old hardware
   D. All of the above are correct

   Correct Answer: A

   Explanation:

   C1–C2 revision posterior fusion for nonunion can be challenging. Certain bone grafting techniques can be used to enhance fusion, one of them is C1–C2 facet joints exposure and carefully **stripping them from any cartilages of scar tissues, and packing the joints with autograft or allograft.** Other options do not enhance fusion.

   (RSS, p. 86)
9. The following is a challenge in recurrent lumbar discectomy:
   A. High risk if incidental durotomy
   B. Nerve roots injury

C. Epidural scar tissue
D. All of the above

Correct Answer: D

Explanation:

All of choices are protentional complication of revision lumbar discectomy. [8]

10. The proper technique to address epidural scar and avoid dura and neural injuries in revision lumbar laminectomy is:
    A. Aggressive scar dissection only caudally
    B. Avoiding the scar entirely and only exposing it laterally
    C. Subperiosteal dissection of the scar
    D. Midline dissection first

    Correct Answer: C

    Explanation:

    Scar dissection in revision lumbar laminectomy surgery is challenging and can cause dura or neural injuries. The dissection should be started at a normal level above or below the scar. Then, the scar is dissected in **subperiosteal manner** and **a minimal non-compressive midline scar tissue can be left to avoid dura or neural injuries.** Subperiosteal dissection is extended laterally to fully expose the prior hardware (if present) and ensure clear visualization of the dura and neural elements.

    (RSS, p. 105)

11. One of the following steps is crucial when removing posterior lumbar pedicle hardware:
    A. Obtain the old operative note to know the type of the hardware
    B. Use a universal spine system set if the type of the hardware is unknown
    C. Use of counter-torque device to remove set screws and limit rotation of the hardware
    D. All of the above

    Correct Answer: D

    Explanation:

    Thorough preoperative planning, including **identification of prior hardware**, is crucial to any revision spine surgery specially when dealing with hardware. If prior operative reports are unavailable, **universal hardware removal systems** from various manufacturers can be utilized. Set screws and cross-links are removed first, with **counter-torque applied to minimize stress** on the pedicle, hardware rotation, and reduce the risk of fracture. If a set screw is stripped, removal systems typically offer tools to reverse-thread into the stripped screw for extraction. Once set screws and cross-links are addressed, the rods and lateral mass screws are removed. The size of each screw is recorded, and the screw tracts are carefully probed with a ball-tip probe to confirm the absence of cortical breaches.

    (RSS, p. 105)

12. Salvage options for fixation in the posterior cervical spine for revision cervical lateral mass screws is:
    A. Alternative lateral mass screw trajectory
    B. Cervical pedicle screws
    C. Trans-facet screws
    D. All of the above

    Correct Answer: D

    Explanation:

    Salvage fixation options in the posterior cervical spine revision fusion include alternative lateral mass screw trajectories, cervical pedicle screws, transfacet screws, and various wiring techniques. The fusion construct can also be extended proximally or distally.

    (RSS, p. 105)

13. A 43-year-old who had multi-level ACDF presented with mechanical neck pain. X-ray showed good cervical lordosis. Cervical CT scan showed pseudoarthrosis at C4–C5 level (below) (Fig. 12.1). What is the best surgical approach for this patient?
    A. C5 corpectomy
    B. C4 corpectomy
    C. Revision C4–C5 ACDF with removal of the cage
    D. C4–C5 lateral mass fusion

    Correct Answer: D

    Explanation:

    The case showed multiple level ACDF with pseudarthrosis at one level (C4–C5). Since the lordosis is maintained, posterior approach is the best option. Anterior revision has more complications rate than new posterior approach. For delayed pseudarthrosis with loss of lordosis or kyphotic angulation, anterior revision focused on restoring structural support and lordosis, with or without posterior stabilization, should be strongly considered.

    (RSS, p. 43)

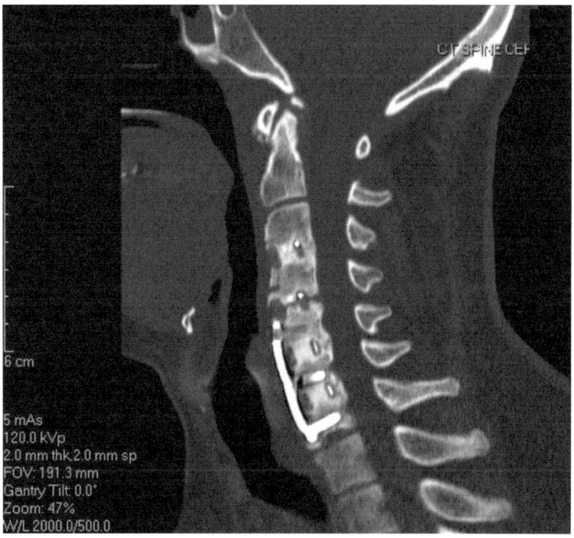

Fig. 12.1 Cervical CT scan showed pseudoarthrosis at C4–C5 level

14. In a revision case of pseudarthrosis after lumbar fusion, which grafting method is most likely to improve fusion rates?
    A. Local bone graft only
    B. Iliac crest autograft
    C. Synthetic graft
    D. Allograft bone

    Correct Answer: B

    Explanation:

    Due to the biological challenges in achieving bony fusion in revision non-union surgery, like the presence of avascular tissue, the use of **iliac crest autograft** or Bone morphogenetic proteins (BMP) is strongly recommended due to their osteoinductive properties.

    (RSS, p. 186)
15. What is the most effective intraoperative strategy to prevent hardware failure in revision spinal fusions?
    A. Use of larger diameter screws
    B. Use of multilevel fixation
    C. Intraoperative navigation for precise screw placement
    D. All of the above

    Correct Answer: D

    Explanation:

    Intraoperative strategy to revise failed pedicle screw includes: The potential to upsize each screw in diameter and length, maximize bony purchase by using other screw trajectory, extend the level of fusions, utilizing neuro-navigation will enhance a proper screw placement and preparing the fusion area carefully.

    (RSS, p. 186)
16. A 52-year-old patient with a history of L4–L5 fusion has severe L3–L4 lumbar degenerative disease and mechanical low back pain. For this patient, the best surgical strategy is:
    A. Decompression at the adjacent level posteriorly
    B. Disc replacement of the adjacent level
    C. Fusion extension to the adjacent segment
    D. Dynamic stabilization that incorporates the adjacent level

    Correct Answer: C

    Explanation:

    Extending fusion to the affected adjacent segment is the best surgical approach for lumbar adjacent segment disease that is highly degenerative and accompanied by mechanical low back pain that could indicate instability. This method effectively addresses extreme instability as well as degeneration. Disc replacement (B), lumbar decompression (A), and dynamic stabilization (D) do not address instability.

    (RSS, pp. 205–206)
17. What is the most critical technical step to ensure successful re-fusion in patient with lumbar fusion pseudarthrosis?
    A. Removal of the existing hardware
    B. Proper preparation of the fusion bed

C. Use of larger interbody cages
D. Use of neuronavigation

Correct Answer: B

Explanation:

The most important intraoperative step in revision surgery to increase the likelihood of re-fusion is **proper fusion bed preparation.** Following instrumentation placement, the fusion bed is prepared by removing all soft tissue and using a high-speed burr to decorticate the lamina's and facet joints' cortical bones.

(RSS, p. 106)

18. A 62-year-old patient presents with mechanical low back pain and radicular pain. He has history of L4–L5 posterior-lateral fusion 3 years ago. New lumbar MRI shows L3–L4 severe degeneration. What is the best surgical strategy to deal with the epidural scar tissues?
A. Start scar dissection at the cranial part
B. Start exposing normal dura then extend dissection toward the scar
C. Use micro dissectors to remove the scar tissue carefully
D. Start the scar dissection at the lateral edges bilaterally

Correct Answer: C

Explanation:

This patient has symptomatic adjacent degenerative disease. Revising such cases carry risks of dura and nerves injuries. One of the proven surgical principles to reduce this risk is to expose normal tissue and extend cranially and caudally to the scar tissue. This approach helps in clearly defining the epidural scar plane, minimizing the risk of inadvertent dural injury. In case of revision lumbar decompression, the previous laminotomy defect is extended cranially to expose normal dura without scar. Then, after outlining the proper depth and the scar area from all direction, the scar tissue can be dissected. The scar is only dissected till satisfactory decompression of the neural tissues. It is safe to leave central non compressive scar over the dura or the nerve.

(RSS, pp. 169–170)

19. A significant amount of epidural venous bleeding occurs when the surgeon performs revision decompression of the lumbar lateral recess. Which approach to hemostasis is the most successful in this case?
A. Applying bipolar electrocautery directly to the bleeding veins
B. Packing the area with thrombin-soaked gelatin sponges
C. Elevating the abdomen
D. Using cottonoid compression

Correct Answer: B

Explanation:

Bleeding is more common in revision lumbar surgeries than in primary lumbar surgeries, especially when working with scar tissue.

Thrombin-soaked gelatin sponges is a very useful tool for controlling epidural venous bleeding. Though bipolar electrocautery (A) may be beneficial, its overuse is dangerous and may cause further tissue damage. The venous pressure would rise rather than fall if the abdomen (C) were raised. While cottonoid compression (D) is helpful, it is not as efficient as sponges soaked in thrombin.

(RSS, pp. 169–170)

20. What indicates the need of osteotomy to correct sagittal imbalance in revision lumbar fusion surgery?
    A. Number of previous fusion levels
    B. Presence of nonunion
    C. Preoperative sacral slope and pelvic tilt
    D. Adjacent segment degeneration degree

    Correct Answer: C

    Explanation:

    As in primary surgery, pelvic tilt and sacral slope parameters are the indicators for correcting sagittal balance by osteotomy in revision lumbar fusion surgery

    These measurements indicate the degree of compensation and imbalance in the spine and pelvis.

    While the extent of previous fusion levels (A), presence of pseudarthrosis (B), and adjacent segment degeneration (D) contribute to the decision-making process, they are secondary to the analysis of pelvic alignment in determining the necessity for osteotomy.

    (RSS, p. 128)

21. The use of an interbody fusion is crucial when performing a revision for recurrent lumbar disc herniation in the following situations:
    A. Large disc fragment recurrence
    B. mechanical back pain with instability
    C. Radiculopathy without instability
    D. Disc extrusion without loss of disc height

    Correct Answer: B

    Explanation:

    Because it treats both the instability and radicular symptoms, interbody fusion is indicated in cases of recurrent lumbar disc herniation when there is mechanical back pain and evidence of spinal instability. For radiculopathy without instability (C) or large disc fragment recurrence (A), decompression alone may be sufficient. Interbody fusion is generally not required for disc extrusion without a significant loss of height (D), unless instability is present.

    (RSS, p. 174).

22. Patient with recurrent C5–C6 disc herniation who underwent ACDF 2 year ago. You decided to perform revision C5–C6 ACDF. One of the following are WRONG regarding revision ACDF:
    A. You will need to dissect through obscured tissue planes
    B. There is increased risk of tracheoesophageal injury
    C. Preoperative evaluation of vocal cord function is preferably needed
    D. All of the Above are correct

    Correct Answer: D

Explanation:

All of the listed points (A, B, and C) are accurate considerations for revision ACDF. Preoperative evaluation of vocal cord function is preferably needed by use of indirect laryngoscopy to identify a preexisting unilateral asymptomatic recurrent laryngeal nerve palsy

(RSS, pp. 41–45)

23. A 60-year-old patient presents with proximal junctional kyphosis at T10 following a T10–L5 fusion. Imaging shows a focal kyphotic deformity at the upper fused level with vertebral collapse. The patient has pain and walking difficulty. When revising this patient, what is the most appropriate surgical strategy?
    A. Physical therapy and bracing
    B. Smith-Petersen osteotomies to extend the fusion to the proximal thoracic spine
    C. Hardware removal
    D. All of the above are valid options

    Correct Answer: B

    Explanation:

    This patient has symptomatic proximal junctional kyphosis and the best surgical strategy is to restore alignment and treat the sagittal imbalance. This can be achieved by Smith-Petersen osteotomies with extension of the fusion levels.

    (RSS, p. 117)

24. What is the primary factor in preventing more adjacent segment degeneration after revision surgery for lumbar adjacent segment disease?
    A. Minimizing the number of fused levels
    B. Dynamic stabilization systems
    C. Sagittal balance correction
    D. Placing interbody fusion at all levels

    Correct Answer: C

    Explanation:

    Restoring sagittal balance is the most crucial step in stopping the adjacent segment from further degenerating. Adjacent segment disease is less likely when the unfused segments are subjected to less mechanical stress due to proper sagittal alignment. Although dynamic stabilization and reducing the number of fused levels can occasionally lessen the degeneration of adjacent segments, they do not address the underlying biomechanical demands that poor sagittal alignment places on adjacent segments. Placing interbody fusion at all levels is unnecessary in preventing adjacent segment diseases.

    (RSS, p. 118)

25. During a revision posterior lumbar fusion surgery, what surgical strategy can be used to minimize the risk of nerve root injury?
    A. Aggressive foraminotomy
    B. Placement of an interbody cage with a smaller footprint
    C. Sequential nerve root retraction
    D. Use of low-energy trigger EMG probe

    Correct Answer: D

Explanation:

The use of low-energy trigger EMG probe in differentiating between scar tissue and normal element is helpful in minimizing nerve root injury.

(RSS, p. 189)

26. A patient with a history of L5–S1 anterior lumbar interbody fusion presents with lower back pain and sagittal imbalance. CT scan shows nonunion and subsidence of the interbody cage.

    Which preoperative measure is most important to improve the outcome of revision surgery?

    A. Preoperative administering of Cefazolin
    B. Preoperative smoking cessation and glycemic control
    C. Using neuromonitoring during the procedure
    D. Intraoperative fluoroscopy for accurate hardware placement

    Correct Answer: B

    Explanation:

    Smoking and poor glycemic control are known modifiable risk factors that increase the risk of nonunion and infections in primary or revision fusion spine surgeries. Controlling them preoperatively improve bone healing.

    (RSS, p. 152)

27. A 48-year-old female undergoes revision ALIF for nonunion at L5–S1. Intraoperative findings reveal significant fibrous tissue in the interbody space. What is the most appropriate next step during surgery?

    A. Place a new interbody cage without further preparation
    B. Perform meticulous removal of fibrous tissue to expose bleeding bone
    C. Insert an interbody graft with no end plate contouring
    D. Skip anterior revision and rely on posterior stabilization alone

    Correct Answer: B

    Explanation:

    Preparation of interbody space and removal of fibrous tissue and exposing bleeding bone is usually safe and critical to creating an optimal fusion bed. This step enhances graft integration and fusion success. End plate preparation and ensuring structural support are vital components of the revision surgery.

    (RSS, p. 153)

28. A 55-year-old man had multilevel spinal fusion for sagittal imbalance with correction by pedicle subtraction osteotomy. Six months later, he presents with worsening back pain and postural deformity. Radiographs show a Cobb angle of 12° at the proximal junction and disruption of the posterior tension band at T6. Which intervention would most likely prevent recurrence if revision surgery is performed?

    A. Transitioning from pedicle screws to hooks at the proximal segment
    B. T7 vertebroplasty
    C. Extending the fusion construct superiorly with rigid instrumentation
    D. Use of hooks over pedicle screws at the upper levels of instrumentation

    Correct Answer: B

Explanation:

Vertebroplasty at the uppermost level reduces stress and prevents vertebral body fractures, a common cause of proximal junctional kyphosis. Use of hooks over pedicle screws at the upper levels of instrumentation lacks substantial clinical evidence. Extending the construct may help correct deformity but does not address the underlying risk factors.

(CN, p. 326)

Spine Surgical Technique

13

1. What is the correct entry point and trajectory for the Magerl technique in cervical lateral mass screw placement?
   A. Center of the lateral mass, perpendicular trajectory
   B. One mm medial and superior to midpoint, 30° lateral, 15° cephalad
   C. Midpoint, perpendicular trajectory
   D. Two mm above midpoint, 0° lateral, 30° cephalad

   Correct Answer: B

   Explanation:

   The Magerl technique uses an entry point 1 mm medial and superior to the midpoint of the lateral mass, with a 30° lateral and 15° cephalad angulation for optimal screw placement and stability (Fig. 13.1).

   (SS, p. 280)
2. Which of the following correctly matches a C1 lateral mass screw entry point with its trajectory?
   A. Tan (2003): Posterior arch midpoint, angled medially and superiorly
   B. Harms Technique: Lateral mass entry, directed straight anteriorly
   C. Lateral Mass Entry: Junction of the posterior arch and lateral mass, angled medially
   D. Posterior Arch Entry: Midpoint of the lateral mass, avoiding the vertebral artery

   Correct Answer: A

   Explanation:

   The following figure summarizes C1 lateral mass screw entry points and trajectories (Fig. 13.2).
3. The term *anatomic* thoracic screw insertion technique means:
   A. Screws following the natural angle of the pedicle in axial plane
   B. Screws following the natural angle of the pedicle in sagittal plane
   C. Screw trajectory that runs parallel to the surface of the superior end plate
   D. Screw trajectory that runs parallel to the surface of the superior facet

   Correct Answer: B

K. F. AlAli, H. T. Hashim, *Spine Surgery and Peripheral Nerve Surgery*,
https://doi.org/10.1007/978-3-031-98543-0_13

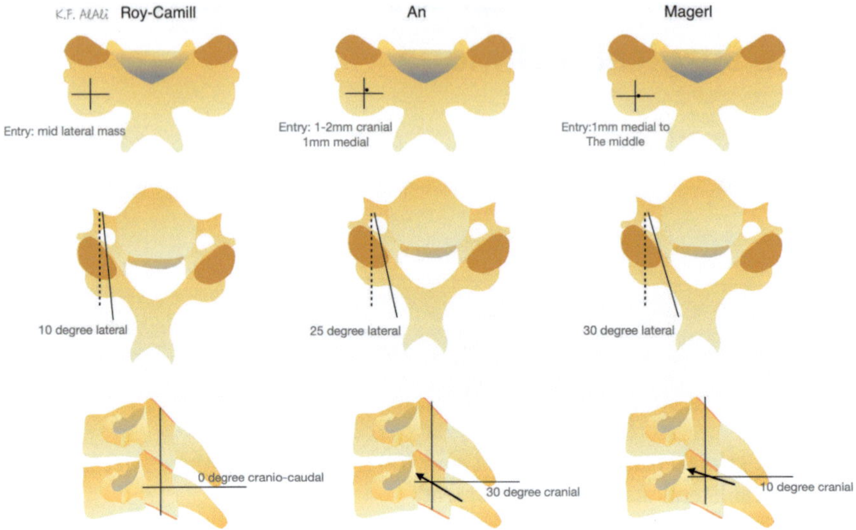

Fig. 13.1 Entry points and trajectories for the Roy-Camill, An, and Magerl technique in cervical lateral mass screw placement

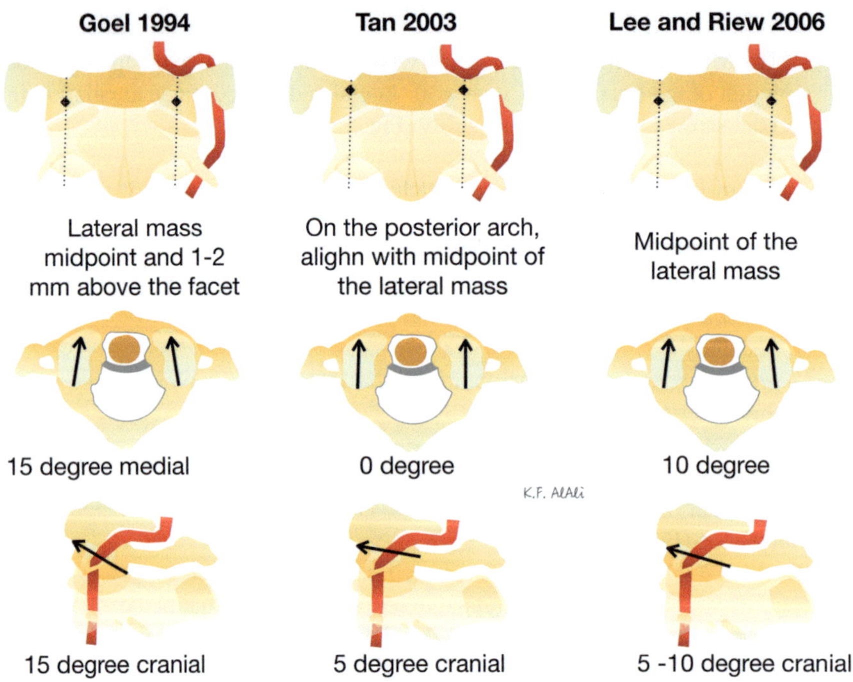

Fig. 13.2 Illustration of C1 lateral mass screw entry points and trajectories methods

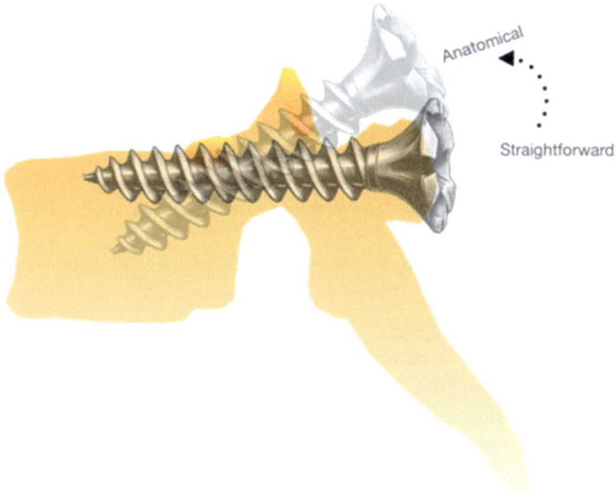

Fig. 13.3 Anatomical vs straightforward trajectories of the thoracic pedicle screw

Explanation:
Anatomical versus Straightforward Thoracic Pedicle Screw Trajectory:
Anatomical Trajectory (Fig. 13.3):

- Follows the natural curvature of the pedicle.
- Requires precise alignment with the pedicle's axis.
- Typically involves a medial angulation and slight cranial tilt.
- Provides better purchase within the pedicle and vertebral body.
- Reduces the risk of pedicle breach.

Straightforward (Straight) Trajectory:

- Easier and faster to execute.
- Involves minimal medial angulation, often aligned straight along the pedicle.
- May result in less optimal screw purchase and increased risk of lateral or medial breach.
- Often used in cases with challenging anatomy or during less complex procedures.
(GB, p. 1792)

4. The typical entry point for a lumbar pedicle screw is:
   A. The junction of the pars interarticularis with the middle of transverse process and mammillary process
   B. The junction between pars interarticularis with superior facet and mammillary process.
   C. 2–3 mm below superior end of the inferior facet of the targeted level
   D. All of the above

   Correct Answer: A
   Explanation:
   The entry point for the pedicle of lumbar spine is the entry point of the pedicle screw is defined as the confluence of any of the four lines (Fig. 13.4):

- Pars articularis
- Mamillary process

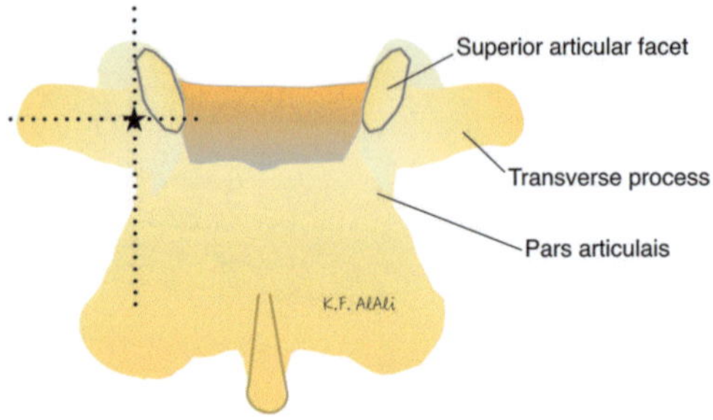

Fig. 13.4 Lumbar pedicle entry point (star) is the transection of vertical line of lateral border of superior facet or in line with the pars articularis and the horizontal line of mid. point of the transverse process. If a laminectomy is done at that level, the pedicle's location is confirmed by palpating with a probe within the spinal canal. Fluoroscopy is used for verification (Table 13.1)

- Lateral border of the superior articular facet
- Mid. point of the transverse process

(GB, p. 1797)

5. The entry point of S1 pedicle screw is:
   A. The superiolateral margin of the inferior L5 facet
   B. The superiomedial margin of the inferior L5 facet
   C. The inferolateral margin of the S1 superior facet
   D. The inferomedial margin of the S1 superior facet

   Correct Answer: C

   Explanation:

   The S1 pedicle screw entry point is the inferolateral margin of the S1 superior facet and directed anteromedially through the pedicle and toward the sacral promontory.

   (CN, p. 322)
6. The entry point of S2-alar-iliac screw is:
   A. Midway between the S1 and S2 neural foramen and at the lateral edge of the foramina
   B. Midway between the S1 and S2 neural foramen and at the medial edge of the foramina
   C. Below S2 neural foramen in the midline
   D. Above S2 neural foramen in the midline

   Correct Answer: A

   Explanation:

   The entry point for S2-alar-iliac screw is midway between the S1 and S2 neural foramen, at the lateral edge of the foramina, in line with the S1 pedicle screw (if placed) (Fig. 13.5).

   (GB, p. 1808)

7. What is the most critical step to avoid during transforaminal lumbar interbody fusion (TLIF) in order to prevent neural injury?
   A. Retraction of the thecal sac
   B. Avoidance of excessive disc space distraction
   C. Excessive nerve root retraction
   D. Overreaming the vertebral endplates
   Correct Answer: C

Table 13.1 Surgical technique: open posterior lumbar pedicle screw fusion

Step	Description
Positioning	Patient is placed prone on a radiolucent Jackson frame with proper padding. Neck is kept in neutral position, arms positioned under 90° abduction, and knees flexed about 30° to reduce sciatic nerve stretch. Pads are positioned to allow the abdomen to hang freely, reducing epidural bleeding
Anesthesia/ Neuromonitoring	General anesthesia is used. Neuromonitoring is generally not required for lower lumbar levels unless significant myelopathy or deformity correction is involved, in which case SSEP and TcMEP neuromonitoring is used
Incision Localization	Long spinal needles are used to identify cranial and caudal ends of the planned incision, 1–2 cm above and below the cranial and caudal targeted pedicle. Lateral X-rays are obtained to confirm correct needle placement and incision location. During surgery, facet joints are marked for reference with an additional X-ray
Approach	Standard posterior midline approach. A midline incision is made over spinous processes, and paraspinal muscles are subperiosteally dissected off the laminae and transverse processes using electrocautery and retractors. Key venous bleeders are controlled with electrocautery
Retractor Placement	Self-retaining retractors (e.g., Weitlaner, cerebellar retractors) are used to maintain exposure. For pedicle screw placement, 90° Zelpi retractors are preferred to optimize visibility of the pedicle entry points
Pedicle Screw Placement	Pedicle entry point is typically at the junction of the pars interarticularis with the middle of transverse process and mammillary process. A burr is used to breach the cortex, and a pedicle finder is used to canulate the pedicle with guidance from preoperative imaging and fluoroscopy for correct angulation a. A ball-tipped probe checks for cortical integrity before screw insertion. Pedicle is tapped, then screw is inserted, with fluoroscopy confirming trajectory
Fusion Bed Preparation	The transverse processes, pars interarticularis, and lateral facet walls are decorticated using a high-speed burr to create a fusion surface. Bone graft material is then packed over these decorticated areas, creating a fusion bed
Rod Insertion and Fixation	After bone grafting, pedicle screws are inserted and confirmed with fluoroscopy. Rods are inserted and secured with set screws to stabilize the spine
Closure Techniques	Hemovac drain is optional. Vicryl 0 or 1.0 for lumbosacral fascia, inverted Vicryl 2.0 or 3.0 for dermal layer, and Monocryl or staples for skin
Postoperative Care	Immediate neurological assessment is conducted, with focus on any new deficits. Drain output is monitored, and the drain is removed when output drops to around 30 mL/8 h. Postop CT for hardware placement is done

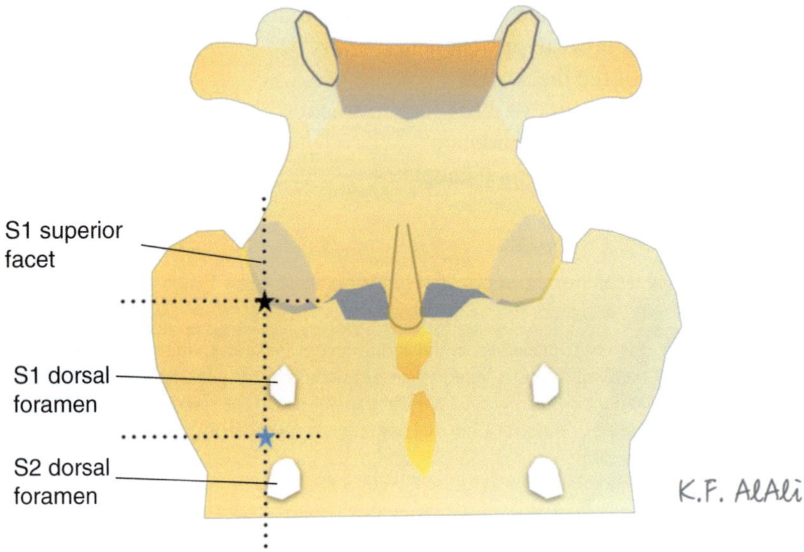

Fig. 13.5 S1 pedicle entry point (black star) is at the lateral border of superior facet of S1 and the inferolateral margin of the S1 superior facet. The entry point for S2-alar-iliac screw (blue star) is midway between the S1 and S2 dorsal neural foramen, at the lateral edge of the foramina, in line with the S1 pedicle screw

Explanation:

In TLIF, the Kambin's triangle is used for accessing the intervertebral disc. It is an anatomical space in the lumbar spine bounded by the exiting nerve root, the superior border of the lower vertebra's pedicle, and the traversing nerve root. This space is usually small, and nerve roots retraction may be needed. Minimizing nerve root retraction is necessary to avoid injuries, especially on the exiting nerve root where dorsal root ganglion is exposed. Extending the exposure more medially will allow minimal traction of dorsal root ganglion and the exciting nerve (Fig. 13.6).

(SSW, p. 1820)

8. Which cervical spine level corresponds to the surface landmark of the hyoid bone?
   A. C2
   B. C3
   C. C4
   D. C5

   Correct Answer: B

   Explanation:

   Surface landmarks for anterior cervical spine are helpful in identifying the appropriate incision's location. However, intraoperative cervical X-ray is mandatory to confirm the level. The followings landmark can be used (Fig. 13.7):

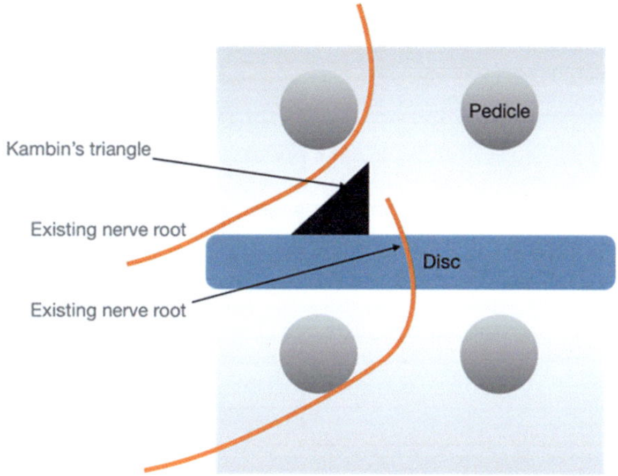

Fig. 13.6 The Kambin's triangle in TLIF

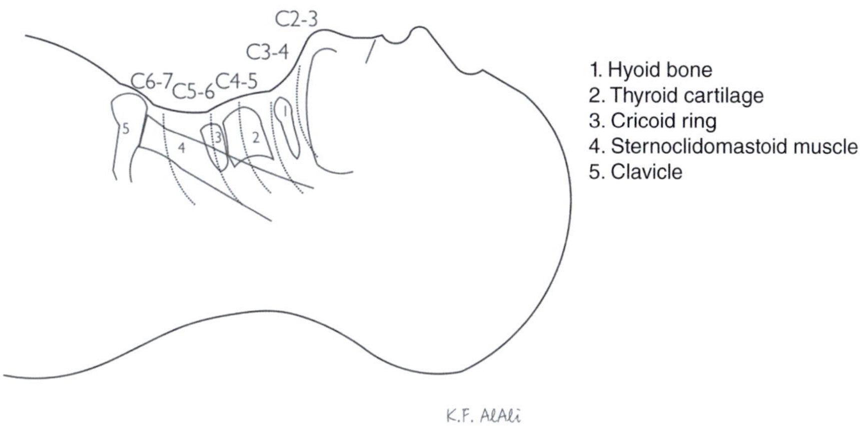

Fig. 13.7 Surface landmark for anterior cervical surgery approach

- Hyoid bone at C3
- Thyroid cartilage at C4-C5
- Carotid tubercle at C6
- Cricoid cartilage at C7

9. What is the main benefit of the extreme lateral interbody fusion (XLIF) method in comparison to other lumbar fusion techniques?
   A. Avoidance of major vascular structures
   B. Direct visualization of the dura
   C. Superior access to the posterior elements
   D. Minimal disruption of the paraspinal musculature
   Correct Answer: D

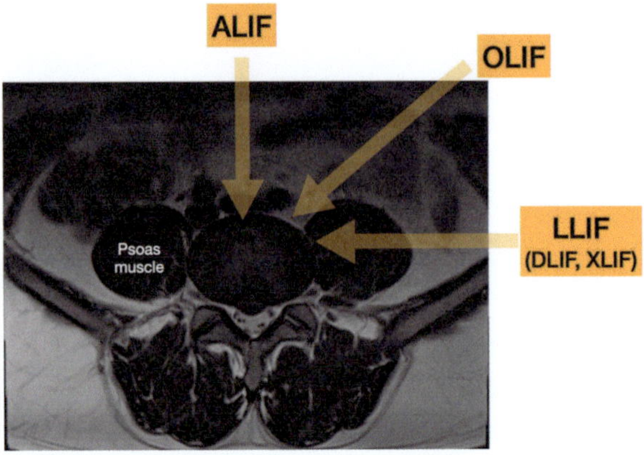

Fig. 13.8 Anterior (ALIF) and lateral lumbar interbody approaches

Explanation:

XLIF (XLIFTM, NuVasive, San Diego, CA) is a trademarked procedure like direct lumbar interbody fusion (DLIF, Medtronic, Memphis, TN). Both are under the generic term lateral lumbar interbody fusion (LLIF).

Oblique lumbar interbody fusion (OLIF, Medtronic, Memphis, TN) is a variation form of LLIF which approach the spine anterior to the psoas muscle, unlike XLIF and DLIF, through the psoas muscle (Fig. 13.8).

All variations of LLIF have the following advantages: minimal disruption of paraspinal musculature, smaller incisions, reduced operative time, lower blood loss, shorter hospital stay, less postoperative pain, improved fusion rates, and the convenience of placing instrumentation through the same incision (Table 13.2).

(GB, p. 1802; BS, p. 1102)

10. A 54-year-old with cervical myelopathy at C5 undergoes ACCF. The surgeon selects a fibular autograft over an iliac crest graft. What is the most likely reason?
    A. Fibular graft has better osteoinductive properties.
    B. Iliac crest graft has higher donor site morbidity and may be too short.
    C. Fibular graft eliminates the need for plating.
    D. Iliac crest graft is less stable in OPLL cases.

    Correct Answer: B

    Explanation:

    For multilevel corpectomies, fibular grafts or cages are often chosen due to their length and strength, as well as to avoid the morbidity associated with harvesting large iliac crest grafts which has high donor site morbidities.

    (RS, p. 748)

11. Which of the following graft materials has a reported fusion rate of 94%–100% and is particularly effective in anterior lumbar interbody fusion (ALIF)?
    A. Allograft
    B. rhBMP-2 (Recombinant BMP)
    C. Ceramics and synthetics
    D. Local autograft

Table 13.2 Trademarked variations of lateral lumbar interbody fusion (LLIF)

Procedure	DLIF (Direct Lateral Interbody Fusion)	XLIF (Extreme Lateral Interbody Fusion)	OLIF (Oblique Lumbar Interbody Fusion)
Approach	Lateral, through the psoas muscle	Extreme lateral, through the psoas muscle	A variation of LLIF in which the spine is approached obliquely, anterior to the psoas muscle
Patient position	Lateral decubitus	Lateral decubitus	Lateral decubitus
Structures avoided	Avoids large posterior muscles; bypasses abdominal organs	Avoids large posterior muscles; bypasses abdominal organs	Avoids posterior muscles; avoids direct psoas approach
Nerve Injury Risk	Moderate (risk to lumbar plexus)	Moderate	Lower risk
Use of Neuromonitoring	Yes, due to psoas traversal	Yes	Sometimes used, but less critical
Limitations	Limited visibility at L4–L5, L5–S1; psoas muscle manipulation	Similar to DLIF, with slightly larger lateral exposure	Requires oblique approach expertise; not always feasible for larger patients
Ideal for Levels	L1–L4	L1–L4	L2–L5, including easier access to L5–S1
Common Complications	Lumbar plexus injury, transient thigh numbness	Lumbar plexus injury, thigh pain	Iliac vein or artery injury, risk of vascular injury
Instrumentation	Require with posterior fixation	Required	Required

Correct Answer: B

Explanation:

The following table summarizes bone graft for lumbar fusion (Table 13.3):

12. The most important determinant of successful outcomes in a lumbar interbody fusion is:
    A. Adequate disc and endplate preparation
    B. Use of expandable cages
    C. Placement of pedicle screws
    D. Number of levels fused

    Correct Answer: A

    Explanation:

    The most critical determinant of a successful lumbar interbody fusion is **adequate disc and endplate preparation**. Ensuring thorough clearance of the disc and meticulous preparation of the endplates significantly enhances the likelihood of achieving solid fusion, as it maximizes the contact surface area for graft placement and reduces the risk of nonunion.

    [21]

13. In lateral lumbar interbody fusion (LLIF), what is the primary structure at risk when accessing the L4–L5 disc space?
    A. The iliac vein
    B. The genitofemoral nerve

Table 13.3 The table summarizes bone graft for lumbar fusion

Graft material	Reported fusion rate (%)	Details	References
Iliac Crest Autograft	97.7	Gold standard but associated with donor site morbidity	RS, p. 900
Allograft	50% –94%	Generally lower fusion rate than autograft; associated with higher revision rates	RS, p. 1124
rhBMP-2 (Recombinant BMP)	94%–100%	High fusion rates observed, especially in ALIF; approved by FDA for anterior lumbar fusion but not for posterior	RS, p. 1095

C. The psoas muscle
D. The lumbar plexus

Correct Answer: D

Explanation:

During LLIF, the approach is lateral and retroperitoneal. It passes through or near the psoas muscle. At L4-L5, the lumbar plexus moves anteriorly. This increases the risk of injury. Neuromonitoring helps reduce this risk by providing real-time nerve feedback.

[21]

14. In the surgical management of high-grade spondylolisthesis, what is the preferred approach?
    A. Anterior-only approach
    B. Posterior-only approach
    C. Combined anterior–posterior approach
    D. None of the above

Correct Answer: D

Explanation:

The management of high-grade spondylolisthesis often involves debate among spine specialists, as there is no universally "preferred" approach. Options include in situ fusion without reduction, partial reduction with instrumentation, or circumferential fusion with instrumentation to stabilize the vertebral column. Due to the unique anatomical challenges and risks associated with high-grade spondylolisthesis, such as nerve injury and instability, the approach is tailored to each patient based on their anatomy, symptoms, and surgeon experience. Circumferential fusion provides structural stability, but some cases may also benefit from in situ fusion or partial reduction depending on individual requirements, confirming that no single approach is universally preferred for all high-grade cases.

(SB, p. 319; RS, p. 557)

15. When performing a minimally invasive transforaminal lumbar interbody fusion (MIS TLIF), which of the following retractors is commonly used?
    A. Caspar retractor
    B. McCulloch retractor
    C. Tubular retractor

D. Taylor retractor

Correct Answer: C

Explanation:

For MIS TLIF, a tubular retractor is used. It requires a smaller incision and less muscle dissection. This reduces tissue damage and speeds up recovery. Serial dilation creates a narrow corridor. This minimizes muscle retraction and lowers the risk of atrophy.

(SSW, p. 1821)

16. For optimal CBT screw placement, what is the ideal trajectory angle in the caudocephalad and mediolateral planes?
    A. 45° caudocephalad, 30° mediolateral
    B. 30–45° caudocephalad, 20° mediolateral
    C. 15–20° caudocephalad, 5° mediolateral
    D. 60° caudocephalad, 40° mediolateral

    Correct Answer: B

    Explanation:

    CBT screws require a 30–45° caudocephalad and 20° mediolateral trajectory for optimal placement. The following table summarizes the approach (Table 13.4; Fig. 13.9):

    (BS, p. 1049)

17. During an anterior cervical discectomy and fusion (ACDF), the preferred graft material to achieve fusion is:
    A. Autograft from the iliac crest
    B. Allograft bone
    C. Titanium cage
    D. Polyetheretherketone (PEEK) cage

    Correct Answer: A

Table 13.4 Surgical technique: Cortical Bone Screw (CBT) Technique

Steps	Details
Purpose	Provides strong fixation through cortical bone, especially for patients with osteoporosis
Timing of screw placement	Performed after decompression and interbody placement to maintain anatomical landmarks
Entry point	Located at the junction of the transverse process base and 3–5 mm medial to the pars edge
Trajectory angle	Caudocephalad: 30–45 degrees; Mediolateral: ~20 degrees ("up and out" toward vertebral body)
Drilling technique	High-speed drill used to create a pilot hole; tap confirms cortical bone engagement
Fluoroscopic guidance	AP and lateral fluoroscopy (or navigation) confirm entry point and trajectory
Pilot hole depth	Approximately 30 mm; adjusted based on patient anatomy and spinal level
Screw specifications	Standard screw: 5–5.5 mm diameter, 30–35 mm length; larger screws (7.5 mm) for S1 level
Avoided levels	Typically not used at S1; medially oriented pedicle screws are preferred for sacral stability
Final steps	Decortication of posterior elements; bone graft placement lateral to rods to avoid nerve compression

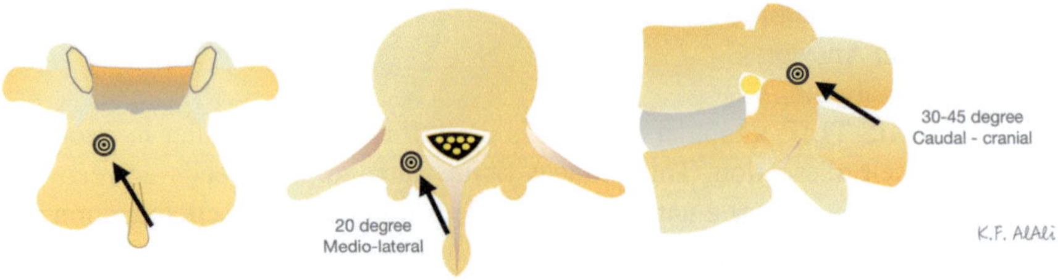

Fig. 13.9 Cortical Bone Screw (CBT) entry point and trajectory technique

Explanation:

Autograft from the iliac crest is still considered the gold standard but associated with donor site morbidity with fusion rate of up to 98%; however, due to donor site morbidities, other bone graft are commonly used with acceptable fusion rate percentage.

(RS, p. 900)

18. What is the starting point for the placement of a transarticular screw in the C2 vertebra?
   A. At the C2 spinous process
   B. 3–4 mm superior and 3–4 mm lateral to the inferior medial aspect of the C2–C3 facet joint
   C. Directly at the C1–C2 facet joint
   D. 1 mm lateral to the midline of the C2 vertebra

   Correct Answer: B

   Explanation:

   The starting point for a transarticular screw is 3–4 mm superior and 3–4 mm lateral to the inferior medial aspect of the C2–C3 facet joint, with a medial trajectory to avoid breaching the C2 isthmus. Insertion is guided by exposing the posterior C1–C2 facet and C2 isthmus. The screw path traverses the C2 inferior articular process, isthmus, superior endplate, C1–C2 facet joint, and C1 lateral mass (Fig. 13.10).

   (SS, p. 279)

19. In a pedicle subtraction osteotomy (PSO) for sagittal imbalance, the bone wedge is typically removed from:
   A. The anterior column
   B. The middle column
   C. The posterior column
   D. Both anterior and middle columns

   Correct Answer: B

   Explanation:

   In the pedicle subtraction osteotomy (PSO), the bone is typically removed from middle and posterior columns; however, the bone removed that is targeting sagittal imbalance is the in the middle columns (Fig. 13.11).

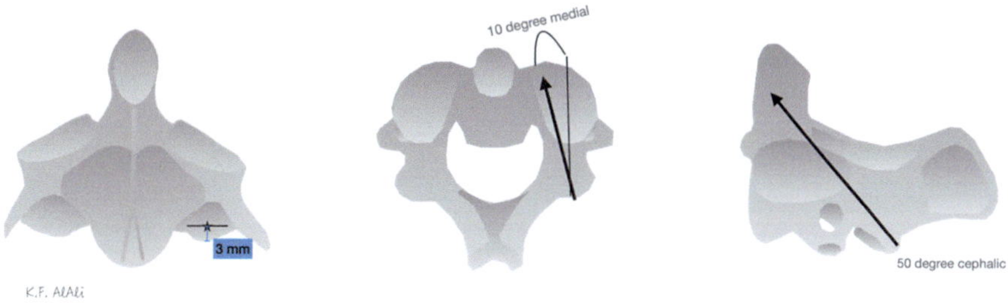

Fig. 13.10 C2 transarticular screw entry point and trajectory

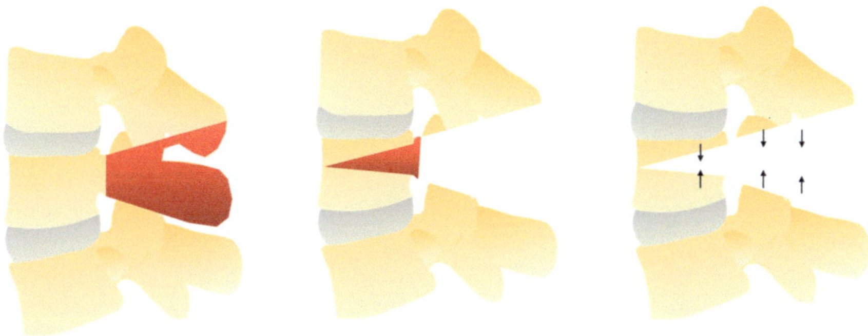

Fig. 13.11 In the pedicle subtraction osteotomy (PSO), the bone is typically removed from middle and posterior columns

20. The following anatomical landmark are important in safe thoracic pedicle screw insertion:
    A. Spinous process
    B. Superior facet joint
    C. Transverse process
    D. B and C

    Correct Answer: D

    Explanation:

    Generally, the entry point of the thoracic spine pedicle is at the junction of the proximal transverse process and lateral to the superior articular facet's midpoint. See next question answer for more details.

    (CN, p. 321)
21. The ideal entry point for a thoracic pedicle screw at T6 is:
    A. At the junction of the transverse process and lamina
    B. 3 mm inferior to the junction of the lateral edge of the superior facet and the transverse process
    C. At the midpoint of the transverse process
    D. At the intersection of a line extending from the medial border of superior articular process and the transverse process

    Correct Answer: B

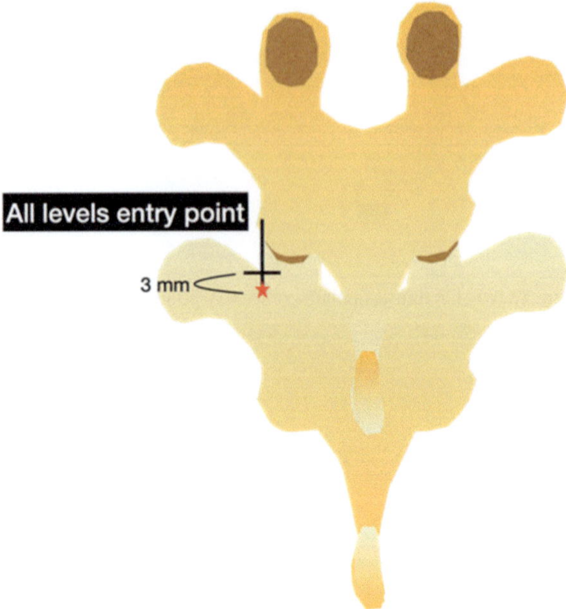

Fig. 13.12 The "all level" thoracic spine pedicle screw entry point

Explanation:

There are different methods to identify entry point for thoracic spine pedicle screw (Fig. 13.12):

- **Anatomic (Freehand) Technique:** It is level-specific. Entry points: Generally, the entry point is at the junction of the proximal transverse process and lateral to the superior articular facet's midpoint. In mid-thoracic levels, the entry is relatively medial and cranial, while it is more lateral and caudal at the upper and lower thoracic regions.
- **Laminotomy-Assisted Palpation:** A small laminotomy is performed to expose the medial and superior aspects of the pedicle. The surgeon palpates the pedicle with a probe, feeling for boundaries to confirm the correct trajectory.
- **Al level entry points:** This technique uses a uniform entry point across levels, allowing for a standardized approach throughout the thoracic spine. The entry point is at 3 mm inferior to the junction of the lateral edge of the superior facet and the transverse process (illustration).

  (GB, p.1794)

22. During a standard left-sided Lateral Lumbar Interbody Fusion (LLIF), why is the left side generally preferred over the right?

    A. Better access to disc space

    B. To avoid complications related to inferior vena cava

    C. To gain access to the L5–S1 disc space

    D. To avoid contact with the ureter

    Correct Answer: B

Table 13.5 Surgical technique: Lateral lumbar interbody fusion (LLIF)

Step	Technique/details
Positioning	Lateral decubitus position, typically left side up, stabilized with axillary rolls
Identify the level	AP and lateral fluoroscopic images; mark vertebral bodies and disc spaces on the skin
Incision	Make a direct lateral incision and a posterolateral incision above the pelvis for retroperitoneal access
Retroperitoneal access	Enter through posterolateral incision to reach retroperitoneal space; avoid peritoneum to prevent bowel injury
Localization	Palpate psoas with finger through retroperitoneal space to guide safe lateral approach trajectory
Blunt muscle dissection	Use Kocher clamps to bluntly dissect through oblique muscles to avoid muscle innervation disruption and pseudohernia
Dilator placement	Insert initial dilator and confirm level with lateral radiograph; stimulate to check proximity to lumbar plexus
Sequential dilation	Gradually insert larger dilators, stimulating each to check for lumbar plexus proximity
Retractor insertion	Place retractor over final dilator, verify placement with AP radiograph, and open blades to access anterior disc space
Disc access	Open retractor blades cranially and caudally for full access, verify position with AP radiograph
Nerve monitoring	Optionally, probe for lumbar plexus to confirm safety distance from retractor blades
Annulotomy	Perform annulotomy and use Cobb elevator to release annulus from endplates, checking with lateral fluoroscopy
Disc removal	Remove disc material using dilators, shavers, curettes, and pituitary rongeurs
Trial and Final Implant	Insert trial cage and confirm positioning; place final graft with bone graft

Explanation:

Some surgeons prefer a left-sided approach because of the abdominal aorta, iliac arteries, and vena cava. The left side might provide better access to disc space; however, that is not the key reason in left-side preferences (Table 13.5).

(RS, p. 368)

23. In the "open door" technique for cervical laminoplasty, a partial-thickncss cut is made:
    A. Bilaterally on both laminae
    B. Only on the dominant hand side
    C. Along one side at the junction of the lamina and lateral mass
    D. Only at the midline of the lamina

    Correct Answer: C

    Explanation:

    The open door technique involves a partial-thickness trough on one side at the junction between the lamina and lateral mass, while a complete cut is made on the other side to create a greenstick fracture on the partially cut side, allowing decompression. There are different variations of cervical laminoplasty, described in Table 13.6:

    (SSW, p. 1665))

Table 13.6 The different variations of cervical laminoplasty

Technique	Description	Fixation Method
Z-Plasty	Involves removing spinous processes and creating Z-shaped cuts in the lamina at the junction of the lateral mass. The laminae are separated to expand the spinal canal	Sutures or wires to secure laminae open
Open-door (Hirabayashi)	Bicortical cut on the "open" side and a more lateral trough on the "closed" side. The door is lifted and held open, creating a greenstick fracture on the partially cut side	Nonabsorbable sutures, bone graft, or titanium miniplates
Double-door (French-Door)	Symmetrical midline opening; laminae are lifted off the spinal cord after bilateral trough cuts	Bone graft, sutures, titanium screws, ceramic or hydroxyapatite spacers
Muscle-sparing	Developed to maintain paraspinal muscle attachments and reduce postoperative neck pain. Includes techniques like myoarchitectonic spinolaminoplasty, preserving muscle attachments to the spinous processes	Not specified, less invasive
En bloc laminoplasty	Preferred for high-recurrence intradural pathologies; laminae are removed and replaced in original positions to reconstruct ligamentous tension band, with minimal scarring	Sutures or miniplates, figure-of-eight stitch

24. During a transforaminal endoscopic lumbar discectomy (TELD), which anatomical landmark is critical for needle placement to safely access the disc space through Kambin's triangle?
    A. The cranial aspect of the caudal vertebral body
    B. The midpoint of the intervertebral disc space
    C. The superior articular process (SAP)
    D. The lateral edge of the spinous process

    Correct Answer: C

    Explanation:

    The SAP serves as a critical landmark for guiding the needle trajectory through Kambin's triangle, which provides safe access to the disc space while avoiding the nerve roots. The axial MRI should be thoroughly reviewed. A line should be drawn from the disc pathology site through the superior articular process (SAP) to the skin surface, with an ideal trajectory as close to the ventral aspect of the SAP as possible. This line will help determine the incision's lateral distance from the midline and the extent of SAP resection required (Fig. 13.13).
25. In the fluoroscopic planning phase of TELD (Table 13.7), how is the cranial-caudal trajectory optimized for safe access to the disc pathology, and what degree of angulation is typically used?
    A. The trajectory connects the midpoint of the intervertebral space with the lateral pedicular line at 5°–10°.
    B. A 15°–20° angle to avoid the retroperitoneum, targeting the lateral recess.
    C. The upper superior articular process (SAP) is aligned with the medial pedicular line at the disc space level, angled at 10°–15°.

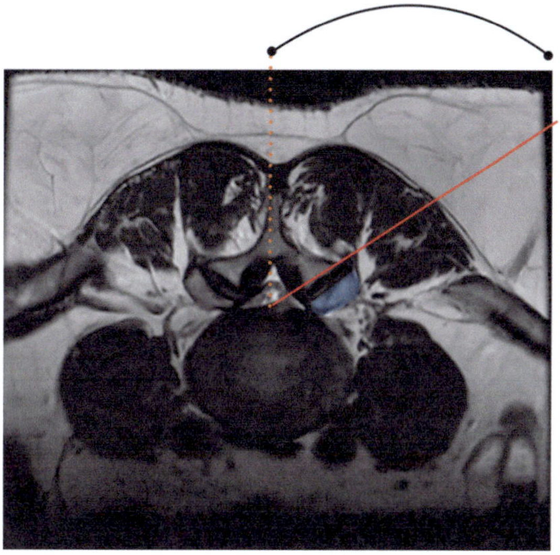

Fig. 13.13 Measurement of the incision in transforminal discectomy. The blue shaded area is the amount needed to be resected from the superior articular surface

D. The cranial pedicle is aligned with the posterior vertebral body line, angled at 5°–15°.

Correct Answer: C

Explanation:

The cranial-caudal trajectory is optimized by angling at 10°–15°, aligning the upper SAP with the medial pedicular line to ensure safe access without retroperitoneal entry.

(ES, pp. 193–202)

26. In the paraspinal (Wiltse) approach to the lumbar spine, which anatomical interval is utilized to access the surgical site?
    A. Interval between the longissimus and iliocostalis muscles
    B. Interval between the multifidus and longissimus muscles
    C. Interval between the multifidus and erector spinae muscles
    D. Interval between the iliocostalis and quadratus lumborum muscles

Correct Answer: B

Explanation:

The paraspinal (Wiltse) approach is a posterolateral lumbar technique. It accesses the spine between the multifidus and longissimus muscles. The lumbodorsal fascia is incised two fingerbreadths from the midline. Blunt dissection or tubular dilators expose the facet joint and interlaminar space. This method removes extraforaminal disc herniations and decompresses stenosis. It avoids resecting the pars interarticularis or facet complex. It also allows pedicle screw placement and intertransverse fusions. Unilateral facet resection creates a direct path for interbody fusion, such as TLIF.

(SS, p. 264)

Table 13.7 Surgical technique: Transforaminal endoscopic lumbar discectomy (TELD)

Step	Details
Approach & Goal	Access disc pathology via Kambin's triangle, a safe corridor under the exiting nerve root. Ideal for treating posterolateral disc herniations and foraminal pathologies without extensive facetectomy or fusion
Required instruments	Endoscopy Cart (video, pump, RF unit, drill) Transforaminal Endoscope Reamers K-wire 18-gauge Spinal Needle Blunt Dissector Micro-punch Grasping Forceps Kerrison Rongeur Bipolar Coagulator Burr C-arm
Positioning	Patient prone on a Wilson frame or with pelvic/thoracic rolls
Fluoroscopic target identification	Pre-op MRI: Plan trajectory from disc pathology through SAP to skin, focusing on a ventral SAP entry **AP X-ray** for midline identification and square endplate view Planning lines drawn on AP X-ray for incision (L3–L5: ~8 cm; L4–L5: ~10 cm; L5–S1: ~12 cm from midline) Trajectory: 10°–15°, ensuring tip aligns with SAP and medial pedicular line
Procedure Steps	1. Insert 18-gauge needle at planned entry site, advance to SAP, and guide into Kambin's triangle 2. Insert K-wire, remove needle, and use dilators for corridor expansion 3. Use reamers for foraminoplasty if needed, creating space without crossing medial pedicle line 4. Insert beveled working channel and secure with AP/lateral X-rays
Intraoperative Monitoring	Keep awake patient feedback for nerve irritation (or EMG in sedated patients) Adjust needle if patient reports discomfort or EMG signals indicate nerve pressure
Visualization	Target areas: SAP, cranial pedicle aspect For foraminal herniations, rotate working channel to protect exiting nerve root For central/posterolateral herniations, resect lateral ligamentum flavum and secure traversing nerve root
Disc Fragment Removal	Use dissector or coagulator probe to mobilize fragments, remove with pituitary rongeurs
Neural Element Mobilization	Rotate bevel to inspect traversing and exiting nerve roots, using a blunt dissector or curved probe for mobilization
Endoscope Removal & Closure	Achieve hemostasis with agents or bipolar cautery Remove endoscope; close with deep dermal or subcuticular stitch as needed

27. In a Smith–Petersen osteotomy (SPO), the bone resected is primarily from:
    A. The posterior elements
    B. The Middle column
    C. Inferior facet joint
    D. All of the above

    Correct Answer: C

    Explanation:

    Smith–Petersen osteotomy (SPO) involves resection of the inferior facet and joint capsule and requires a mobile, non-fused anterior column for effective results. This procedure offers limited deformity correction, typically allowing for about 5–10 degrees of adjustment.

    (GB, p. 1356)
28. In scoliosis surgery, the Ponte osteotomy is performed at the level of:
    A. The apex of the curve
    B. The end vertebrae
    C. The neutral vertebrae
    D. Every level where screws are placed

    Correct Answer: A

    Explanation:

    Ponte osteotomy also known as extension osteotomy is similar to the Smith–Peterson osteotomy. It involves resection of inferior and superior facets, ligamentum flavum, and sometimes the spinous process. It is commonly used in scoliosis and the resection is usually at the apex of the curve (Table 13.8).

    (RS, p. 532)
29. A 58-year-old patient with a thoracic spine tumor at T7–T8 is scheduled for decompression via a costotransversectomy approach. The surgeon plans to achieve optimal exposure of the anterior spinal canal without compromising stability. Which of the following steps is most critical for maintaining stability while allowing access to the tumor?
    A. Dissecting the rib head without resecting the transverse process
    B. Resection of the inferior rib along with the adjacent transverse process at T7
    C. Removing the transverse process only, avoiding rib dissection to minimize muscle disruption
    D. Ligation of the intercostal vessels and resection of the facet join

    Correct Answer: B

    Explanation:

    In costotransversectomy, the resection of the adjacent rib and transverse process provides a wider lateral corridor to the anterior canal, which is essential for effective decompression and tumor access while preserving stability. Only removing the transverse process or avoiding rib resection limits exposure.

    (SSW, p. 1686)
30. The major difference between the lateral extracavitary approach and the costotransversectomy is:
    A. A larger lateral resection of the inferior rib is performed in lateral extracavitary approach

Table 13.8 Types of spinal osteotomies

Osteotomy type	Description	Surgical approach	Typical correction	Other names
Smith–Petersen Osteotomy (SPO)	Resection of the inferior facet and joint capsule, often in the lumbar spine. Requires a mobile anterior column	Posterolateral	5–10°	Opening wedge, Chevron Osteotomy
Ponte Osteotomy	Resection of inferior and superior facets, ligamentum flavum, and sometimes the spinous process, commonly used in scoliosis	Posterior	10–15°	Extension Osteotomy
Pedicle Subtraction Osteotomy (PSO)	Wedge resection of the vertebral body including the posterior elements and pedicles	Transpedicular	25–35°	Closing wedge, Transpedicular
Extended Pedicle Subtraction Osteotomy (EPSO)	Similar to PSO, but includes additional resection of the endplate and adjacent intervertebral disc for increased correction	Transpedicular with extended resection	35–40°	
Vertebral Column Resection (VCR)	Complete removal of a vertebral body and its adjacent intervertebral discs, often in severe deformity cases	Anterior or combined posterior and anterior	40–60°	

B. A Larger vertebral body is performed in costotransversectomy approach
C. Spinal nerve root is scarified in lateral extracavitary approach
D. Spinal nerve root is scarified in costotransversectomy approach

Correct Answer: A

Explanation:

In lateral extracavitary approach, a larger lateral resection of the inferior rib is performed. The following tables outlines both techniques (Tables 13.9 and 13.10; Fig. 13.14):

(SSW, p. 1686)

31. While performing costotransversectomy for T7–T8 discectomy, the rib that is needed to be resected is:

A. 7th rib
B. 8th rib
C. Both 7th and 8th ribs
D. No ribs needed to be resected

Correct Answer: B

Explanation:

In costotransversectomy , the bony resection starts by locating the rib adjacent to the lower vertebral body (for example, rib 8 for a T7–T8 disc). The rib

Table 13.9 Surgical technique: costotransversectomy

Step	Description
Purpose	Provides a lateral corridor for improved access to the anterior spinal canal, especially for thoracic disc herniations, fractures, tumors, infections, and deformities
Developers	Initially developed by Hulme and Menard
Positioning	Prone or partial lateral position; allows versatile access and positioning based on specific requirements
Incision type	Longer than transpedicular, typically curvilinear or paramedian to allow wide exposure; spans multiple segments above and below the affected region, or longer midline incision
Bony and muscular dissection	Involves significant dissection of trapezius and erector spinae to expose ribs and transverse processes; rib removal typically begins with identifying and freeing the rib near the target vertebra Specific muscles dissection as above can be avoided with midline incision which require muscle retraction as a bulk
Landmarks	Key landmarks include the pedicle, neurovascular bundles of the resected rib, and the pleura. The pleura is retracted with malleable retractors to prevent injury
Disc removal	Pedicle drilled just inferior to the affected disc; herniated disc exposed from its lateral aspect and removed in stages, from lateral to central regions
Closure	Involves careful inspection of the pleura for tears; small pleural tears closed with sutures, larger tears with chest tube placement
Risks	Risks include increased postoperative pain, radicular artery damage, and potential pneumothorax

Table 13.10 Surgical technique: lateral extracavitary

Step	Description
Purpose and origin	Developed in 1976 by Larson for traumatic thoracic spine injuries; modified from Capener's 1954 technique for tuberculous spondylitis. Offers extensive visualization of anterior spinal canal
Incision types	Either a hockey-stick incision centered over the affected level, a curvilinear incision with medial convexity or long midline incision
Comparison to costotransversectomy	**Involves a larger lateral resection of the rib**, allowing a lower viewing angle toward the canal compared to costotransversectomy
Procedure details	Begins with resecting the inferior rib and transverse process to expose the canal; hemilaminectomy may follow, allowing ligation and rotation of nerve root for better thecal sac exposure
Disc removal and vertebral drilling	After lateral removal, central nucleus pulposus and remaining herniated material are retracted and removed. Portions of vertebral body may be drilled to improve disc access; rib struts can be used for grafting
Closure	Closure follows costotransversectomy techniques, with pleural inspection, irrigation, and potential chest tube placement for pleural injuries

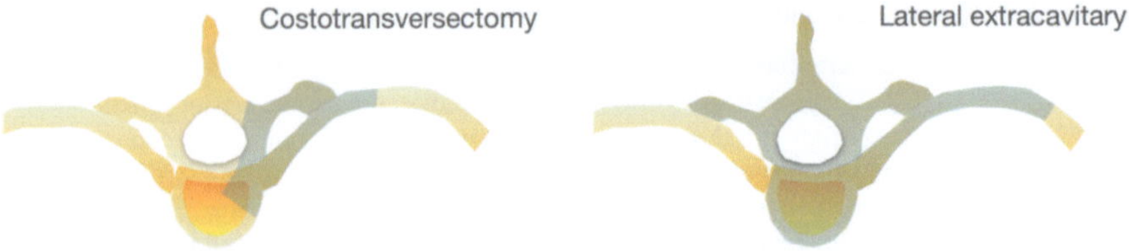

Fig. 13.14 Resection area (shaded area) in costotransversectomy compared to lateral extracavitary approach

is then carefully dissected away from the surrounding fascia and pleura before resection.

(SSW, p. 1686)

32. A 65-year-old male with T6 osteomyelitis undergoes costotransversectomy. During surgery, the pleura is disrupted. What is the best next step?
    A. Ignore the tear if small
    B. Suture the tear and continue
    C. Cover with a hemostatic agent
    D. Place a chest tube after surgery

    Correct Answer: D

    Explanation:

    A chest tube is required to prevent pneumothorax when the pleura is disrupted during a costotransversectomy. This step is essential to manage any air or fluid accumulation that could lead to respiratory complications postoperatively.

    (SSW, p. 1686)

33. In performing an anterior cervical foraminotomy, the key landmark for identifying the nerve root is:
    A. The uncinate process
    B. The vertebral artery
    C. The pedicle
    D. The dorsal root ganglion

    Correct Answer: A

    Explanation:

    The key landmark for identifying nerve root when doing foraminotomy during anterior cervical discectomy and fusion is the uncinate process. The following table summarizes the anterior foraminotomy:

34. The best sign to ensure adequate decompression when performing anterior cervical foraminotomy is
    A. Loss of cerebrospinal fluid (CSF) from the foramen
    B. A "blush" of blood from the neural foramen
    C. Absence of any bleeding from the foramen
    D. Easy pass of Woodson instrument

    Correct Answer: C

Table 13.11 Surgical technique: anterior cervical foraminotomy

Step	Description
Exposure	As ACDF exposure
PLL preservation	Keep the posterior longitudinal ligament (PLL) intact during foraminotomy to provide protection until decompression is completed
Uncinate process thinning	Use a burr to thin the medial posterior uncinate process; ensure awareness of vertebral artery location based on preoperative imaging to prevent inadvertent injury
Microscope positioning	Angle the microscope toward the foramen for enhanced visualization during decompression
Contralateral decompression	It is easier to perform contralateral decompression with a Kerrison rongeur and curette for complete access to the foramen; however, drill can be used as well
Nerve hook assessment	Use a nerve hook to assess decompression adequacy. Guide the hook at a 45-degree angle along the posterior uncinate to prevent nerve injury, as the nerve exits ventrolaterally
Sign of adequate decompression	**A "blush" of blood** from the neural foramen often signals that decompression is adequate
PLL removal	Once decompression is complete, excise the PLL with a Kerrison rongeur to clear the disc space
Final check for compression	After disc resection and endplate decortication, use a nerve hook to identify any residual compression sources, especially posterior osteophytes at the cranial and caudal edges of the disc space

Explanation:

The following table summarizes the anterior foraminotomy (Table 13.11): (RS, p. 746)

35. When utilizing the L5–S1 mini-open anterior lumbar interbody fusion (ALIF) approach, the most common vessel retraction is performed on:
    A. The aorta and vena cava for right-sided approaches
    B. The aorta and vena cava for left-sided approaches
    C. The iliac vessels for right-sided approaches
    D. The iliac vessels for left-sided approaches

    Correct Answer: D

    Explanation:

    At the L5–S1 level, the central two-thirds of the disc space can typically be accessed without substantial mobilization of the iliac vessels. However, in instances where the left iliac vessels cross obliquely over the central to left side of the disc space, gentle mobilization is necessary. In these cases, the vessels are carefully displaced from the sacral promontory using Kittner dissectors.

    (EM, p. 168)

36. A patient experiences recurrent radiculopathy after posterior cervical foraminotomy. Which intraoperative factor most likely contributed to this outcome?
    (a) Failure to remove the medial 50% of the inferior articular process
    (b) Overuse of a Kerrison rongeur during facet joint thinning
    (c) Insufficient irrigation leading to thermal injury of nerve roots
    (d) Incomplete identification of the exiting nerve root trajectory

    Correct Answer: A

Explanation:

Recurrent radiculopathy is usually caused by inadequate neural foramen decompression. This occurs when the medial 50% of the inferior articular process is not removed, leaving residual compression on the nerve root. The other factors are less commonly implicated in recurrent symptoms.

(EM, pp. 61–69)

37. When performing posterior cervical foraminotomy, which step ensures safe decompression without increasing the risk of nerve root injury?
    (a) Removing the lateral lamina completely to expose the nerve root
    (b) Thinning the inferior articular process until translucent before removal
    (c) Visualizing the dural sac before identifying the pedicle
    (d) Using a Kerrison to aggressively remove uncovertebral joint osteophytes

    Correct Answer: B

    Explanation:

    Thinning the inferior articular process of the vertebra above until it is translucent ensures that bone removal is precise and minimizes the risk of inadvertently injuring the nerve root. This approach also avoids unnecessary manipulation of surrounding structures (Table 13.12; Fig. 13.15).

    (EM, pp. 61–69)

38. In a pedicle screw-based dynamic stabilization system, the flexible connecting device is typically made of:
    A. Titanium
    B. Polycarbonate urethane (PCU)
    C. Polyethylene terephthalate (PET)
    D. Cobalt–chromium alloy

    Correct Answer: C

    Explanation:

    In pedicle screw-based dynamic stabilization systems, such as Dynesys, the flexible connecting device or cord is typically made of **polyethylene terephthalate (PET)**. This material is chosen for its strength to constrain spinal motion and flexibility to reduce the load on adjacent segments.

    (SSW, p. 1798)

39. A 72-year-old with a type II odontoid fracture needs odontoid screw fixation. The surgeon struggles to see the odontoid fracture due to the mandible. What is the best way to improve visualization?
    A. Reposition the patient's head in slight flexion to lower the mandible.
    B. Place a radiolucent plate with an insufflation bag under the neck to adjust the cervical spine angle.
    C. Increase the retractor angle to improve anterior exposure of the odontoid process.
    D. Perform a partial dissection of the longus colli muscle for additional retraction.

    Correct Answer: B

Table 13.12 Surgical technique: posterior cervical foraminotomy

Step	Key points
Positioning	Patient is positioned prone on a reversed OR table with a Mayfield head holder and chest bolsters Table inclined 20°–30° reverse Trendelenburg; Mayfield adjusted for neck flexion to reduce redundant skin and facilitate facet exposure Shoulders taped for radiographic localization
Neuromonitoring	Neuromonitoring generally unnecessary
Incision localization	Use external occipital protuberance, C2, and C7 spinous processes for incision landmarks Use a lateral C-arm X-ray prepped with a metallic marker on the skin Confirm levels intraoperatively with a lateral C-arm and spinal needle on the facet
Approach	Midline incision for bilateral; unilateral can use 2 cm lateral or midline incision Subperiosteal dissection to expose facet joint and lateral mass-laminar junction Expose more than 50% of the facet while considering the lateral edge location
Retractor placement	McCulloch retractor or alike with blade laterally and hook on the interspinous ligament
Decompression technique	Address compressive elements: superior articular process (SAP) and uncovertebral osteophyte/disk herniation Medial facet resection (50%) to uncover nerve root Burr thinning of inferior articular process of vertebra above until translucent; bone removed with curette or Kerrison rongeur Venous bleeding managed with gelfoam packing
Discectomy	Remove extruded fragments; manipulate nerve root if needed for intraforaminal herniations Cranial pedicle resection possible for access with microsurgical instruments
Closure	No drain required Deep muscle and fascial layers closed with Vicryl figure-of-eight sutures; dermal and skin layers closed with Vicryl and subcuticular Monocryl sutures
Postoperative care	Detailed neurological exam post-op Optional soft collar for less than 2 weeks Resume range of motion as tolerated

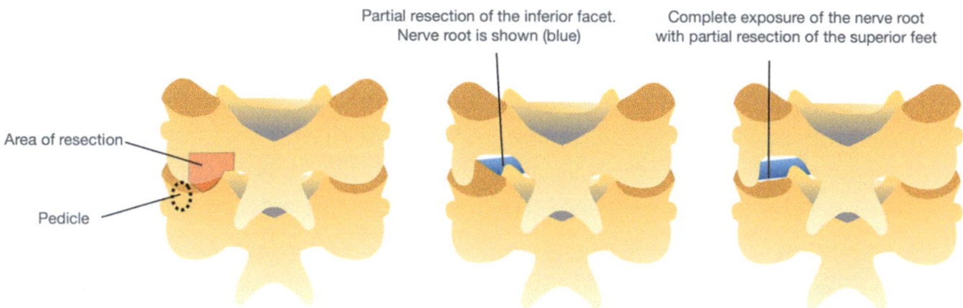

Fig. 13.15 Steps of nerve root exposure in posterior cervical foraminotomy. The nerve root is illustrated as blue

Explanation:

Using a radiolucent plate with an insufflation bag under the neck helps adjust the cervical angle and gently translates the spine anteriorly, improving the alignment and visualization of the odontoid without altering head positioning or muscle dissection, which would increase risk.

(SSW, p. 1884)

40. During odontoid screw fixation, which of the following patient factors would most likely necessitate reconsideration of the technique due to increased risk of improper screw placement and potential complications?
    A. Mild osteopenia affecting C1 and C2
    B. Oblique fracture in the plane of screw insertion
    C. Reduced mobility in the C1–C2 articulation
    D. Midline odontoid fracture displacement of 1–2 mm

    Correct Answer: B

    Explanation:

    An oblique fracture in the plane of the screw insertion (posterior–superior to anterior–inferior fracture) presents a challenge for maintaining secure fixation and proper alignment, increasing the risk of misplacement or failure to properly stabilize the fracture. Other conditions like mild osteopenia and minor midline displacement are typically manageable in the context of odontoid screw fixation, but oblique fractures in the screw path can significantly compromise the procedure's effectiveness (Table 13.13).

    (SSW, p. 1884)

41. The primary indication for a transpedicular approach to a thoracic disc herniation is:
    A. Central disc herniation
    B. Calcified disc herniation
    C. Laterally located disc herniation
    D. Disc herniation with significant kyphosis

    Correct Answer: C

    Explanation:

    Laminectomy is generally considered an unsuitable option for managing thoracic disc herniations. Instead, posterior techniques—such as the transpedicular, Stillerman transfacet pedicle-sparing, transcostovertebral, costotransversectomy, and lateral extracavitary approaches—are often preferred for **lateral**, non-calcified, extradural disc herniations. They usually cause instability and require instrumentation and fusion. In contrast, anterior approaches, including transthoracic, retropleural, and transsternal techniques, are better suited for centrally located, calcified, or intradural disc herniations, as they provide superior ventral exposure. Both posterior and anterior approaches have comparable complication rates.

    (SSW, p. 1681)

Table 13.13 Procedure: anterior odontoid screw placement

Steps	Details
Preoperative assessment	**Imaging**: AP, lateral, and open-mouth odontoid views, plus thin-cut CT **Challenges**: Any deformity of body figure that may obstruct screw trajectory like short neck, barrel chest, or kyphotic alignment; scout CT views can help assess possible instrument paths **Contraindications**: Severe osteopenia, chronic nonunion, posterior displacement, complex fracture patterns, irreducible canal compromise or fracture patterns that extend from posterior–superior to anterior–inferior (see below) 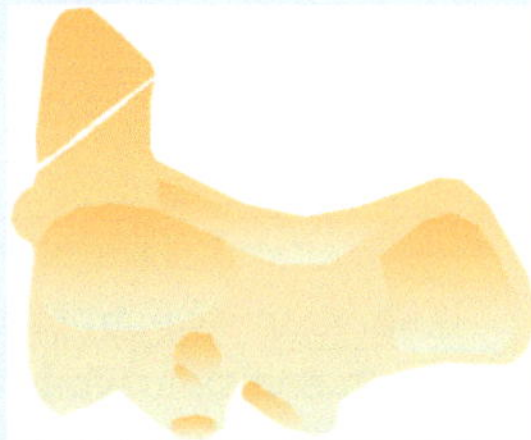 Posterior–superior to anterior–inferior fracture (same as plane of the screw insertion) is contraindicated
Positioning	**Setup**: Supine on a radiolucent table with a shoulder roll for neck extension, which aids in achieving the proper screw trajectory **Stabilization**: Gardner–Wells tongs with 10 lbs of traction stabilize the head and assist with fracture reduction or Mayfield head clamp if fracture is reduced **Fluoroscopy**: AP and lateral fluoroscopy
Surgical technique	**Approach**: Standard anterior cervical approach— **Instrumentation**: K-wire is inserted to mark the trajectory, using AP and lateral fluoroscopy for guidance. Avoid advancing the K-wire past the cortex initially to prevent penetration of the brainstem **Screw Placement**: A cannulated screw is placed over the K-wire, achieving bicortical purchase when feasible
Instrumentation details	**Measurement**: Screw length is measured using the K-wire for bicortical purchase, which helps compress the fracture site without exceeding safe depths **Guidewire Technique**: During drilling, slightly retract the K-wire to avoid pushing it into the brainstem. Drilling is completed under biplanar fluoroscopy, and a partially threaded screw is passed over the K-wire to compress the fracture **Verification**: By fluoroscopic views confirm depth and positioning
Postoperative management	**Stabilization**: cervical collar for 6–12 weeks **Early Mobilization**: Encourage early movement to aid recovery **Follow-up Imaging**: CT: immediate post op and 6–12 months post-op should show fracture healing and preservation of C1–2 motion without translation

42. A 60-year-old patient with a lateralized T8–T9 disc herniation is scheduled for a transfacet pedicle-sparing decompression. During the procedure, the surgeon notes difficulty accessing the disc space without affecting the pedicle. Which of the following adjustments would best improve access to the herniation while maintaining the pedicle-sparing intent?
    A. Shift the surgical approach to the contralateral side to improve the viewing angle.
    B. Increase the depth of facet joint drilling to penetrate the lateral aspect of the foramen.
    C. Adjust the surgical approach to a more lateral entry point on the facet joint to expose the disc space.
    D. Change to a transpedicular approach for a more direct path to the disc.

    Correct Answer: C

    Explanation:

    In the transfacet pedicle-sparing approach, modifying the entry point to a more lateral position on the facet joint can improve access to the lateral disc herniation without compromising the pedicle, allowing better visualization and decompression while preserving structural integrity. Switching to a transpedicular approach, while direct, would defeat the pedicle-sparing intent (Table 13.14).

    (SSW, p. 1681)

43. During a C6 anterior cervical corpectomy and fusion (ACCF), the surgeon encounters ossification of the posterior longitudinal ligament (OPLL) firmly adherent to the dura. Which of the following techniques would be most appropriate to safely proceed with decompression?
    A. Use a high-speed burr to completely resect the ossified PLL and decompress the spinal cord directly.
    B. Leave a small bone island adherent to the PLL to avoid direct manipulation of the ossified tissue.
    C. Perform a posterior approach to reach the PLL and remove it without dura involvement.
    D. Use a Kerrison rongeur to remove the PLL and reduce compression at the midline level.

    Correct Answer: B

    Explanation:

    In cases with OPLL, leaving a small bone island attached to the PLL minimizes the risk of dural tears or neurologic injury, as the ossified PLL may be tightly adherent to the dura. This approach avoids aggressive resection and helps reduce potential complications during ACCF (Table 13.15).

    (RS, p. 748)

44. During a transoral decompression of C1–C2, the surgeon encounters difficulty visualizing the anterior arch of the atlas. Which of the following adjustments is most likely to improve surgical visualization while minimizing risks?
    A. Increasing the length of the posterior pharyngeal mucosal incision to 6 cm
    B. Applying traction with Caspar posts to the C1 vertebra

Table 13.14 Surgical technique: transpedicular approach for thoracic disc

Step	Description
Purpose and origin	Provides lateral access to the spinal canal ventral to the spinal cord, primarily for thoracic disc herniations. Developed by Patterson and Arbit in 1978 as a modification of Carson's 1971 technique
Positioning	Prone on gel rolls or a Wilson frame to ensure stability
Incision and exposure	Vertical midline incision centered over the level of interest; unilateral exposure is performed to minimize trauma to contralateral paravertebral muscles
Dissection technique	Dissection proceeds through the thoracodorsal fascia, followed by subperiosteal dissection to expose the lateral facets on the affected side using Cobb elevators
Pedicle localization	Pedicle located 1–2 mm below the edge of the inferior facet of the superior vertebra. For example, for T7–T8 herniation, the T8 pedicle is drilled, located just below the T7 inferior facet
Bone removal	A pneumatic drill and 2-mm Kerrison rongeurs are used to perform a lateral laminotomy to visualize the lateral edge of the thecal sac, extending bone removal to the medial facet and ventral pedicle
Pedicle drilling	Pedicle interior is drilled with protection provided by the superior and medial cortex; performed with an operating microscope to maintain precision
Disc access and removal	After pedicle resection, lateral disc space and spinal canal are visible. The lateral herniated disc is incised, and disc material is removed centrally. Medial herniated tissue is displaced back into the disc space using a down-biting curet
Closure	Closure is similar to standard posterior lumbar or cervical procedures, following careful inspection of the dura
Surgical technique:	**transfacet pedicle-sparing approach**
Purpose and origin	Developed by Stillerman and colleagues, this approach offers access to thoracic disc herniations while sparing the pedicle, reducing the structural impact on the vertebra
Positioning	Prone, similar to the transpedicular technique
Incision and exposure	A midline linear incision is made. Standard dissection and subperiosteal exposure are performed to reveal the ipsilateral facet joint
Fluoroscopic verification	AP fluoroscopy is used to confirm the correct spinal level and facet joint alignment during exposure and preparation
Bone removal	The medial aspect of the facet joint is drilled with a pneumatic drill to access the neural foramen, without resecting the underlying pedicle, which is preserved
Foramen and disc space access	Upon reaching the neural foramen, blunt dissection is used to access the disc space at the inferior aspect of the foramen. The exiting nerve root, often located at the superior foramen, is typically not encountered except in higher levels
Disc removal	The annulus is identified, and disc material is removed similarly to other posterior approaches, allowing decompression without extensive bone resection
Advantages	Avoids pedicle resection, preserving vertebral structure while providing adequate access to the disc space and reducing the risk to the nerve root, especially in lower thoracic levels

Table 13.15 Surgical technique: Anterior Cervical Corpectomy and Fusion (ACCF)

Step	Description
Positioning	Supine an ipsilateral anterior cervical incision, usually right side
Level confirmation	After exposure, Caspar distraction posts are placed in the vertebral bodies above and below the levels to be removed to confirm and stabilize the surgical level
Discectomy and osteophyte removal	Discectomies are performed at levels cranial and caudal to the corpectomy. Osteophytes are removed to improve visualization of uncovertebral joints for centering the resection
Vertebral body resection	A 5-mm midline trough is created using a Leksell rongeur and burr for controlled resection of the vertebral body. The width of resection is 15–18 mm to accommodate the graft
Posterior cortex removal	After debulking, a curette removes the thin posterior cortex, directed anteriorly to avoid damage to the dura. The PLL is then excised with a Kerrison rongeur, unless it is adherent due to OPLL (ossification), where complete resection may risk dural tear
Endplate preparation	Endplates are prepared by removing cartilage with a burr to expose subchondral bone, enhancing fusion potential. Measurements for graft or cage size are taken
Graft selection and insertion	Graft options include iliac crest bone graft for smaller defects, fibular graft/cage for larger reconstructions or a cage filled with graft. Cervical traction (~30 lbs) is applied for graft placement, and its position is verified fluoroscopically
Plating	A plate spanning the corpectomy region is secured with screws in vertebral bodies above and below the graft to increase stability. Final plate position is confirmed with fluoroscopy
Postoperative immobilization	Patients may use a semirigid orthosis for 6–10 weeks based on construct stability. Activities involving cervical spine twisting, bending, and overhead lifting are restricted until fusion is confirmed

C. Using a Mayfield retractor and hyperextending the neck with a shoulder roll
D. Extending the incision laterally to improve exposure of the lateral masses

Correct Answer: C

Explanation:

Neck hyperextension using a shoulder roll combined with a Mayfield retractor improves visualization in the confined transoral field. This adjustment enhances the surgical view by expanding the interdental distance and aiding direct access to the anterior atlas without altering the incision's midline focus.

(RS, p. 325)

45. A surgeon performing a transoral approach for odontoid resection makes a 4-cm midline incision. During dissection, they encounter resistance while trying to access the medial edge of the C1–C2 facet. What precaution should the surgeon take to avoid a critical vascular complication at this stage?
   A. Use a high-speed burr to thin the lateral masses.
   B. Limit dissection strictly to the midline and avoid extending beyond the facet joint's medial edge.
   C. Increase cervical traction to improve exposure of the vertebral artery.
   D. Extend the mucosal incision laterally to ensure complete exposure of the transverse foramen.

Correct Answer: B

Explanation:

Staying within the midline and limiting dissection near the C1–C2 facet joint's medial edge is crucial, as extending laterally increases the risk of vertebral artery injury, a potentially life-threatening complication of the transoral approach (Table 13.16).

(RS, p. 325)

46. During a lumbar laminectomy for stenosis, the surgeon prepares to remove the ligamentum flavum. Which of the following techniques is essential to minimize the risk of dural tears and nerve root injury during ligamentum flavum removal?
    A. Retract the ligamentum flavum laterally with a Kerrison rongeur before resecting.
    B. Use a forward-angled curette to detach the ligamentum flavum from the caudal lamina and lift it from the dura.
    C. Insert a Penfield 4 under the ligamentum flavum and use sharp dissection.
    D. Remove the ligamentum flavum by grasping with forceps and applying traction inferiorly.

    Correct Answer: B

Table 13.16 Surgical technique: transoral approach for upper cervical spine

Step	Description
Antibiotic use	Broad-spectrum antibiotics are administered preoperatively to cover both gram-positive and gram-negative bacteria. Antibiotics are continued for 3 days post-surgery to minimize infection risk
Incision and approach	A vertical incision (3–5 cm) is made through the posterior pharyngeal mucosa, centered around 1 cm below the C1 anterior tubercle. Careful midline dissection is essential to avoid damaging lateral structures, e.g., vertebral artery
Exposure limitations	Exposure is limited by factors such as interdental distance, neck extension, and conditions like TMJ stiffness or basilar invagination. Minimum recommended interdental distance is 25 mm for sufficient surgical access
Mandibulotomy (optional)	To increase exposure, a mandibulotomy may be performed, involving a midline incision on the lower lip and osteotomy between the central incisors. Titanium plates are pre-drilled for later reattachment to prevent malocclusion
Risks and complications	Risks include infection, wound dehiscence, and vascular injury. Infection risk is high due to pharyngeal flora exposure. Venous hemorrhage is manageable, but arterial injuries can be severe (vertebral artery), sometimes requiring urgent intervention
Infection management	Infection risk can be reduced by minimizing bone graft use and maintaining sterile conditions. Nasogastric (NG) tube placement postoperatively helps prevent wound contamination by reducing oral secretions
Postoperative airway care	Due to swelling or hemorrhage risk, some patients may need an endotracheal tube for 24 h post-surgery. Nasogastric tube is retained for 5–7 days to allow mucosal healing and prevent aspiration or reflux
Wound closure issues	Difficulty with closure, especially if the incision reaches C3, is managed by ensuring graft placement within vertebral boundaries or by creating lateral flaps for adequate tissue coverage

Explanation:

Using a forward-angled curette to carefully detach the ligamentum flavum protects the dura by controlling the detachment process in a medial-to-lateral direction. Then the rest of the flavum can be removed by Kerrison rongeur in piecemeal fashion. This minimizes the risk of dural injury and ensures safe removal (Table 13.17).

(RS, p. 364)

47. During the interlaminar lumbar endoscopic discectomy approach, which of the following BEST describes the correct sequence and approach for accessing the ligamentum flavum and epidural space safely?
    A. Begin with a medial skin incision at the interlaminar space; advance a dilator to the ligamentum flavum; insert the working sleeve facing laterally, and use a punch to make a single incision through the ligamentum flavum.
    B. Perform an incision 2 cm lateral to the interlaminar space; advance the dilator to the inferior edge of the cranial lamina; rotate the working sleeve to expose the ligamentum flavum; incise in a single step and enter the epidural space.
    C. Position the dilator at the ligamentum flavum with AP and lateral fluoroscopic confirmation; insert the working sleeve with its opening medially; incise the ligamentum flavum layer-by-layer using a punch, and monitor for color change to confirm depth.

Table 13.17 Surgical technique: lumbar posterior exposure and laminectomy

Step	Description
Positioning	Prone with abdomen free to allow venous drainage, reducing plexus pressure around the cauda equina. Use padding for bony prominences to prevent injury
Incision and exposure	Midline incision at the target spinal level. Dissect erector spinae and multifidus muscles from bony structures using electrocautery, elevating paraspinal muscles subperiosteally to minimize blood loss
Avoiding structures	Avoid facet joint capsules and interspinous ligaments in areas that require preserved motion postoperatively. For wider exposure, dissect to the transverse processes if necessary
Ligamentum flavum removal	**Detach the ligamentum flavum with a curette at the caudal edge of the lamina, lifting it with an elevator to protect the dura**, then remove it with a Kerrison or pituitary rongeur
Hemostasis	Control bleeding from epidural veins using bipolar cautery, cottonoids, Surgicel, or Gelfoam
Discectomy preparation	For discectomy, gently retract the traversing nerve root medially and use a Penfield 4 to identify the disc space above the pedicle
Laminectomy	Use a high-speed burr to thin lamina or a rongeur to remove it, protecting dura from accidental injury
Lateral recess and foramen exploration	Explore lateral recesses and foramen to ensure adequate nerve root decompression. Remove ligamentum flavum and osteophytes carefully, preserving <50% of the facet joint for stability
Closure	Muscle are approximated, fascia is closed with Vicryl 0.0 to decrease dead space and then subcutaneous tissue and skin

D. Make a midline incision at the interlaminar space; place the dilator directly against the superior articulating process; insert the working sleeve laterally and puncture the ligamentum flavum directly with a Kerrison rongeur.

Correct Answer: C

Explanation:

Proper technique involves using fluoroscopic confirmation to guide the dilator to the ligamentum flavum. The working sleeve should face medially, and the ligamentum flavum should be incised layer-by-layer while monitoring for color change, indicating final depth (Table 13.18).

(ES, p. 237)

48. In an interlaminar lumbar endoscopic discectomy, while addressing a large axillary disc herniation, which approach should be taken to minimize tension on the traversing nerve root?
   A. Incise the ligamentum flavum as laterally as possible to increase exposure to the lateral canal and allow for fragment extraction without retracting neural structures.
   B. Incise the ligamentum flavum as medially as possible to expose the axilla, removing part of the extruded disc to release tension on the traversing root.
   C. Place the working sleeve obliquely toward the lateral edge of the spinal canal, retract the ligamentum flavum laterally, and proceed with direct removal of the herniated disc fragments.
   D. Use a posterior longitudinal ligament incision, rotate the working cannula 360 degrees for maximal retraction of the nerve root, and perform disc removal from a lateral entry.

   Correct Answer: B

Table 13.18 Surgical technique: interlaminar endoscopic lumbar discectomy

Step	Description
Preoperative planning	Review anteroposterior radiograph for interlaminar space width and MRI for disc herniation location and size
Patient positioning	Prone on Jackson table with hips and knees flexed to widen interlaminar window. Surgeon stands on side of the operated site with C-arm opposite
Portal entry	Make an 8–10 mm midline skin incision at the interlaminar space. Insert 6.9 mm dilator until it reaches the ligamentum flavum
Working sleeve and endoscope	Insert an 8 mm working sleeve along the dilator, then insert a 25°, 6.9 mm-diameter endoscope
Ligamentum Flavum Incision	Incise the ligamentum flavum layer-by-layer with a punch. Apply gentle pressure to stretch tissue before each cut
Accessing epidural space	Enlarge ligamentum flavum opening laterally. Remove epidural fat and gently dissect any epidural scars from neural structures
Disc fragment removal	Mobilize the traversing nerve root medially, use a pituitary rongeur to remove disc herniation, and rotate the cannula as needed for safe decompression
Annuloplasty	Perform annuloplasty with radiofrequency probe on the annular tear to minimize recurrence
Decompression confirmation	Ensure free pulsation and mobility of nerve root to confirm adequate decompression
Closure	Close the wound with a single skin suture

Explanation:

For large axillary herniations, incising the ligamentum flavum medially allows better access to the axilla, relieving tension on the nerve root and reducing the risk of injury. This approach ensures safer nerve root retraction during disc removal.

(ES, p. 237)

49. In a transforaminal lumbar interbody fusion (TLIF), which structure is most critical to protect while preparing the disc space?
    A. Dorsal root ganglion
    B. Ventral nerve root
    C. Axilla of the nerve root
    D. Lateral recess

    Correct Answer: D

    Explanation:

    During TLIF, the disc space is approached through Kamben triangle. This space is usually small and nerve roots retraction maybe needed. Minimizing nerve root retraction is necessary to avoid injuries specially on the exiting nerve root where dorsal root ganglion is exposed (Table 13.19).

    (SSW, p. 1820)

50. What is the typical percentage of the facet joint that can be safely removed without causing instability?
    A. 25%
    B. 40%
    C. 50%
    D. 75%

    Correct Answer: C

    Explanation:

    This concept of "safe 50% facetectomy" originating from a cadaveric study in 1992 [22]. Using 12 cadaveric cervical spines, this study investigated the stability of the cervical spine following laminectomy and graded facet joint resections in an in vitro model. The study determined that facetectomies exceeding 50% result in significant segmental hypermobility, highlighting the significance of preserving at least half of the facet joint during cervical spine decompression to maintain stability. Stability was evaluated using biomechanical tests on intact spines, then after C5 laminectomy, and finally after progressive C6 foraminotomies involving 25%, 50%, 75%, and 100% facet positions.

    [22]

51. Which of the following muscles should be dissected off the spinous processes to expose the lamina during posterior cervical laminectomy and fusion?
    A. Semispinalis cervicis
    B. Rhomboid major
    C. Splenius cervicis
    D. Levator scapulae

    Correct Answer: A

Table 13.19 Surgical Technique: Open TLIF (Transforaminal Lumbar Interbody Fusion)

Step	Description
Positioning	Prone on a radiolucent Jackson table to decompress the abdomen and reduce epidural bleeding. A Foley catheter, sequential compression devices, and stockings are applied, and fluoroscopy is used to confirm the affected level
Exposure	Midline incision is extended to the dorsal lumbar fascia over the disc space. Subperiosteal dissection proceeds past the facet joints and transverse processes on the side intended for decompression and bone grafting
Decompression	Based on the pathology, a laminectomy, facetectomy, or both may be performed. Bone is removed from pedicle to pedicle using a high-speed drill or osteotome, exposing the neural foramen and nerve roots. Minimal retraction is applied to protect the traversing and exiting nerve roots
Pedicle screw placement	Pedicles are cannulated before disc space preparation, though screws are not inserted on the ipsilateral side until the intervertebral graft is positioned. Cannulation is done under direct visualization, confirmed with fluoroscopy or navigation
Disc preparation	An aggressive discectomy is performed within the annulus to prevent vascular injury. Disc space distractors are used to expand the space, and the endplates are meticulously scraped to remove cartilage while preserving bone. The posterior vertebral lip is removed for direct access, and distraction is maintained via a temporary rod if necessary
Interbody fusion	Various structural grafts are available, with a preference for structural allograft. After packing locally harvested autograft, the graft (e.g., cage) is placed anteriorly and contralaterally within the disc space. Bone graft substitutes like BMP-2 or tricalcium phosphate may be used to enhance fusion
Final fixation and closure	After graft placement and verification with fluoroscopy, the temporary distraction rod is removed, and ipsilateral pedicle screws are inserted. Compression across the screws induces lordosis and locks the graft. The wound is closed in multiple layers, and no external orthosis maybe required postoperatively

Explanation:

Semispinalis cervicis starts from the transverse processes of the upper thoracic vertebrae. It attaches to the spinous processes of C2-C5. It helps in neck extension.

52. In comparison to the lumbar spine pedicle, which of the following statements about thoracic pedicle screws is correct?
    A. The pedicle is consistently wider than in the lumbar spine.
    B. The medial wall of the pedicle is thinner in the thoracic spine.
    C. The thoracic pedicles are aligned in the axial plane with the vertebral bodies.
    D. The transverse process has no role in guiding screw placement.

    Correct Answer: B

    Explanation:

    The thoracic pedicle is narrow and has a thin wall. This makes pedicle screw placement more difficult. It is riskier than in the lumbar spine. The challenge increases in patients with spinal deformities.

    [23]

53. During sacroiliac joint fusion (SIJF), the anterior approach provides several unique advantages. Which of the following is the PRIMARY benefit of using the anterior approach for SIJF?
    A. It offers a full view of the entire articular surface of the SI joint for complete joint decortication.
    B. It allows simultaneous bilateral access to the SI joint for complex bilateral fusion.
    C. It reduces operative time and blood loss compared to lateral and posterior approaches.
    D. It provides access to the anterior and cranial aspects of the joint while preserving the primary posterior ligamentous stabilizers.

    Correct Answer: D

    Explanation:

    The anterior approach for SIJF is primarily used to access the anterior and cranial aspects of the joint while preserving the posterior ligamentous structures that provide stabilization. This approach utilizes a standard ilioinguinal technique, which spares the posterior SI ligaments, making it particularly beneficial for maintaining posterior stability.

    (RS, p. 405)
54. During ACDF, careful planning of Caspar pin placement is critical. Why should the Caspar pin in the cranial vertebral body be placed slightly further from the endplate?
    A. To allow adequate endplate preparation by providing space for burring without pin obstruction
    B. To provide a stable anchor point and avoid interference with screw insertion in the later plating stage
    C. To increase distraction force at the disc space for achieving better lordotic alignment
    D. To maintain a safer distance from the nerve root during pin insertion, thereby preventing iatrogenic nerve injury

    Correct Answer: A

    Explanation:

    The Caspar pin in the cranial vertebral body is placed further from the endplate to allow room for burring and preparation of the endplate, ensuring smooth access for endplate work without interference from the pin itself. This is particularly important for creating optimal contact surfaces for graft placement.

    (EM, p. 3)
55. In ACDF, why might a modified Trendelenburg position of the OR table be used when operating with a microscope?
    A. To align the cervical spine in a more flexed position, which helps avoid excessive angulation of the microscope
    B. To provide a gravity-assisted view that pulls soft tissues downward, improving exposure to deeper cervical levels
    C. To achieve a more upright line of sight by aligning the cervical spine vertically, improving ergonomics and minimizing the need for microscope angulation

D. To prevent excessive blood pooling in the neck area and reduce intraoperative blood loss

Correct Answer: C

Explanation:

Using a microscope, reverse Trendelenburg tilts the OR table. This aligns the cervical spine vertically. It gives the surgeon a better line of sight. Less microscope angulation is needed. It improves visualization of lower cervical levels (Table 13.20).

(EM, p. 3)

Table 13.20 Surgical technique: anterior cervical discectomy and fusion (ACDF)

Step	Description
Positioning	Supine with the head on a foam donut. A roll under the scapula increases neck extension, and shoulders are taped down to improve visualization. Arms are secured with foam padding
Anesthesia	General endotracheal anesthesia is used. In cases involving C4 or above, nasotracheal intubation may be considered. Eyes are protected and the tube is taped to prevent pressure on the face
Incision localization	Identify incision site using surface landmarks: hyoid bone (C3), thyroid cartilage (C4–C5), carotid tubercle (C6), and cricoid cartilage (C7). Incision location is confirmed with preoperative lateral x-rays
Approach	A transverse incision is made in a natural skin crease, starting at midline and extending laterally. The platysma is divided, omohyoid muscle is identified and divided if necessary, and the SCM is retracted laterally
Dissection	Blunt dissection is used to create a plane between the carotid artery laterally and the esophagus medially. The pretracheal fascia is then dissected to expose the anterior spine
Level confirmation	A bent spinal needle is placed into the vertebral body, and a lateral x-ray confirms the correct level. The longus colli muscle is elevated and retracted bilaterally, and lateral osteophytes are removed to improve visualization
Retractor placement	Trimline retractor is places and secured underneath longus colli muscles. Caspar pins are placed, slight distraction is applied, and an annulotomy is performed
Decompression	The disc is removed with curettes and pituitary rongeurs. Anterior osteophytes are thinned for decompression and proper graft seating
PLL removal	If needed, the posterior longitudinal ligament (PLL) is resected for full decompression. A nerve hook is used to free the PLL from the dura underneath A Kerrison rongeur removes the PLL, and foraminal decompression is performed to ensure nerve root visualization and decompression. The nerve root is coursed ventrolaterally. Hook is used to ensure decompression and usually a "gush" of blood indicates satisfactory decompression
Graft insertion	Graft or cage size is determined using sizers, and autograft/allograft is inserted. Additional bone graft is packed around the graft as needed
Plate Placement	An anterior plate is selected and placed over the vertebral bodies with screws angled medially to avoid vertebral arteries. Fluoroscopy is used to confirm positioning, and screws are inserted to secure the plate
Closure	Hemostasis is achieved, a drain is optional, and the platysma is sutured with interrupted vicryl sutures. Skin is closed with running monocryl sutures, and dressings are applied

56. During a cervical total disc replacement (TDR) procedure, the surgeon notices that the distraction pins are slightly angled rather than parallel to the C5–C6 disc space. This results in asymmetric disc space opening and challenges with centering the implant. Which action should the surgeon take to correct this?
    A. Continue with implant placement as-is, compensating for the angle by adjusting the implant's position in the coronal plane.
    B. Remove the pins, reinsert them under fluoroscopic guidance to achieve parallel alignment with the disc, then proceed with distraction.
    C. Increase the distraction force on the pins to even out the disc space and align the endplates.
    D. Rotate the C-arm to visualize the pins from a different angle, then use this new view to guide implant positioning.

    Correct Answer: B

    Explanation:

    For cervical TDR, parallel distraction is essential to ensure even opening of the disc space and proper implant positioning. Removing and reinserting the pins under fluoroscopic guidance allows the surgeon to correct alignment issues, facilitating precise and symmetric placement of the TDR implant (Table 13.21).

    (SS, p. 320)

57. During occipital-cervical fusion surgery, after placing the occipital plate with three screws in the midline, the surgeon prepares to insert the rods for fixation. However, when attempting to align the rods, the assistant notices that the occipital plate is not flush against the occiput. What is the MOST appropriate next step to ensure correct alignment and stability?
    A. Continue with rod placement, applying additional force to press the occipital plate against the skull.
    B. Insert longer screws to force the plate against the skull, improving fixation strength.
    C. Increase the distraction force on the rods to bring the plate into alignment with the occiput.
    D. Remove the occipital screws, contour the plate further, and reposition it flush against the occipital bone.

    Correct Answer: D

    Explanation:

    Proper contouring of the occipital plate is essential to ensure it sits flush against the occiput, providing stable fixation without applying excessive force. Removing the screws, adjusting the plate, and repositioning it is the safest and most effective option (Table 13.22).

    (EM, p. 83)

58. During a posterior thoracic fusion procedure, the surgeon encounters excessive bleeding from the paraspinal muscles and intercostal vessels despite using standard cautery techniques. What adjustment in surgical technique could potentially reduce further blood loss during the exposure phase?
    A. Increase retractor repositioning to improve visualization.

Table 13.21 Surgical technique: cervical total disc replacement (TDR)

Step	Description
Patient positioning	Supine with a small rolled towel under the neck to maintain a stable, slightly lordotic alignment. Shoulders are taped down with cloth tape to improve visualization of the lower cervical levels, especially at C6–C7 if needed. The OR table may be rotated 180° to facilitate C-arm use and positioning around anesthesia equipment
Fluoroscopic check	Preoperative fluoroscopy is used to confirm visualization of the operative level and parallel alignment of vertebral endplates. The neck position should match the preoperative neutral lateral radiograph to maintain proper sagittal alignment
Incision localization	The incision location is determined with fluoroscopy. A transverse incision is typically used, similar to the Smith–Robinson approach. The longus coli muscles are exposed to the lateral aspect of the uncinate joints, and midline is confirmed using fluoroscopic guidance
Distraction pin placement	Fluoroscopic guidance is used to place distraction pins parallel to the disc at the operative level. This ensures anatomical alignment of the TDR and enables accurate preservation of motion
Discectomy and decompression	A thorough discectomy is performed with careful removal of osteophytes and foraminal decompression to prevent recurrent radiculopathy due to foraminal stenosis. Minimal bone resection is done, and the endplates are prepared according to the specific TDR device requirements
TDR implant placement	The TDR device, selected based on height similar to an adjacent healthy disc, is centered in the coronal and sagittal planes to maximize endplate coverage
Hemostasis	Bone wax is used to achieve meticulous hemostasis, minimizing the risk of blood loss and reducing the potential for postoperative heterotopic ossification
Preparation for Conversion	Throughout the procedure, the team should be prepared to convert to ACDF if needed, ensuring the flexibility to adapt the surgical plan as necessary

Table 13.22 Surgical technique: occipitocervical fixation and fusion

Step	Description
Positioning	Prone as per C1–C2 posterior fusion guidelines. Use C-arm to confirm final head positioning. Prep posterior iliac crest if autograft will be harvested
Anesthesia/ Neuromonitoring	Maintain mean arterial pressure >80 mm Hg in myelopathy cases. Neuromonitoring is used, particularly in cases involving myelopathy, as detailed in neuromonitoring guidelines
Incision localization	Mark the external occipital protuberance (EOP) and midline spinous processes at intended fusion levels. Incision starts 2 cm above the EOP and continues distally along the midline
Surgical approach	Identify key landmarks (EOP, C2 spinous process) and the midline median raphe. Use electrocautery and self-retaining retractors to maintain orientation to the midline. Divide ligamentum nuchae and trapezial fascia, then perform subperiosteal dissection of paraspinal muscles from caudal to cephalad, maintaining tension with repositioned retractors
Occipital instrumentation	Place occipital screws along the midline where bone is thickest. Use bicortical screw purchase for increased pullout strength. Maximum safe screw length within 2 cm lateral to EOP is 8 mm. Generally, three midline screws are placed

(continued)

Table 13.22 (continued)

Step	Description
Fixation Sequence	Insert cervical screws first to determine the width of the occipital plate. Contour the plate to fit flush against the skull. Pilot holes are drilled through the plate for screws. Bleeding from venous sinus (if ventral cortex is breached) can be controlled by screw tamponade
Rod placement	Measure rod length using the Bovie cord technique. If complex deformity correction is needed, use a rod template to bend the final rod accurately. This avoids weakening the rod from multiple bends
Bone decortication and grafting	Decorticate occipital bone just distal to the plate, proximal to the foramen magnum, as well as C1 and/or C2 lamina. Place structural iliac crest or rib autograft to span the occiput to the cervical spine
Decompression techniques	Indirect posterior reduction of basilar invagination may be performed using gentle bilateral distraction under neuromonitoring and fluoroscopy. A suboccipital craniectomy may be done if additional decompression of the foramen magnum is required, thinning bone with a burr and expanding with a Kerrison rongeur

B. Pack off portions of the wound with sponges and release retractor tension periodically.
C. Extend the incision laterally to minimize muscle tension.
D. Increase the length of the incision to expose additional segments.

Correct Answer: B

Explanation:

Minimizing retractor repositioning and releasing retractor tension periodically helps reduce paraspinal muscle necrosis and subsequent bleeding. Additionally, packing off portions of the wound with sponges helps absorb blood and minimizes further blood loss.

(EM, p. 137)

59. Regarding epidural free fat graft during lumbar discectomy, the following is CORRECT:
A. There is evidence that it decreases nerve root fibrosis.
B. There is evidence that it aggregates nerve root fibrosis
C. It can cause nerve root compression or cauda equina syndrome.
D. None of the above.

Correct Answer: C

Explanation:

Autogenous free fat grafts are sometimes used in the epidural space to reduce post-op scar formation, though opinions on their effectiveness vary. Some find it beneficial, while others believe it may worsen scarring. In some cases, the graft is undetectable during later surgeries. Rarely, fat grafts can cause nerve root compression or cauda equina syndrome within days of surgery, with one case reported 6 years post-op.

(GB, p. 1258)

60. Which structure is avoided to prevent retrograde ejaculation duringL5-S1 anterior lumbar interbody fusion (ALIF) exposure?
   A. Superior hypogastric plexus
   B. Inferior hypogastric plexus
   C. Medial and lateral hypogastric plexus
   D. All of the above

   Correct answer: A

   Explanation:

   The superior hypogastric plexus is a sympathetic plexus. It lies near the L5 vertebral body and anterior L5-S1 disc. It is at risk during anterior L5-S1 exposure. In men, injury can cause retrograde ejaculation and possible sterility. Erection remains unaffected as it is controlled by parasympathetic pathways.

   (SS, p. 41)

61. All of the structures are encountered in the Wiltse approach minimally invasive extraforaminal lumbar discectomy of L4-L5 level, EXCEPT:
   A. Intertransversarii ligament
   B. Inferior facet of L4
   C. Superior facet of L5
   D. L5 pars articularis

   Correct Answer: D

   Explanation:

   In minimally invasive L4–L5 extraforaminal discectomy, key structures are visible. These include the intertransversarii ligament and the inferior facet of L4. The superior facet of L5 and the pars articularis of L4 are also identified (Table 13.23; Figs. 13.16 and 13.17).

   (MISS, p. 333)

62. What imaging finding would most contraindicate vertebroplasty?
   A. Fracture with retropulsed bone fragments into the spinal canal
   B. Severe vertebral body compression with less than 20% height remaining
   C. Adjacent level degeneration with endplate edema
   D. Chronic fracture with evidence of sclerosis

   Correct Answer: A

   Explanation:

   Any spinal canal compression likc tumor or retropulsed bone fragment is a contraindication for vertebroplasty or kyphoplasty. The cement might push the compressing element back and can cause more canal compromisation and yet neurological deficit. Some of the other contraindication of vertebroplasty or kyphoplasty are: completely healed Fractures, sepsis, osteomyelitis, discitis, or epidural abscess, spinal Instability, focal neurologic deficits, iodine allergy, severe vertebral body collapse, significant canal compromise due to tumor or retropulsed bone, and partial or total destruction of the posterior vertebral body wall.

   (GB, p. 1214)

Table 13.23 Surgical technique: minimally invasive extraforaminal (far lateral) lumbar discectomy

Step	Description
Positioning	Prone under general anesthesia; Wilson's frame used for spinal flexion to widen interlaminar space; C-arm fluoroscope positioned for lateral view and used for level localization
Incision	2-cm incision made 4–5 cm lateral to midline on side of disc herniation; tubular retractor is docked at the superior part of the facet joint of the targeted level and walked to the pars interarticularis of the cranial vertebra (e.g., L4 in L4–L5 disc herniation), see image below
Dilation	K-wire inserted toward the transverse process and pedicle of the superior vertebra; sequential dilators placed over K-wire; tubular retractor connected to articulating arm holder, ensuring firm downward pressure on the retractor
Endoscopic setup (optional)	25-degree endoscope inserted into tubular retractor for visualization; endoscope orientation adjusted for anatomical accuracy (medial anatomy at the top of video screen, lateral at the bottom) Most of the surgeons use the microscope
Bone exposure	The following structures must be seen: Intertransversarii ligament, Inferior facet of cranial vertebra Superior facet of the caudal vertebra and pars articularis of the cranial vertebra Soft tissue cleared with cautery and curette; small portion of the superior part of the facet joint of the targeted level and pars of the cranial vertebra are removed with drill and Kerrison rongeur to expose the lateral neuroforamen
Nerve and disc decompression	Nerve root identified and gently retracted cranially. The disc herniation is located with a nerve hook and removed with rongeurs
Irrigation and closure	Surgical field irrigated with antibiotic solution; hemostasis ensured; tubular retractor removed, allowing muscle to close naturally; fascia and subcutaneous tissues closed with sutures, skin approximated with skin glue
Alternative approach	Cranial approach: docking the tubular retractor at pars and transverse process of the cranial vertebral and remove small part of both
Postoperative care	Routine postoperative care; most patients discharged the same day with pain management and stool softeners

63. Targeted mean arterial pressure (MAP) during surgery for cervical spondylotic myelopathy is:
    A. 50 mm Hg or higher
    B. 60 mm Hg or higher
    C. 70 mm Hg or higher
    D. 80 mm Hg or higher

    Correct Answer: D

    Explanation:

    It has been shown that keeping mean arterial pressure (MAP) during complex spine surgery or surgeries with spinal cord stenosis or compression at 80 mm Hg or higher prevents spinal cord ischemia.

    (SS, p. 208)

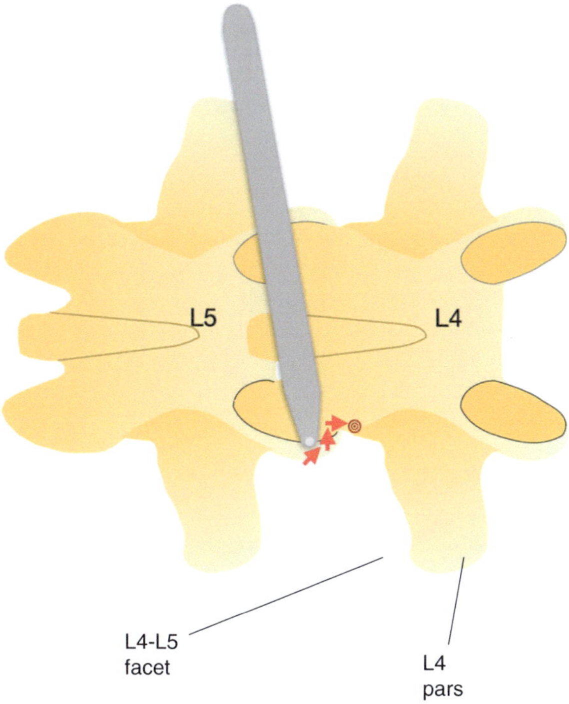

Fig. 13.16 The tubular dilators are docked at the superior part of the facet joint of the targeted level and walked to the pars interarticularis of the cranial vertebra (e.g., L4 in L4–L5 disc herniation). Then the tubular retractor is fixed when seeing the superior part of the facet joint of the targeted level and walked to the pars interarticularis of the cranial

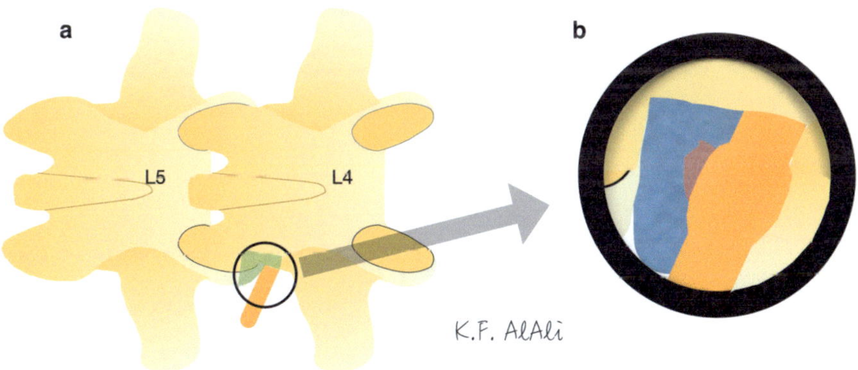

Fig. 13.17 (**a**) showing the area of the bone resection to expose the herniated disc and the nerve. (**b**) Microscopic view after the bone resection of the field showing the disc, the herniated disc compressing the dorsal nerve ganglion

Spine Complications

14

1. Which of the following is a common intraoperative complication of spine surgery?
   A. Myocardial infarction
   B. Incidental durotomy
   C. Pulmonary embolism
   D. Deep vein thrombosis
   Correct Answer: B
   Explanation:
   Incidental durotomy with CSF leakage has varying incidence from 1% to 17% based on the type and location of spinal surgery. Risk factors for incidental durotomy include revision surgery for spinal stenosis, ossification of the posterior longitudinal ligament or ligamentum flavum, and older age.
   The best approach is a watertight primary closure of the dura. Key principles for successful repair include adequate surgical exposure, precise hemostasis, magnification for clear visualization, and a watertight suture closure. The repair's integrity should be tested using a Valsalva maneuver to check for CSF leaks. In minimally invasive surgery, watertight repair is challenging and use of dural sealant is usually effective.
   Tears in the cervical spine are rare, and those occurring during anterior cervical surgery may be challenging to repair due to limited exposure. In such cases, a dural sealant or onlay patch may be used instead.
   A closed lumbar subarachnoid drainage system can be employed postoperatively to divert CSF, particularly if primary repair is not feasible or as an adjunct following repair.
   (SS, p. 212)
2. What is the most common complication following spine fusion for adolescent idiopathic scoliosis?
   A. Urinary tract infection
   B. Pulmonary embolism

K. F. AlAli, H. T. Hashim, *Spine Surgery and Peripheral Nerve Surgery*,
https://doi.org/10.1007/978-3-031-98543-0_14

C. Surgical site infection
D. Instrumentation failure

Correct Answer: C

Explanation:

For adolescents with idiopathic scoliosis, the rate of complications after spinal fusion varies from 5% to 23%. Due to long surgical field and time, surgical site infections are a common postoperative complication, occurring between 0.17% and 9%.

[18]

3. A patient with a history of chronic obstructive pulmonary disease undergoes a thoracolumbar fusion. Postoperatively, he develops shortness of breath and hypoxia. What is the most likely complication?
A. Heart failure
B. Pulmonary embolism
C. Pneumonia
D. Atelectasis

Correct Answer: D

Explanation:

Following spine fusion surgery, **atelectasis** is the most frequent respiratory complication. Clinical manifestations include fever, tachycardia, and tachypnea as a result of the collapse of peripheral lung alveoli. The main goals of treatment are efficient pain management and lung expansion methods, such as coughing, chest physical therapy, CPAP, suctioning, deep breathing exercises, incentive spirometry, early mobilization, and frequent bed shifting. (SS, p. 226)

4. What is the most common reason for 30-day readmission after spine surgery?
A. Surgical site infections
B. Systemic infections
C. Venous thromboembolism
D. Neurological complications

Correct Answer: A

Explanation:

Surgical site infection is defined as an infection that occur within 30 days of surgery if no implant is used or within 365 days if an implant is present. It is the most common reason for 30-day readmission after spine surgeries. It is classified as superficial (suprafascial) or deep (subfascial) and as acute (within 3 weeks of surgery) or chronic/delayed (beyond 4 weeks).

(BS, p. 442)

5. One of the following is a risk factor for surgical site infections in spine surgery:
A. Use of robotic or intraoperative CT scan
B. Use of intraoperative neuromonitoring
C. Increased total anesthesia time
D. All of the above are risk factors

Correct Answer: C

Explanation:

The risk factors for surgical site infections in spine surgery are divided into patient specific and surgical factors:

Patient-specific factors: Obesity, diabetes mellitus, malnutrition, smoking, society of anesthesiologists (ASA) score >2 and comorbid conditions like chronic liver disease.

Surgical factors: Increased surgery and anesthesia time, blood loss, use of instrumentation, dural tear and CSF leak, prolonged hospital stay, revision surgery, and type of surgical approach, posterior approaches may have higher infection rates compared to anterior approaches.

(SB, p. 502)

6. A patient presents with new rapid-onset neurological deficits following lumbar decompression surgery. What is the most likely cause?
   A. Epidural hematoma
   B. Meningitis
   C. Steroid-induced myopathy
   D. Recurrent disc herniation

   Correct Answer: A

   Explanation:

   New neurological symptoms following spine surgery can be caused by:

   Ioatrogenic nerve injury, deformity correction, acute vascular etiology (intraoperative hypotension or disruption of key segmental blood vessels), surgical positioning (brachial plexopathy, compressive neuropathy of ulnar or peroneal nerves, lower extremity compartment syndrome, or cervical cord injury, especially in patients with cervical stenosis), postoperative bleeding (**epidural hematomas**, usually rapid onset).

   Meningitis, steroid-induced myopathy, or recurrent disc herniation all can cause new neurological symptoms; however, their onset is usually late in the postoperative course and not immediate.

   (SS, p. 224)

7. Which complication in the postoperative period after lumbar spine surgery is significantly associated with mortality within 2 years?
   A. Cardiac complications
   B. Gastrointestinal complications
   C. Pneumonia
   D. Spinal cord complications

   Correct Answer: A

   Explanation:

   In an analysis of 767 patients who underwent lumbar spine surgery, the incidence cardiac complications were: cardiac 13%, compared to pulmonary 7%, gastrointestinal 6.7%, neurological 8.2%, hematological 17.5%, and urologic 10.3%. **Cardiac and pulmonary complications were significantly associated with a higher risk of death within 2 years**. [19]

8. What preoperative factor is crucial in reducing the incidence of surgical site infections in patients having spinal surgery?
   A. Postoperative glycemic control
   B. Immediate cessation of smoking before surgery
   C. Decolonization of MRSA carriers
   D. All of the above

Correct Answer: C

Explanation:

The prevention of spinal surgery site infections requires a thorough implementation of preoperative, intraoperative, and postoperative methods.

Preoperative measures:

- **Patient selection:** Improve modifiable risk variables such as blood glucose management and HbA1c in diabetic patients at least 3 months prior to surgery (not just during the postoperative period).
- **Comorbidity management**: Assess and enhance the condition of individuals with cardiac, pulmonary, or renal disorders.
- **Smoking cessation** is advised at least 4–6 weeks before to and after surgery.
- **MRSA Screening:** Employ nasal swabs and decolonize carriers using mupirocin ointment and chlorhexidine showers.
- **Nutrition:** Treat malnutrition, specifically hypoalbuminemia.

Intraoperative measures:

- Prophylactic antibiotics: Provide within 30 min before the incision and re-administer every 4 h. MRSA carriers should receive vancomycin.
- **Sterile technique:** Use chlorhexidine gluconate (ChloraPrep) or iodine povacrylex (DuraPrep) for dermal preparation, adhere to rigorous sterile protocols, and ensure hemostasis.

Betadine irrigation, when diluted to concentrations between 0.5% and 4%, effectively reduces the risk of infection.

- **Topical Vancomycin**: Consider for long incisions and long surgery.
- **Sealed closure**: Assure precise closure of the fascial layer. Employ subfascial drains if dead space is present.
- Negative-Pressure Wound Therapy: Recommended for high-risk patients.

Postoperative measures:

- Vigilantly monitor high-risk wounds and swiftly manage any persistent leakage extending beyond 14 days.
- Early mobilization to avoid nosocomial infections and minimize hospital duration.

(BS, p. 443)

9. A patient with a baclofen pump will undergo scoliosis correction surgery. What is the main concern regarding the baclofen pump during the perioperative period?
   A. Baclofen withdrawal
   B. Pump malfunction due to mechanical damage
   C. Infection at the pump site
   D. Pump programming errors

   Correct Answer: A

   Explanation:

   Abrupt discontinuation of baclofen is a risk for the serious withdrawal symptoms.

   Baclofen withdrawal syndrome may occur if the pump is not refilled on schedule or malfunctions (e.g., during scoliosis surgery), including issues with the catheter. Symptoms may include rebound spasticity, spasms, itching, headaches, drowsiness, confusion, hallucinations, seizures, tachycardia, unstable blood pressure, and fever. Treatment involves reintroducing intrathecal baclofen. In severe cases, baclofen can be administered via lumbar puncture or an external catheter.

(SSW, p. 1290)

10. One of the following is a common complication of intradural extramedullary spinal tumor resection:
    A. Cerebrospinal fluid leak
    B. Pulmonary embolism
    C. Neurological deficit
    D. All of the above

    Correct Answer: A

    Explanation:

    CSF leak is a recognized complication following intradural extramedullary spinal tumor resections. Watertight dura closure is crucial to prevent this complication.

    Dural closure technique: The dura is usually closed using a running 4-0 silk or 6-0 Prolene suture. To confirm watertight closure, a Valsalva maneuver at 35 mm Hg is done. A dural allograft may be placed over the suture line if needed. The paraspinal muscles are closed in layers along with the deep and superficial fascia and the skin.

    (SSW, p. 2032)

11. Regarding postoperative cervical kyphosis:

    11a. What type of surgery commonly causes postoperative cervical kyphosis?
    A. Anterior cervical discectomy and fusion
    B. Anterior cervical corpectomy
    C. Posterior cervical laminectomy
    D. Occipitocervical fusion

    11b. Postlaminectomy cervical kyphosis is usually caused by:
    A. Disruption of the anterior tension band
    B. Disruption of the posterior tension band
    C. Disruption of both anterior and posterior tension bands
    D. Disruption of interspinous and spinous process ligaments

    Correct Answers: 11a: C, 11b: B

    Explanation:

    Posterior cervical surgeries carry a risk of postoperative kyphosis more than anterior techniques like ACDF and corpectomy, which are both used to correct kyphosis in cervical degenerative disc diseases.

    Postlaminectomy kyphosis is usually due to disruption of the posterior tension band. For that in a patient with cervical myelopathy and pre-existing kyphosis, posterior approaches, especially laminectomy, is usually avoided, and anterior approaches are recommended. Laminoplasty is intended to reduce the postlaminectomy kyphosis; however, anterior approaches have the least risk of kyphosis and the advantages of possible correction of any pre-existing kyphosis.

    (SSW, p. 1661)

12. Which nerve is most often injured from a prone position?
    A. Median nerve
    B. Ulnar nerve
    C. Radial nerve
    D. Common peroneal nerve

    Correct Answer: B

    Explanation:

    The ulnar nerve is the most commonly injured nerve in the prone position during spinal surgeries, followed by the common peroneal nerve. Both nerves are superficial and susceptible to compression from the prone position. To prevent nerve injury, routine padding of the elbow to protect the ulnar nerve and the knee to protect the peroneal nerve while avoiding knee and elbow hyperextension is necessary. Most of the postoperative nerve injuries are neuropraxia improved with conservative management.

    (SS, p. 210)
13. What specific risk is connected to using bone morphogenetic protein (BMP) during spine fusion surgery?
    A. Seroma formation
    B. Heterotopic ossification
    C. Dural tear
    D. Vertebral osteomyelitis

    Correct Answer: B

    Explanation:

    Heterotopic bone ossification is when new bone forms at areas where fusion is not intended. These locations can be extradiscal, ectopic, or heterotopic.

    It is thought to occur when bone morphogenetic protein (BMP) seeps into the epidural space from its carrier. It can occur in up to 75% of the cases, especially when posterior techniques like transforaminal lumbar interbody fusion are used.

    While most cases are asymptomatic, symptomatic cases have been reported following TLIF surgeries.

    (DI, p. 1149)
14. What is the primary concern with the breach of the anterior cortex of the lumbar vertebral body during pedicle screw placement?
    A. Abdominal posterior hernia
    B. Splenic injury
    C. Sympathetic chain injury
    D. Retroperitoneal hematoma

    Correct Answer: D

    Explanation:

    Anterior to the lumbar spine are retroperitoneal structures like the abdominal aorta, inferior vena cava, sympathetic chain, pancreas (upper lumbar region), small intestine, and colon. Sympathetic chain injury is rare in lumbar pedicle screw surgery.

In a retrospective review of 2800 screws from 165 patients, it was found that breaches of ≤4 mm did not pose significant risk to adjacent vital structures. [20]

15. What lumbar procedure commonly causes sympathetic chain injury?
    A. Posterior lumbar interbody fusion
    B. Transforaminal lumbar interbody fusion
    C. Oblique lumbar interbody fusion
    D. Anterior lumbar interbody fusion

    Correct Answer: C

    Explanation:

    Sympathetic chain injury commonly occurs in oblique lumbar interbody fusion. It is underestimated and manifests as a difference in body temperature in lower extremities with increased temperature in the injured side. It can be associated with anhidrosis, abnormal sensation, skin discoloration, and swelling.

    [57]
16. A 32-year-old underwent transoral odontoidectomy. On post-operative day 5, he presents with nose discharge and fever. What of the following complications needs to be rolled out immediately?
    A. Pharyngeal abscess
    B. Meningitis
    C. Retropharyngeal infected hematoma
    D. Rapid onset pneumonia

    Correct Answer: B

    Explanation:

    Transoral odontoidectomy can cause dural tear and CSF leak; if not treated, it can lead to meningitis.

    (GB, p. 1773)
17. Which of the following factors is LEAST likely to have contributed to the development of clinically significant heterotopic ossification in a patient with cervical artificial discs?
    A. Obesity
    B. Male sex
    C. Lower endplate coverage by the artificial device
    D. Younger age at the time of surgery

    Correct Answer: D

    Explanation:

    Risk factors for heterotopic ossification are obesity, with a BMI ≥30, male sex; lower endplate coverage by the total disc device; and older age.

    [24]
18. A 58-year-old male patient presents after 7 years of C5–C6 cervical total disc replacement. He reports stiffness in his neck, with reduced mobility. On flexion-extension radiographs, you observe bone formation ventral to the C5–C6 level without restricting the motion at the operated segment.

    Based on the McAfee and Mehren grading system, what grade of heterotopic ossification (HO) does this patient likely have? (Fig. 14.1)

A. Grade 1
B. Grade 2
C. Grade 3
D. Grade 4

Correct Answer: B

Explanation:

McAfee and Mehren grading system for heterotopic ossification:

- Grade 1: Bone is present around the vertebral body but not in the intervertebral disc space.
- Grade 2: Bone extends into the disc space but does not significantly limit movement between the vertebrae.
- Grade 3: Bone restricts the range of motion, but some movement is still possible at the prosthesis.
- Grade 4: A complete bony bridge has formed, causing segmental ankylosis with no motion at the treated level.

[24]

19. In occipito-cervical fusion, the surgeon observed bleeding from the occipital midline region while inserting the occipital plate and cervical screws. Which of the following is the MOST likely cause of this complication, and what is the optimal course of action?
    A. Vertebral artery injury; apply hemostatic agents and continue fixation.
    B. Occipital venous sinuses injury; use the inserted screw as a tamponade.
    C. Epidural venous plexus injury: Pack the area with hemostatic material and avoid further drilling.
    D. Cortical vein and dura damage; repair with exploration to evacuate the possible subdural bleeding and apply a dural patch and abort the fusion surgery.

    Correct Answer: B

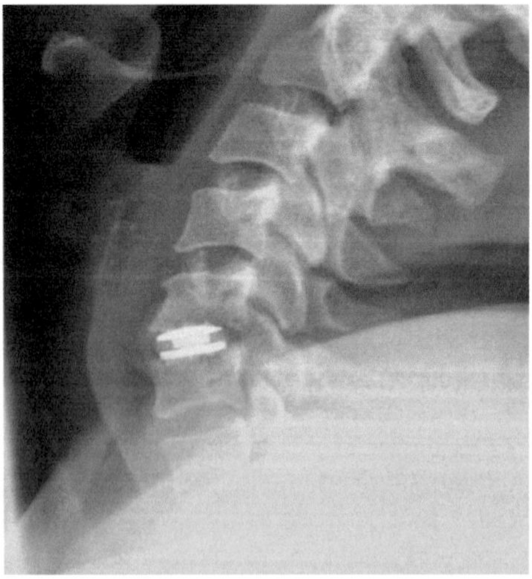

Fig. 14.1 Case 18 X-ray

Explanation:

Occipital suns present in approximately 65% of the patients. It is the smallest venous sinus, running in the midline of the occipital bone from the falx cerebelli and caudally to the level of the foramen magnum [58]. During occipital-cervical fusion, bicortical screws may pierce the ventral cortex of the occipital, puncturing the occipital venous sinus, resulting in bleeding. An efficient method of stopping the bleeding in this case is to use the screw itself as a tamponade.

(EM, p. 83)

20. What is the complication associated with excessive retraction of the dural sac during posterior lumbar interbody fusion (PLIF)?
    A. Arachnoiditis
    B. Conus medullaris syndrome
    C. Cauda equina syndrome
    D. Incidental durotomy

    Correct Answer: C

    Explanation:

    Nerve root injury and cauda equina syndrome are the most devastating complications associated with PLIF. It is due to excessive nerve root and dura retraction because of the posterior near midline approach. Modifications such as superior facet removal (like in TLIF) to access the disc space more laterally have been shown to decrease dura retraction and reduce neural injuries. (RS, p. 903)
21. During L4–L5 lumbar discectomy, which vascular structure can be injured:
    A. Abdominal aorta
    B. Inferior vena cava
    C. Right common iliac artery
    D. Left common iliac artery

    Correct Answer: D

    Explanation:

    The left common iliac artery has a medial course and close relation with the L4–L5 disc level and is more susceptible to

    Injury. At the upper lumbar levels (L1–L4), the vascular structures at risk are the aorta and the inferior vena cava.

    (CN, p. 309).
22. Complete the blank space: The proximal junctional kyphosis (PJK) is defined by ____ increase in kyphosis at the proximal junction, typically measured between the uppermost instrumented vertebra and the vertebra two levels above it.
    A. 5°
    B. 10°
    C. 15°
    D. 20°

    Correct Answer: B

Explanation:

Proximal Junctional Kyphosis (PJK) is a complication that can occur after long-segment spine fusions, specifically following adult spinal deformity cases. The incidence is between 11% and 52.9%. PJK is defined by a ≥10° increase in kyphosis at the proximal junction, typically measured between the uppermost instrumented vertebra and the vertebra two levels above it.

23. A 66-year-old patient with osteoporosis had T10 to S1 fusion for spinal deformity. Postoperatively, she experiences increasing back pain. Imaging indicates a 15° increase in kyphosis at the proximal joint accompanied with a T9 compression fracture. What is the probable diagnosis, and which risk factors contributed to her condition?
   A. Proximal Junctional Failure; advanced age, osteoporosis, and fusion to the sacrum
   B. Proximal Junctional Kyphosis; ligamentum flavum disruption and excessive sagittal realignment
   C. Proximal Junctional Kyphosis; pedicle screw failure and posterior instrumentation rigidity
   D. Proximal Junctional Failure; vertebral body fracture caused by improper implant size

   Correct Answer: A

   Explanation:

   Proximal junctional failure (PJF) is a severe form of PJK characterized by structural failures such as vertebral fractures or posterior ligament disruption, often leading to increased pain, deformity, and the need for surgical correction.

   Risk factors for PJK and PJF include advanced age, osteoporosis, posterior ligament damage, rigid instrumentation, and fusion extending to the sacrum. Excessive sagittal realignment and forces from correction surgeries are also associated with higher rates of PJK. Preventative measures, such as preserving the posterior ligament complex, using less rigid fixation at the proximal junction, and employing techniques like vertebroplasty, may reduce the risk of PJK.

   (CN, p. 326)

24. During a transoral decompression procedure at C1–C2, a surgeon performs a lateral C1–C2 facet dissection. Which of the following complications might occur as a result?
   A. Instability due to disruption of capsules
   B. Vertebral artery injury
   C. Postoperative obstructed airway due to extensive dissection
   D. Wound dehiscence due to compromised mucosal integrity

   Correct Answer: B

   Explanation:

   Dissection beyond the medial edge of the C1–C2 facet joint risks encountering the vertebral artery, which typically lies 20 mm from the midline. This could lead to severe bleeding, requiring immediate control measures such as tamponade or embolization.

   (RS, p. 325)

25. A 54-year-old male has thoracic spine severe stenosis decompression. He develops paraparesis immediately after the surgery. MRI shows spinal cord hyperintense T2 signal at the surgical site. What is the most likely etiology?
   A. Epidural hematoma
   B. White cord syndrome
   C. Transverse myelitis
   D. Surgical site infection

   Correct Answer: B

   Explanation:

   White cord syndrome is a rare complication after spinal cord decompression surgery and results from reperfusion injury after release of chronic compression. It is characterized by immediate or delayed neurological deficits postoperatively, such as worsening weakness or paralysis. MRI findings of T2 hyperintense signals at the surgical site are consistent with spinal cord edema or infarction, hallmark features of white cord syndrome.

   Epidural hematoma: Typically presents with compression of neural structures on imaging and is associated with T2 hyperintensities within the spinal cord itself.

   Transverse myelitis: An inflammatory condition affecting the spinal cord that might occur postoperatively but usually not immediately.

   Surgical site infection: Causes localized pain, fever, and systemic symptoms rather than immediate neurological deficits or intramedullary hyperintensities on MRI.

   White cord syndrome is managed with measures such as corticosteroids to reduce inflammation, maintaining adequate perfusion with mean arterial pressure (MAP) augmentation, and early rehabilitation.

   (GB, p. 1308)

26. Which vertebral level is closest to its exiting nerve root and carries the highest risk during pedicle screw placement?
   A. T1–T2
   B. T3–T4
   C. T6–T9
   D. T11–T12

   Correct Answer: A

   Explanation:

   The thoracic spine has relatively smaller pedicles, making it more prone to nerve root injury during pedicle screw insertion. At T6–T9, the distance between the pedicle and nerve root inferiorly is the largest compared to other thoracic levels. T1–T2 level has the smallest distance, making this level more prone to nerve injury during pedicle screw insertion.

   (CN, p. 304)

27. True or false, spinal surgery wound drains decrease the incidence of postoperative epidural hematoma:
   A. True
   B. False

Correct Answer: B

Explanation:

Postoperative wound drains, whether placed subfascially or suprafascially, are commonly used. Multiple studies have demonstrated no significant difference in the incidence of postoperative epidural hematoma between patients with drains and those without.

(CN, p. 305)

28. During craniocervical junction surgeries, which vertebral artery segment is at higher risk for injury during
    A. V2 and V3 segments
    B. V3 and V4 segments
    C. V4 and V5 segments
    D. V4 segment only

    Correct Answer: B

    Explanation:

    Of the four segments of the VA, the two pertinents to the CCJ are the V3 and V4 because of their course at the craniocervical junction.

29. According to the Gertzbein classification, what grade is assigned to a pedicle screw medial breach measuring 3 mm?
    A. Grade 0
    B. Grade 1
    C. Grade 2
    D. Grade 3

    Correct Answer: C

    Explanation:

    Gertzbein classification of pedicle screws evaluates the extent of medial pedicle breaches, as medial violations over 4 mm have been associated with increased risk of neurological deficits (Table 14.1).

    (GB, p. 1799)

30. While cannulating the C1 lateral mass using Tan entry point, the surgeon encountered significant arterial bleeding. The proper explanation of this complication is:
    A. High-riding vertebral artery
    B. Presence of ponticulus posticus anomaly
    C. Use of 4 mm or larger drill
    D. Presence of incomplete C1 posterior arch

    Correct Answer: B

Table 14.1 Gertzbein classification of pedicle screws medial breach

Grade	Breach distance (mm)
0	No breach
1	Less than 2 mm
2	2–4 mm
3	Greater than 4 mm

Explanation:

The V3 segment of the vertebral artery passes ventromedially, anterior to the thickened lateral edge of the dorsal atlanto-occipital membrane, which forms an arch over the artery. This arch is sometimes ossified and is known as the ponticulus posticus. Recognizing this condition preoperatively is critical, as unawareness could result in catastrophic injury of the vertebral artery during placement of lateral mass screws in C1 if Tan entry point is used (posterior arch). After traversing this region, the artery pierces the dura mater and enters the vertebral canal (Fig. 14.2).

(RP. Vertebral artery)

31. During canulating C2 pedicle using Harms technique, the surgeon encountered significant arterial bleeding due to a high-riding vertebral artery. The definition of a high-riding vertebral artery is:
    A. C2 internal height of more than 2 mm
    B. C2 isthmus height of equal or less than 5 mm

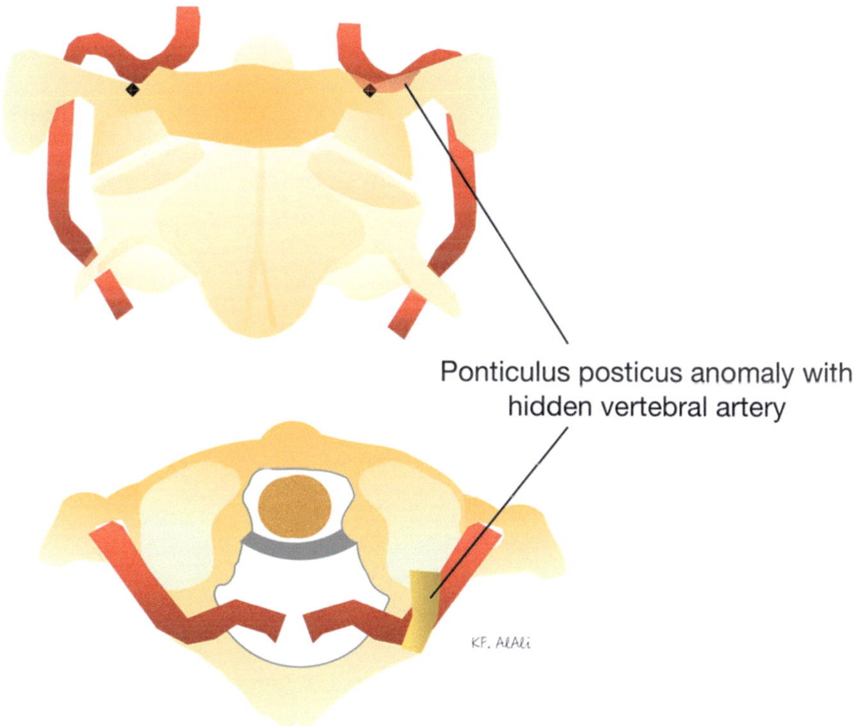

Fig. 14.2 Left-sided vertebral artery: Normal course of V3 vertebral artery on the top of the C1 arch. Right-sided vertebral artery: Showing the calcified arch at the dorsal atlanto-occipital membrane over the V3 course, forming ponticulus posticus anomaly with the hidden vertebral artery segment where Tan C1 lateral mass screw entry point (cube) results in vertebral artery injury

C. C2 internal width of more than 2 mm
D. C2 isthmus height of equal or more than 6 mm

Correct Answer: B

Explanation:

The vertebral artery is at risk during C2 pedicle screw placement. This risk is determined by two primary factors: the size of the pedicle and the presence of a "high-riding" vertebral artery. A high-riding vertebral artery occurs when the vertebral artery groove is positioned too medially and too high within the C2 pedicle isthmus, usually when the **isthmus height is equal to or less than 5 mm** and/or has an internal height of ≤2 mm, making screw insertion unsafe.

Surgeons must carefully evaluate the vertebral artery's course preoperatively for each patient to determine the feasibility of pedicle screw placement. If the trajectory is unsuitable, a shorter pars screw can be placed in C2, which typically provides sufficient fixation (Fig. 14.3).

(CN, pp. 315–316)

32. All of the following are intraoperative measures used to prevent vertebral artery injury in cervical corpectomy, EXCEPT:
    A. The midpoint between the longus colli muscles is identified as a midline landmark.
    B. During foraminal decompression, one should limit the exposure to the uncovertebral joint.
    C. Tilt the microscope to an oblique trajectory when resecting the vertebral body.
    D. Limit the resection of the vertebral body to 16 mm.

    Correct Answer: C

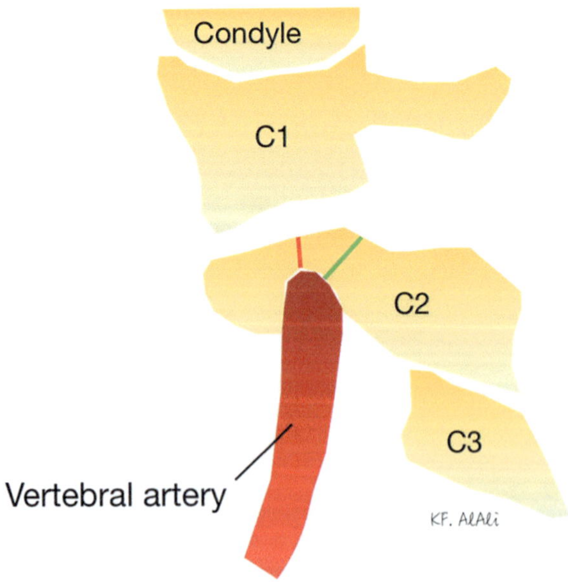

Fig. 14.3 Illustration showing high-riding vertebral artery occurs when the vertebral artery groove is positioned too medially and too high within the C2 pedicle isthmus; usually when the **isthmus height is equal or less than 5 mm** (green line), it is the thinnest part of C2 isthmus and/or has an internal height of ≤2 mm. The internal height is the shortest distance between the transverse foramen and the surface of C2 superior articular surface (red line)

Explanation:

Accurate orientation is critical to avoid the laterally positioned vertebral artery during anterior cervical decompression. The midline is established by identifying the midpoint between the longus colli muscles, along with the uncovertebral joints bilaterally. For foraminal decompression, exposure should be limited to the uncovertebral joint, which typically spares the vertebral artery. During corpectomies, resection of the vertebral body should be restricted to 16 mm to avoid encroaching on the artery. Additionally, when using a microscope, care must be taken to maintain a **straight trajectory** to prevent inadvertent oblique corpectomy that could endanger the artery.

(CN, p. 316)

33. All of the following are risk factors for anterior iliac crest harvesting, EXCEPT?
    A. Pain
    B. Peritoneal perforation
    C. Obturator nerve injury
    D. Hernia

    Correct Answer: C

    Anterior iliac crest complications can include pain, infection, cosmetic deformity, peritoneal perforation, iliac defect with abdominal herniation, and injuries to the ilioinguinal, iliohypogastric, and lateral femoral cutaneous nerves.

    (RS, p. 1081)

34. Regarding the pain after anterior iliac crest harvesting, one of the following is correct:
    A. Incidence varies
    B. No specific risk factors in these patients
    C. Pain usually resolved in a few weeks in most patients
    D. All of the above are correct

    Correct Answer: D

    Explanation:

    Persistent donor site pain from anterior iliac crest harvesting occurs in 2% to 40% of cases. No significant differences in health-related outcomes have been observed between patients who received autografts and those who did not. By 6 weeks postoperatively, most patients experience resolution of the donor site pain.

    (RS, p. 1082)

35. To prevent adjacent disc disease after anterior cervical discectomy and fusion, the plate should be at least:
    A. 1 mm away from the adjacent disc space
    B. 3 mm away from the adjacent disc space
    C. 5 mm away from the adjacent disc space
    D. 7 mm away from the adjacent disc space

    Correct Answer: C

    Explanation:

    To ensure optimal placement, the anterior cervical spine plate should be aligned centrally along the midline of the vertebral body, situated between the uncovertebral joints. The cranial and caudal edges of the plate should correspond with the midpoint of the vertebral body. Additionally, maintaining a distance of at least 5 mm from adjacent disc spaces is recommended to reduce the potential for adjacent segment disease.

(CN, p. 320)

36. In thoracic spine pedicle screw technique, medial breach is considered safe if:
   A. less than 2 mm
   B. less than 4 mm
   C. between 2–4 mm
   D. All medial breaches are unsafe.

   Correct Answer: A

   Explanation:

   In the thoracic spine, a trajectory that is too medial risks violating the spinal canal and causing spinal cord injury, while a lateral trajectory can cause pleural or vascular injuries. Pedicle breaches are a recognized complication, with medial breaches considered safe if **less than 2 mm**, likely safe between 2 and 4 mm. A lateral breach of the thoracic pedicle up to 6 mm is generally considered acceptable, though this may vary depending on individual anatomical differences.

   (CN, p. 321)

37. According to Gertzbein classification of pedicle screw breech, Grade 2 is:
   A. Breach of >2 mm
   B. Breach of 1–2 mm
   C. Breach of 2–4 mm
   D. Breach of >4 mm

   Correct Answer: C

   Explanation:

   Gertzbein classification for pedicle screws breaches is summarized in the following table (Table 14.2): (GB, p. 109)

38. The S1 pedicle screw has a risk for pullout due to:
   A. Wide pedicle
   B. Large cancellous bony component
   C. Caudal orientation in the sagittal plane
   D. All of the above

   Correct Answer: B

Table 14.2 Gertzbein classification for pedicle screw breaches

Grade	Description	Clinical implications
A	No breach	Safe, no breach detected
B	Breach ≤2 mm	Generally considered safe
C	Breach >2 and ≤4 mm	Likely safe; clinical correlation recommended
D	Breach >4 and ≤6 mm	Potentially unsafe; risk of neurovascular injury
E	Breach >6 mm	High risk of neurovascular or structural injury

Explanation:

S1 has a large cancellous bone component, which makes it prone to pullout. To enhance stability, screws are often positioned to engage as much cortical bone as possible, which can sometimes result in anterior screw breach.

(CN, p. 322)

39. Regrading pseudoarthrosis in spinal fusion:

39a. The gold standard imaging modality to assess pseudoarthrosis in spinal fusion is:

A. CT spine
B. Dynamic X-ray (flexion and extension)
C. MRI spine
D. A and B

39b. All of the following are CT radiographic signs of pseudoarthrosis in spinal fusion EXCEPT:

A. Hollowing around the pedicle screw
B. Cage subsidence
C. Broken pedicle screw
D. Unilateral formation of a bony bridge on the posterolateral area

39c. All of the following are signs of pseudarthrosis in spine fusion in dynamic X-ray (flexion and extension), EXCEPT:

A. Translation of the vertebral body >3 mm
B. Angular motion of the vertebral body >5°
C. Any degree of translation of the vertebral body
D. ≥2-mm change in interspinous distance

39d. One of the following is a surgical strategy to treat pseudarthrosis in spine fusion:

A. Change the fusion approach
B. Use of different grafting material
C. Use of large screw diameter
D. All of the above

Correct Answers: 39a: A, 39b: D, 39c: C, 39d: D

Explanation:

Pseudarthrosis, or nonunion, is a common complication of lumbar spine surgery, particularly in multilevel fusions, with rates ranging from 5% to 35%. Symptoms include recurrent pain, instability, and neurologic issues, though diagnosis can be challenging due to overlap with other conditions like infection or adjacent segment disease.

CT Signs of pseudarthrosis:

- Hollowing around the pedicle screw
- Cage subsidence
- Broken pedicle screw
- Broken or dislodged rod
- Lack of continuous bone bridge formation (trabecular bone) in the intended fusing area (e.g., posterolateral, interbody)

Dynamic X-ray (flexion and extension) signs:

- Motion >3 mm or angular motion >5°
- ≥2 mm change in interspinous distance

CT is the preferred imaging modality for assessing fusion, offering higher sensitivity than plain radiographs. Bridging trabecular bone can be detected in 95% of thin-section CT scans compared to 4% with plain films.

Management is primarily surgical and includes regrafting, stabilization, and potentially changing the fusion approach, like adding interbody fusion if not done and removing loose screws and placing larger screws.

(CN, pp. 327–328) (DI, p. 1139)

40. All of the following are risk factors for pseudoarthrosis in spinal fusion EXCEPT:
    A. Smoking
    B. Poor preparation or decortication of the fusion surface
    C. Poor sagittal balance
    D. Strong compression force

    Correct Answer: D

    Explanation:

    Pseudoarthrosis in spinal fusion is associated with factors such as poor surgical preparation, inadequate bone grafting, smoking, malnutrition, osteoporosis, steroid intake and sagittal misalignment.

    (CN, p. 327)

41. Patient underwent lateral lumbar transpsoas approach. Postoperatively, the patient complained of severe superior anterior thigh pain and numbness. The most injured structure is:
    A. T12 subcostal nerve
    B. Iliohypogastric nerve
    C. Femoral branch of genitofemoral nerve
    D. Lateral anterior femoral cutaneous nerve

    Correct Answer: B

    Explanation:

    The iliohypogastric nerve (supplied by L1) runs anterior to the quadratus lumborum muscle, with its anterior branch traveling between the transversus abdominis and internal oblique muscles, making it vulnerable to injury during surgical approaches or from heat transfer via monopolar cautery. The ilioinguinal nerve takes a more posterior path but may move ventrally and inferiorly before piercing the transversus abdominis to enter the inguinal canal. Injury to these sensory nerves can lead to numbness or painful neuroma.

    (CN, p. 332)

42. All of the following are risk factors for cage subsidence in lateral lumbar interbody fusion (LLIF), EXCEPT:
    A. Older age
    B. T score less than −2.5 on femoral neck bone densitometry
    C. Use of recombinant human bone morphogenetic protein-2 (rhBMP-2)
    D. Cage under-sizing

Correct Answer: D

Explanation:

Subsidence, a significant complication of lateral lumbar interbody fusion (LLIF) and other procedures relying on indirect decompression, occurs in 0.3–22% of cases. Risk factors are:

- Patient factors: Advanced age and low bone density (T-score <−2.5)
- Surgical factors:

  Graft Oversizing: Overly tall grafts (>12 mm) increase endplate injury and subsidence risk, with studies recommending 10-mm maximum heights.

  Narrow Cage Widths: The second most common factor, though exceeding working channel limits raises neurovascular injury risks.

  Poor fluoroscopic visualization can contribute to trajectory errors and elevate endplate stress when placing the cage.

  Use of RhBMP-2: May accelerate bone remodeling, potentially increasing early subsidence risk.
- Anatomical factors:

  Specific anatomical challenges, such as the high iliac crest at L4–L5, increase risk by altering entry angles and elevating endplate stress.

  (CN, p. 333)

43. Regarding the risk of spinal cord ischemia during thoracic spine surgery:

43a. Which one of the following factors does NOT increase the risk of spinal cord ischemia?

A. Right-sided surgery at the thoracic spine
B. Multiple ligations of arteries
C. Intraoperative hypotension
D. Anemia

43b. The ideal mean arterial pressure (MAP) during thoracic surgery with stenosis is

A. 60 mm Hg or higher
B. 70 mm IIg or higher
C. 80 mm Hg or higher
D. 90 mm Hg or higher

43c. The watershed area in the thoracic spine is at:

A. T1–T6
B. T3–T7
C. T4–T9
D. T9–T12

Correct Answers: 43a: A, 43b: C, 43c: C

Explanation:

During thoracic surgery, the risk of spinal cord ischemia can be minimized, but preoperative measures include stabilizing blood pressure, adequate intravascular volume, and appropriate hemoglobin/hematocrit levels. Additionally, it has been shown that keeping **mean arterial pressure** (MAP) during complex spine surgery or surgeries with spinal cord stenosis or compression at 80 mm Hg or higher prevents spinal cord ischemia.

During thoracic surgery, multiple arterial ligations could include the artery of Adamkiewicz. The largest radicular artery (also known as arteria radicularis magna), typically originates from the left side in approximately 80% of individuals. Therefore, the **risk of injuring the artery is high when operating in the left side of the thoracic region.** It arises between T5–T8 in 15%, T9–T12 in 75%, and L1–L2 in 10% of cases. The area of the thoracic spine that lies between the vertebral arteries and the artery of Adamkiewicz is the watershed area, and it is more susceptible to watershed infarcts due to the variability in arterial supply, typically at **T4–T9 levels.**

(SS, p. 208) (CN, pp. 304–305)

44. Which factor most significantly increases the risk of vertebral compression fractures in lytic spinal tumors treated with radiosurgery?
    A. Stereotactic radiation dosage per fraction is 20 Gy or more.
    B. Single-fraction radiosurgery with a maximum dosage of 10 Gy.
    C. Radiosurgery at the cervicothoracic junction.
    D. Absence of preexisting spinal deformity.

    Correct Answer: A

    Explanation:

    High-dose radiosurgery fractions (≥20 Gy) are significantly correlated with an increased risk of spinal compression fractures, especially in individuals with preexisting lytic tumors or kyphotic deformities. Additional factors, including lesion location and preexisting abnormalities, influence risk but are less significant than high-dose radiation exposure.

    (BS, pp. 1396–1397)

45. What is the recommended maximum single-fraction dose to the spinal cord to reduce the risk of myelopathy, according to radiosurgery literature?
    A. 20 Gy
    B. 14 Gy
    C. 10 Gy
    D. 24 Gy

    Correct Answer: C

    Explanation:

    Radiation-induced myelopathy is an uncommon yet severe consequence. A maximum dose of 14 Gy has shown efficacy in preventing toxicity; nevertheless, single-fraction doses of 10 Gy and multi-fraction doses up to 20 Gy carry a myelopathy risk of under 1%.

    (BS, pp. 1396–1397)

46. What is the most common non-neurological complication of radiosurgery to the cervical and thoracic spine?
    A. Thyroiditis
    B. Radiation-induced esophagitis
    C. Non-specific chest pain
    D. Lung interstitial disease

    Correct Answer: B

Explanation:

Radiation-induced esophagitis is the most common side effect of radiosurgery of the cervical and thoracic spine, typically presenting as dysphagia and odynophagia. Most cases are self-limiting; however, significant esophageal strictures may occur. Mild cases are treated with a gradual transition to a soft diet and topical anesthetics to relieve symptoms. Strictures may require dilation, but repeated procedures increase the risk of esophageal perforation.

(CM, pp. 358–359)

47. What is the principal mechanism of radiation-induced esophagitis?
    A. Direct thermal injury to esophagus wall
    B. Esophageal secondary bacterial infection
    C. Inflammatory mucosal damage
    D. All of the above

Correct Answer: C

Explanation:

Radiation therapy induces esophagitis primarily by eliciting an inflammatory response that damages the esophageal mucosa. The radiation causes the generation of reactive oxygen species and other inflammatory mediators, damaging basal cells of the epithelium.

[32]

48. What is the most common complication of posterior cervical foraminotomy?
    A. Dural tear
    B. Postoperative kyphosis
    C. C5 palsy
    D. Persistent radiculopathy

Correct Answer: D

Explanation:

Persistent radiculopathy is the most common complication and concern after posterior cervical foraminotomy. It is usually caused by insufficient decompression of the nerve root. Dural tear, kyphosis, and C5 palsy may occur; however, their incidence is rather lower.

[33]

49. The most common complication of the lateral transpsoas approach is:
    A. Vascular injury
    B. Ureteral injury
    C. Thigh numbness
    D. Iliopsoas weakness

Correct Answer: D

Explanation:

Iliopsoas weakness is the most common complication of the lateral transpsoas approach. It occurs due to irritation or injury to the lumbar plexus. The second most common complication is thigh numbness. Vascular injury, ureteral injury, and bowel injury are less common but serious complications.

[34]

50. In an endoscopic transforaminal lumbar discectomy, the most common complication arises from:
    A. Excessive removal of the annulus
    B. Insufficient decompression of the neural elements
    C. Acute leg dysesthesia
    D. Surgical site infection

    Correct Answer: C

    Explanation:

    The most common complication following lumbar transforaminal endoscopic decompression is dysesthesia due to dorsal root ganglion irritation. It affects around 21.5% of patients. The patient typically has an acute onset of dysesthetic leg pain after an initial pain-free period lasting 5–10 days postoperatively. It is generally transient and can be managed with neuropathic medications such as pregabalin or gabapentin or with epidural injections.

    Although insufficient decompression and excessive annulus removal can result in suboptimal outcomes, and surgical site infection is a recognized complication, these are less common.

    [35]

51. Regarding C5 palsy following a cervical laminectomy and fusion procedure for myelopathy

    51a. Which of the following is the most acceptable etiology?
    A. Thermal injury from using monopolar coagulation
    B. Tethering of the nerve root with subsequent traction from posterior migration of the cord after decompression
    C. Nerve root ischemia from manipulation
    D. C5 nerve root has a shorter course and is angled more caudally

    51b. It typically occurs:
    A. Postoperative day 1 to 5
    B. Postoperative day 6 to 14
    C. Postoperative day 15 to 30
    D. Can occur post-operative time

    51c. All of the following are unique anatomy of C5 that contribute to C5 palsy, EXCEPT:
    A. Shorter rootlets
    B. Horizontal course
    C. Small cross-sectional area
    D. Larger transverse foramen of C5

    Correct Answers: 51a: B, 51b: A, 51c: D

    Explanation:

    C5 palsy is characterized by new-onset deltoid weakness, with or without biceps involvement, typically occurring 1–3 days postoperatively after decompressive cervical spine surgery. It is defined as a motor decline of at least one grade in deltoid strength within 6 weeks post-surgery. The incidence is 6% of cervical decompression cases and occurs unilaterally in 92% of cases. The leading etiology is thought to be **traction from posterior migration of the spinal**

cord after decompression, exacerbated by C5's unique anatomy, including shorter rootlets, a horizontal course, and a small cross-sectional area.

Risk factors include a decreased preoperative C4–C5 foraminal diameter (<2 mm), spinal cord rotation, and posterior surgical approaches, though demographic or surgical variables (e.g., number of levels or graft type) have not been consistently implicated. No effective preventative measures are established, though prophylactic foraminotomies have shown mixed results.

Management is usually expectant, as recovery is likely; 48% resolve within 3 months, and severe cases may take up to 6 months. Recovery rates are higher with posterior approaches (89%) than anterior ones (75%). Physical therapy to maintain joint mobility and prevent contractures is critical. For persistent palsy, interventions like nerve or tendon transfers or joint fusion may be necessary.

(GB, p. 1306)

52. Regarding recurrent lumbar disc herniation:

52a. What is the definition of recurrent lumbar disc herniation?

A. Reherniation at the same surgical level and either on the ipsilateral or contralateral side after at least 6 months of a pain-free period.
B. Reherniation at the same surgical level and either on the ipsilateral or contralateral side after at least 3 months of a pain-free period.
C. Reherniation at the same surgical level and on the ipsilateral side only after at least 6 months of a pain-free period.
D. Reherniation at the same surgical level and on the ipsilateral side only after at least 3 months of a pain-free period.

52b. What is the approximate recurrence rate of herniation at the same level?

A. 2%
B. 6%
C. 15%
D. 25%

52c. All of the following are risk factors for recurrent lumbar disc herniations, EXCEPT:

A. Smoking
B. Obesity
C. Female sex
D. Occupational lifting

Correct Answers: 52a: A, 52b: B, 52c: C

Explanation:

Recurrent lumbar disc herniation is defined as the recurrence of herniation at the same surgical level after at least 6 months of being pain-free, occurring either on the ipsilateral or contralateral side. The reported incidence varies widely, ranging from 5% to 23%. Most of the surgeons quote an incidence of 6–10%. Contributing risk factors include age, male sex, BMI, smoking, diabetes, obesity, intraoperative techniques, type of herniation, disc height index, large annular defects (≥6 mm), occupational lifting, trauma, and limited discectomy during the initial surgery.

[8]

53. What is the most common complication of vertebroplasty for osteoporosis compression vertebral fracture?
   A. Cement leakage
   B. Infection
   C. New vertebral fracture
   D. Hematoma

   Correct Answer: A

   Explanation:

   Cement extravasation is the most common complication in vertebral augmentation surgeries. It occurs in up to 87.9% of vertebroplasty cases and 9% of kyphoplasty cases. The majority are asymptomatic; nonetheless, extravasation may lead to severe complications, including pulmonary embolism, neurological impairment, or spinal cord injury. Kyphoplasty has a lower extravasation rate due to its low-pressure injection system, allowing for more viscous cement. Preventive measures include high-quality imaging, careful needle placement, and the use of well-opacified cement.

   Additional complications include rib and pedicle fractures, which occur at low rates and are often linked to patient positioning during the procedure.

   (BS, p. 1171)

54. A 62-year-old patient who underwent multilevel lumbar laminectomy complicated by incidental durotomy. The dura was closed with watertight closure. What would you order for his postoperative activity?
   A. Bed rest 4–7 days
   B. Normal post-op mobilization
   C. Head of the bed elevation 40° when laying down
   D. Prone position for the first 24 h postoperatively

   Correct Answer: B

   Explanations:

   In incidental durotomy, a watertight primary closure using nonabsorbable sutures, with or without a patch graft, is recommended to prevent pseudomeningocele or CSF fistula. Care must be taken to avoid entrapping nerve roots in the closure, and a cottonoid may be placed over the defect to protect nerve roots from aspiration. In cases where the tear is inaccessible, such as on the anterior dura or nerve root sleeve, alternative strategies include using fat or muscle grafts, fibrin glue, or blood patches. Watertight closure of fascia, fat, and skin is often advocated, and drainage options vary based on surgical preferences.

   CSF diversion, such as using a drain placed at a different spinal level, may be utilized in more complex cases. While bed rest for 4–7 days is often advised to facilitate healing, normal mobilization is acceptable if a watertight repair is achieved. In cases of postoperative leaks, noninvasive management with resuturing under local anesthesia, Trendelenburg positioning, and daily drainage has been successful. Broad-spectrum antibiotics and vigilant wound care are also crucial in such scenarios.

   (GB, p. 1261)

55. A 32-year-old patient had bilateral visual loss after two levels of transforaminal lumbar interbody fusion. The following are risk factors for this condition, EXCEPT:
    A. Surgery in the prone position
    B. Lack of tight glycemic control
    C. Use of reverse Trendelenburg position
    D. Overuse of crystalloid

    Correct Answer: C

    Explanation:

    Postoperative visual loss is a rare but devastating complication, most commonly caused by ischemic optic neuropathy (ION), particularly posterior ION. It is frequently associated with significant blood loss (≥2 L), prolonged operative time (≥6 h), or anesthetic duration (>5 h), often leading to hypotension and impaired blood flow. Risk factors include prone positioning, Trendelenburg positioning, hemodilution, cellular hypoxia, and poor glycemic control. Six independent risk factors for POVL include male gender, obesity (BMI ≥30), use of the Wilson frame, prolonged anesthesia, excessive blood loss, and imbalanced fluid replacement favoring crystalloids over colloids.

    Since the blindness is often permanent and no effective treatments exist, prevention through meticulous surgical and anesthetic management is critical.

    (GB, p. 1262)

56. Routine use of BMP in anterior cervical spine surgery should be avoided due to, EXCEPT
    A. Risk of pseudoarthrosis
    B. Risk of dysphagia
    C. Risk of postsurgical hematoma
    D. Increased risk of infection

    Correct Answer: A

    Explanation:

    Bone morphogenetic protein (BMP) use in the cervical spine, specifically in anterior approaches, has been linked to increased risks of dysphagia, prevertebral swelling, hematoma, reintubation, and infections. Due to these risks, the U.S. Food and Drug Administration (FDA) issued a warning in 2008 regarding BMP use in cervical spine procedures. Therefore, routine application of BMP in the cervical spine is not recommended.

    (RSS, p. 106)

57. Post cervical laminectomy kyphosis can cause dysphagia due to:
    A. Increased pharyngeal space and overworked of swallowing muscles
    B. Collapse of pharyngeal space and inefficient coordination of swallowing muscles
    C. Inability to maximally extend the neck
    D. Osteophyte compression of the pharyngeal space

    Correct Answer: B

Explanation:

Dysphagia is also a common symptom of post-cervical laminectomy kyphosis, typically resulting from the collapse of the pharyngeal space and impaired coordination of the swallowing muscles.

(NSE, p. 72)

15 Other Spine Conditions MCQs

1. All of the following are features of low back pain from ankylosing spondylitis, EXCEPT:
   A. Age at onset ≤40 years
   B. Pain not relieved when supine
   C. Morning back stiffness
   D. Pain <3 months duration
   Correct Answer: D
   Explanation:
   Back pain in usually >3 months of duration
   (GB, p. 1229)
2. The typical radiographic Paget's disease affected vertebral is called:
   A. Ivory vertebra
   B. Paget's vertebra
   C. Victory vertebra
   D. Von-Paget Helsing vertebra
   Correct Answer: A
   Explanation:
   Paget's disease is characterized by increased bone absorption and increased osteoblastic activity, producing weak bone appearing in imaging as vertebra with increased opacity, Ivory vertebra.
   (GB, p. 1362)
3. Spine Paget's disease commonly affect:
   A. Cervical
   B. Thoracic
   C. Lumbar
   D. Sacral
   Correct Answer: C
   (GB, p. 1362)

K. F. AlAli, H. T. Hashim, *Spine Surgery and Peripheral Nerve Surgery*,
https://doi.org/10.1007/978-3-031-98543-0_15

4. A 23-year-old presented with thoracic back pain for 2 years. Thoracic X-ray is shown (Fig. 15.1). What is the best next step in management?
   A. Rheumatoid factor test
   B. HLA-B27 genetic test
   C. MRI thoracic spine
   D. Physiotherapy referral
   Correct Answer: C
   Explanation:
   Imaging shows increased thoracic kyphosis. When a patient is young with chronic back pain and thoracic kyphosis, Scheuermann's syndrome needs to be ruled out by MRI of the thoracic spine. (GB, p. 1375)
5. All of the following are features of Scheuermann's syndrome, EXCEPT:
   A. Endplate irregularities
   B. Anterior narrowing of disc space
   C. Schmorl's nodes
   D. Pars articularis defect
   Correct Answer: D
   (GB, p. 1375)

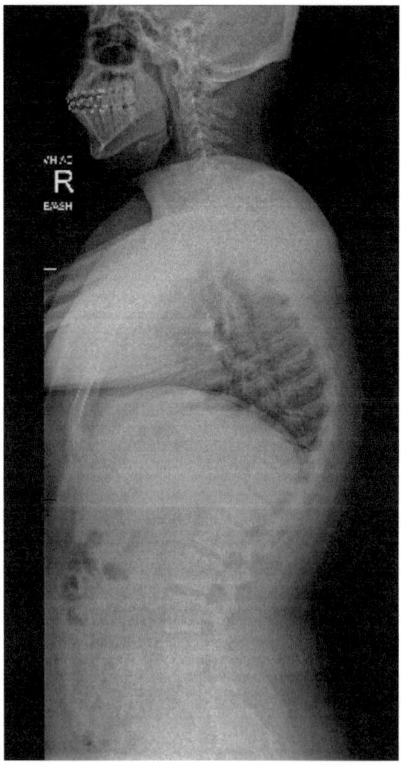

Fig. 15.1 Case 4 thoracic X-ray

6. A 28-year-old female presents with acute onset of back pain, followed by progressive weakness and numbness in both legs over 12 hours. She also reports urinary retention. Her medical history includes a recent viral illness and autoimmune hypothyroidism. MRI of the thoracic spine is shown (Fig. 15.2). What is the likely diagnosis?
   A. Transverse myelitis
   B. Systemic autoimmune diseases
   C. Multiple sclerosis
   D. Intramedullary neoplasm
   Correct Answer: A
   Explanation:
   Transverse myelitis is an idiopathic, post-infectious, or autoimmune disease affecting the spine. It has a rapid progression course, like in this case.
   (GB, p. 195)
7. Which of the following statements regarding diffuse idiopathic skeletal hyperostosis (DISH) involving the cervical spine is true?
   A. It typically affects the posterior longitudinal ligament.
   B. It is associated with HLA-B27 positivity.
   C. It can lead to dysphagia due to anterior osteophyte formation.
   D. It results in ligamentum flavum ossification.
   Correct Answer: C

Fig. 15.2 Case 6 MRI of the thoracic spine

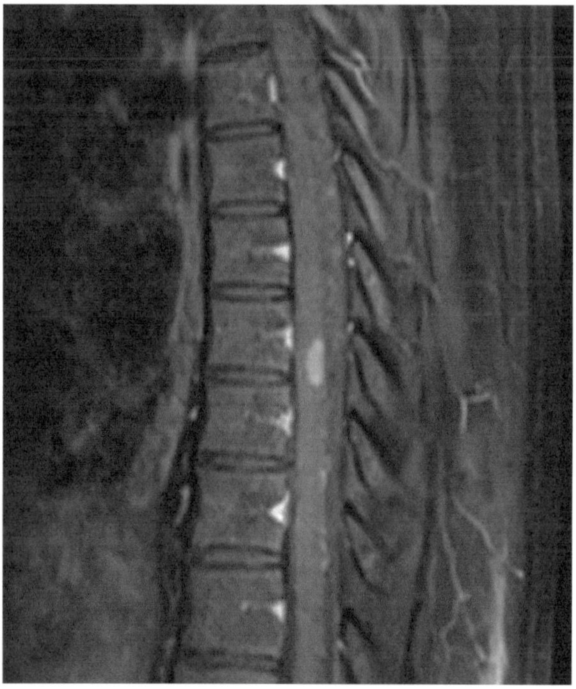

Explanation:

Diffuse idiopathic skeletal hyperostosis (DISH) is characterized by **flowing osteophyte formation** along the anterior longitudinal ligament, which can compress the esophagus, leading to **dysphagia**. This condition typically affects older individuals and is more common in the cervical and thoracic spine. Dysphagia occurs due to the mechanical obstruction caused by the large anterior osteophytes.

(**SS,** p. 683)

8. Rheumatoid arthritis can lead to cervical spine involvement. The most common cervical spine manifestation is:
   A. Atlantoaxial subluxation
   B. Basilar invagination
   C. Subaxial subluxation
   D. Uncovertebral joint arthrosis

   Correct Answer: A

   Explanation:

   Rheumatoid arthritis can affect the cervical spine. The most common location is **atlantoaxial subluxation**. Chronic inflammation weakens the **transverse ligament** of the atlas. It causes atlantoaxial instability.

   (GB, p. 1376)
9. Systemic sclerosis (scleroderma) can lead to cervical spine involvement. The most common cervical spine manifestation is:
   A. Intervertebral disc calcification
   B. Facet joint arthritis
   C. Osteoporotic compression fractures
   D. Ligamentous ossification

   Correct Answer: A

   Explanation:

   Scleroderma induces dystrophic calcinosis that can cause intervertebral disc calcification, leading to spinal canal stenosis and spinal instability.

   [63]
10. Tuberous sclerosis complex (TSC) can have spinal manifestations. Which of the following is NOT typically associated with TSC?
   A. Cortical tubers
   B. Subependymal nodules
   C. Dural ectasia
   D. Shagreen patches

   Correct Answer: C

   Explanation:

   Tuberous sclerosis is a group of autosomal dominant neurocutaneous disorders that can affect spine with hamartomas, ependymoma, vertebral bone lesions, and dural-based lesions. It has specific clinical features, dural etasia is not of them.

   (GB, p. 644)

11. In patients with ankylosing spondylitis, which of the following is the most common cause of spinal cord injury?
    A. Disc herniation
    B. Epidural abscess
    C. Fracture through an ankylosed segment
    D. Transverse myelitis

    Correct Answer: C

    (GB, p. 1365)
12. Which of the following is NOT a typical feature of spinal involvement in psoriatic arthritis?
    A. Asymmetric sacroiliitis
    B. Syndesmophyte formation
    C. Non-marginal vertebral body syndesmophytes
    D. Bamboo spine appearance

    Correct Answer: D

    Explanation:

    Psoriatic arthritis affects the joints of the spine. Bamboo spine appearance is not a typical feature

    (SS, p. 671)
13. In patients with sarcoidosis, spinal cord involvement is most commonly due to:
    A. Granulomatous vertebral osteomyelitis
    B. Dural ectasia
    C. Epidural lipomatosis
    D. Direct spinal cord granuloma

    Correct Answer: A

    Explanation:

    In sarcoidosis, spinal cord involvement—though rare—most commonly results from direct granulomatous inflammation of the spinal cord (i.e., intramedullary granulomas). These lesions can cause progressive myelopathy and may mimic neoplastic or infectious etiologies on imaging.

    (SS, p. 666)
14. Which of the following is NOT a common spinal manifestation of hemochromatosis?
    A. Osteopenia
    B. Osteoarthritis
    C. Chondrocalcinosis
    D. Asymmetric sacroiliitis

    Correct Answer: D

    Explanation:

    Hemochromatosis can affect bone and cartilage. In the spine, it affects vertebral bodies and discs. Asymmetric sacroiliitis is not a feature.

    [64]
15. In patients with osteogenesis imperfecta, which spinal pathology is most common?
    A. Atlantoaxial instability
    B. Thoracic kyphosis

C. Lumbar hyperlordosis
D. Spondylolisthesis
Correct Answer: B
Explanation:
Osteogenesis imperfecta frequently affects the spine, causing fractures leading to deformities, commonly in the thoracic spine.
[65]

16. Which of the following is a typical spinal manifestation of acromegaly?
A. Facet joint hypertrophy
B. Spinal stenosis
C. Diffuse idiopathic skeletal hyperostosis (DISH)
D. All of the above
Correct Answer: D
Explanation:
In acromegaly, excess growth hormone leads to characteristic spinal changes including facet joint hypertrophy, spinal stenosis, and sometimes diffuse idiopathic skeletal hyperostosis (DISH). These manifestations result from abnormal bone and soft tissue overgrowth, particularly in the vertebral joints and ligaments, and may present clinically as back pain, radiculopathy, or myelopathy. Early recognition is important as these changes can progress if the underlying endocrine disorder remains untreated.
[66]

17. In patients with Marfan syndrome, which of the following spinal conditions is most commonly observed?
A. Scoliosis
B. Spinal epidural hematoma
C. Cauda equina syndrome
D. Syringomyelia
Correct Answer: A
Explanation:
In patients with Marfan syndrome, the most commonly observed spinal condition is scoliosis, which affects up to 60% of individuals with the disorder. This connective tissue disorder, caused by mutations in the fibrillin-1 gene, leads to ligamentous laxity and skeletal overgrowth, contributing to spinal deformities such as scoliosis and kyphosis. While other spinal issues like dural ectasia may also occur, conditions such as spinal epidural hematoma, cauda equina syndrome, and syringomyelia are rare and not characteristic features of Marfan syndrome.
[67]

18. Which of the following is NOT a typical feature of spinal involvement in Langerhans cell histiocytosis (LCH)?
A. Vertebra plana
B. Osteoblastic lesions
C. Epidural extension of the lesion
D. Painful scoliosis
Correct Answer: B

Explanation:

Langerhans cell histiocytosis is a benign condition that usually affects young patients, characterized by spine lesions that cause lytic lesions. It can cause vertebral plana features, and in severe cases, it causes deformities and lesion extension to the epidural space

(DI, p. 760)

19. In patients with polycystic kidney disease, which spinal abnormality is most commonly associated?
    A. Dural ectasia
    B. Syringomyelia
    C. Spinal stenosis
    D. Spondylolisthesis

    Correct Answer: A

    Explanation:

    Dural ectasia is the widening of the dura causing scalloping of the vertebral bodies. It associated with Marfan's syndrome, polycystic kidney disease, homocystinuria, and Ehlers–Danlo syndrome.

    (DI, p. 178)

20. In patients with primary hyperparathyroidism, which of the following spinal conditions is most commonly observed?
    A. Osteoporotic fractures
    B. Diffuse idiopathic skeletal hyperostosis (DISH)
    C. Osteoid osteoma
    D. Ankylosing spondylitis

    Correct Answer: A

    Explanation:

    In patients with primary hyperparathyroidism, the most commonly observed spinal condition is osteoporotic fractures, particularly involving the thoracolumbar spine. Elevated parathyroid hormone levels lead to increased bone resorption, reduced bone mineral density, and skeletal fragility, making patients more susceptible to compression fractures and kyphotic deformity.

    (DI, p. 968)

21. Which of the following is NOT a typical spinal manifestation of Gaucher's disease?
    A. H-shaped vertebrae
    B. Osteopenia
    C. Epidural hematoma
    D. Kyphoscoliosis

    Correct Answer: C

    Explanation:

    Gaucher's disease is a lipid storage disease resulting from deficiency of lysosomal glucocerebrosidase. It is characterized by H-shaped vertebrae, osteopenia, and deformities.

    (DI, p. 213)

22. Which of the following is NOT a common spinal manifestation of Wilson's disease?
   A. Premature disc degeneration
   B. Osteochondritis dissecans
   C. Kyphoscoliosis
   D. Osteoporosis

   Correct Answer: B

   Explanation:

   Wilson's disease is a rare, autosomal recessive disorder caused by abnormal copper accumulation. In the spine, it can cause premature disc degeneration, kyphoscoliosis, and osteoporosis.

   [68]
23. What is the most common spinal manifestation of hemophilia?
   A. Pseudotumor formation
   B. Epidural hematoma
   C. Subdural hematoma
   D. Hemarthrosis

   Correct Answer: B

   Explanation:

   Spontaneous spinal epidural hematoma is a rare complication of hemophilia, but the most common manifestation of hemophilia in the spine. It most commonly occurs after the fourth or fifth decade of life.

   [69]
24. The following is an indication for surgical treatment of Diffuse idiopathic skeletal hyperostosis (DISH)
   A. Severe mechanical neck pain
   B. Dysphagia
   C. Cervical radiculopathy
   D. All of the above

   Correct Answer: B

   Explanation:

   DISH can cause dysphagia and airway obstruction. Excision of osteophytes using the Smith–Robinson approach, typically without fusion, is considered when conservative treatment fails to resolve these rare issues.

   (SS, p. 683)
25. A 40-year-old male presents with rapidly progressing weakness in both legs, facial weakness, and mild sensory changes in his hands. Lumbar puncture shows albuminocytologic dissociation, and NCV studies indicate slowing. Which of the following clinical features would most cast doubt on the diagnosis of Guillain–Barré Syndrome (GBS)?
   A. Facial weakness
   B. Symmetric progression
   C. Persistent bowel or bladder dysfunction
   D. Increased CSF protein not more than 50 mg/dL

   Correct Answer: C

Explanation:

Persistent bowel or bladder dysfunction is rare in GBS and would raise suspicion for other diagnoses, such as spinal cord pathology. GBS typically presents with symmetric weakness, cranial nerve involvement, and albuminocytologic dissociation in the CSF.

(GP, pp. 193–195)

26. Which of the following features is most characteristic of the Miller–Fisher variant of Guillain–Barré Syndrome?
    A. Ataxia, ophthalmoplegia, and areflexia
    B. Ascending paralysis with absent deep tendon reflexes
    C. Severe sensory loss with pain
    D. Bilateral lower extremity weakness with facial diplegia

    Correct Answer: A

    Explanation:

    The Miller–Fisher variant of GBS is characterized by ataxia, ophthalmoplegia, and areflexia. This variant is associated with anti-GQ1b antibodies and is less common than the typical ascending paralysis form of GBS.

    (GP, pp. 193–195)

27. A 35-year-old woman presents with progressive leg weakness and sensory loss over three weeks. Electrodiagnostics show slowed nerve conduction velocity, and CSF shows elevated protein without pleocytosis. Which finding would most strongly suggest Guillain–Barré Syndrome over other potential causes?
    A. Cranial nerve involvement
    B. Marked asymmetry of weakness
    C. Sharp sensory level
    D. Persistent fever at the onset of neuritic symptoms

    Correct Answer: A

    Explanation:

    Cranial nerve involvement, especially facial diplegia, is seen in up to 50% of GBS cases. Asymmetric weakness, sharp sensory level, and persistent fever are features that cast doubt on the diagnosis of GBS.

    (GP, p. 193–195)

28. A 42-year-old woman presents with a 2-year history of widespread aching pain in her shoulders, lower back, and thighs, accompanied by severe fatigue and difficulty sleeping. She reports feeling unrefreshed in the morning and has trouble concentrating at work. Physical examination reveals multiple tender points, but no joint swelling or warmth.

    28a. What is the most likely diagnosis?
    A. Rheumatoid arthritis
    B. Osteoarthritis
    C. Fibromyalgia
    D. Diabetic polyneuropathy

    28b. What distinguishes this condition from regional myofascial pain syndrome?
    A. This condition involves trigger points with radiating pain.
    B. This condition is characterized by widespread pain and abnormal pain processing.

C. Regional myofascial pain syndrome requires 4 kg/cm^2 pressure to elicit tenderness.
D. This condition is a localized pain syndrome.

28c. Which of the following is the most common symptom reported by patients with fibromyalgia?
A. Cognitive dysfunction
B. Muscle spasms
C. Mood disturbance
D. Fatigue

28d. Which condition is considered a central pain sensitivity syndrome that commonly coexists with this condition?
A. Osteoporosis
B. Irritable bowel syndrome
C. Gout
D. Peripheral neuropathy

28e. Which demographic group is most likely to develop fibromyalgia?
A. Children under 10 years
B. Males aged 20–30 years
C. Females aged 30–55 years
D. Elderly males over 65 years

Answers: 28a: C, 28b: B, 28c: D, 28d: B, 28e: C

Explanation:

This case exemplifies fibromyalgia, distinct from rheumatoid arthritis (joint swelling) or osteoarthritis (joint-specific). Fibromyalgia features widespread pain and abnormal pain processing, unlike the localized trigger points of myofascial pain syndrome. Fatigue affects 90% of patients, making it the most prevalent symptom. Irritable bowel syndrome, a central sensitivity syndrome, commonly coexists. The condition primarily impacts females aged 30–55 years. Acute trauma, like cervical whiplash, can trigger it. Tenderness outside joint locations differentiates it from arthritis on examination. Central sensitization with expanded receptive fields drives its amplified pain perception. Pregabalin effectively addresses sleep disturbance and neuropathic pain.

Part II

Peripheral Nerve Surgery

16 Peripheral Nerves Anatomy and Physiology

1. Identify structures 1–23 and A, B, and C (Fig. 16.1):

   Correct Answers:

   1: C5 vertebra, 2: C5 nerve root, 3: C6 nerve root, 4: C7 nerve root, 5: C8 nerve root, 6: T1 nerve root, 7: dorsal scapular nerve, 8: nerve to subclavius, 9: long thoracic nerve, 10: superior trunk, 11: middle trunk, 12: inferior trunk, 13: lateral pectoral nerve, 14: axillary nerve, 15 radial nerve, 16: lower subscapular nerve, 17: thoracodorsal nerve, 18: upper subscapular nerve, 19:

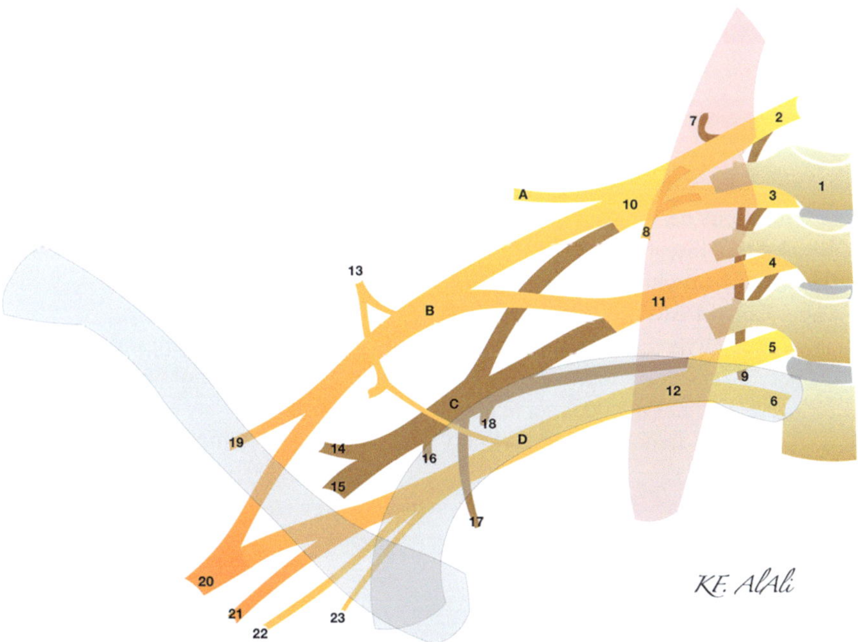

Fig. 16.1 Case 1 diagram

K. F. AlAli, H. T. Hashim, *Spine Surgery and Peripheral Nerve Surgery*,
https://doi.org/10.1007/978-3-031-98543-0_16

Fig. 16.2 Case 2 diagram

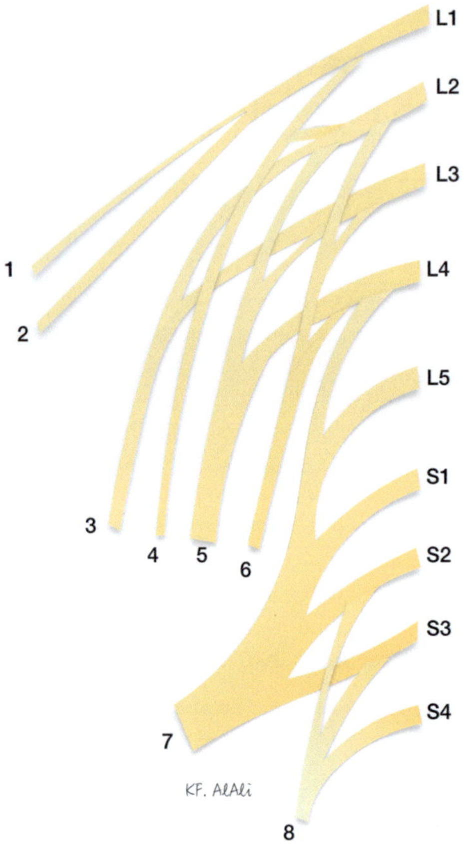

musculocutaneous nerve, 20: median nerve, 21: ulnar nerve, and 22: medial cutaneous nerve of forearm, medial cutaneous nerve of arm

A: suprascapular nerve, B: lateral cord, C: posterior cord, and D: medial cord

2. Identify structures 1–8 (Fig. 16.2):

   Correct Answers:

   1: Iliohypogastric nerve, 2: ilioinguinal nerve, 3: Lateral femoral cutaneous nerve, 4: Genitofemoral nerve, 5: Femoral nerve, 6: Obturator nerve, 7: Sciatic nerve, and 8: Pudendal nerve
3. The lateral femoral cutaneous nerve is a branch from which spinal levels?
   A. L2–L3
   B. L4–L5
   C. S4–S5
   D. C8–T1

   Correct Answer: A

   Explanation:

   The lateral femoral cutaneous nerve arises from the lumbar plexus, specifically the posterior divisions of the L2 and L3 nerve roots.(NB, p. 782)

4. In the brachial plexus, the medial cord gives rise to all of the following nerves EXCEPT:
   A. Medial pectoral nerve
   B. Medial cutaneous nerve of the forearm
   C. Ulnar nerve
   D. Thoracodorsal nerve
   Correct Answer: D
   (NB, p. 777)
5. Which of the following nerves passes through both the greater and lesser sciatic foramina?
   A. Pudendal nerve
   B. Sciatic nerve
   C. Superior gluteal nerve
   D. Inferior gluteal nerve
   Correct Answer: A
   Explanation:
   The pudendal nerve comes from the sacral plexus, S2, S3, and S4. It leaves the pelvis through the lower greater sciatic foramen. It crosses over the sacrospinous ligament near the ischial spine. Then, it re-enters the pelvis through the lesser sciatic foramen.
6. The Alcock's canal contains the following nerve:
   A. Pudendal nerve
   B. Sciatic nerve
   C. Superior gluteal nerve
   D. Inferior gluteal nerve
   Correct Answer: A
   Explanation:
   The pudendal re-enters the pelvis and follows the internal pudendal vessels. It moves anterosuperiorly through Alcock's canal (pudendal canal). This canal forms from the fascia of the obturator internus muscle. Inside, the nerve splits into branches. First, it gives off the inferior rectal nerve. Next, it sends out the perineal nerve. Finally, it continues as the dorsal nerve of the penis or clitoris.
   (EPN, p. 204)
7. Regarding the autonomic innervation of peripheral nerves, which neurotransmitter is primarily released by postganglionic sympathetic fibers supplying sweat glands?
   A. Norepinephrine
   B. Acetylcholine
   C. Dopamine
   D. Epinephrine
   Correct Answer: B
   Explanation:
   Although most postganglionic sympathetic fibers release norepinephrine, those that innervate eccrine sweat glands are an important exception — they

release acetylcholine. This cholinergic innervation activates muscarinic receptors on sweat glands, leading to perspiration. This is a unique feature of the sympathetic nervous system and explains why anticholinergic medications can reduce sweating.

8. The brachial plexus roots passed between:
   A. Anterior scalene and middle scalene muscles
   B. Middle scalene and posterior scalene muscles
   C. Anterior scalene and posterior scalene muscles
   D. Two heads of anterior scalene muscles

   Correct Answer: A

   Explanation:

   The roots of the brachial plexus (C5–T1) emerge between the anterior and middle scalene muscles in the neck, forming part of the interscalene triangle along with the subclavian artery.

   (EPN, p. 86)
9. Damage to which nerve would result in loss of the cremasteric reflex, and what spinal levels does it involve?
   A. Iliohypogastric nerve
   B. Genitofemoral nerve
   C. Femoral nerve
   D. Obturator nerve

   Correct Answer: B

   Explanation:

   The genital branch of the genitofemoral nerve supplies the cremaster muscle. This muscle controls testicular movement. It helps regulate temperature by lifting the testicle on the same side. The cremasteric reflex can be tested by touching the inguinal area lightly. This should cause the testicle to rise on the same side.

   (EPN, p. 187)
10. The peroneal component of the sciatic nerve originates from which divisions of the sacral plexus, and what is its primary function?
    A. Anterior divisions; plantar flexion
    B. Anterior divisions; dorsiflexion
    C. Posterior divisions; plantar flexion
    D. Posterior divisions; dorsiflexion

    Correct Answer: D

    Explanation:

    Before the sciatic nerve forms, the ventral rami split. The tibial nerve comes from the anterior divisions. **The common peroneal nerve comes from the posterior divisions**. This setup seems unusual. The tibial nerve supplies posterior compartment muscles. The common peroneal nerve supplies the anterior ones.

    (EPN, p. 139)

11. The sacral plexus originates from the spinal nerves of:
    A. L5–S2
    B. L4–S4
    C. L4–S3
    D. S1–S4
    Correct Answer: C
    Explanation:
    The sacral plexus is formed by the lumbosacral trunk (L4–L5) and the anterior rami of S1 to S4, making L4–S4 the correct range. This plexus lies on the anterior surface of the piriformis muscle.
    (MPN, p. 42)
12. The dorsal scapular nerve arises from which root/trunk of the brachial plexus, and what muscle does it innervate?
    A. C5 root; Rhomboid major
    B. C6 root; Levator scapulae
    C. Upper trunk; Serratus anterior
    D. Middle trunk; Subscapularis
    Correct Answer: A
    Explanation:
    The dorsal scapular nerve arises from the C5 nerve root of the brachial plexus, before the formation of trunks. It typically pierces the middle scalene muscle and travels posteriorly to innervate the rhomboid major, rhomboid minor, and sometimes the levator scapulae. It plays a key role in retracting and stabilizing the scapula.
    (MPN, p. 85)
13. The nervi nervorum are:
    A. Small nerves that innervate the vasa vasorum
    B. Autonomic fibers innervating the meninges
    C. Nerves supplying the connective tissue of peripheral nerves
    D. Sensory fibers within muscle spindles
    Correct Answer: C
    Explanation:
    Nervi nervorum are tiny nerve fibers. They supply the outer layers of larger nerves. They provide sensation to the nerve sheaths. These fibers detect pain and irritation. They help in nerve protection and response. When compressed, they may cause nerve pain.
    (CA, p. 528)
14. The differences between abductor pollicis longus and abductor pollicis brevis in:
    A. The longus is innervated by a recurrent branch of the median nerve
    B. The longus is located in the hand
    C. The longus is more superficial
    D. The longus adducts the thumb in a radial direction
    Correct Answer: D

Explanation:

The abductor pollicis longus and abductor pollicis brevis are different. The longus is in the forearm, but the brevis is in the hand. The longus is innervated by the posterior interosseous nerve. The brevis gets its nerve supply from the recurrent branch of the median nerve. The longus abducts the thumb in a radial direction. The brevis moves the thumb away from the palm. The longus is deep in the forearm. The brevis is more superficial in the hand.

(MPN, p. 38)

15. Which nerve provides cutaneous innervation to the medial aspect of the leg and foot?
    A. Saphenous nerve
    B. Superficial peroneal nerve
    C. Sural nerve
    D. Deep peroneal nerve

    Correct Answer: A
16. Which nerve root contributes to the sensory innervation of the lateral foot, and which peripheral nerve transmits these fibers?
    A. L3; Saphenous nerve
    B. L5; Deep peroneal nerve
    C. S1; Sural nerve
    D. S2; Tibial nerve

    Correct Answer: C
17. The following illustration is showing the feet dermatomes. Identify the rest of the sensory innervations [1–6] (Fig. 16.3).

    Answers:

    1: Lateral plantar nerve. 2: Sural nerve. 3: Calcaneal nerve. 4: Medial plantar nerve. 5: Deep peroneal nerve. 6: Superficial peroneal nerve
18. Regarding the neural crest origin of peripheral nerves, which cells responsible for myelination are derived from neural crest cells?
    A. Schwann cells
    B. Oligodendrocytes
    C. Astrocytes
    D. Microglia

    Correct Answer: A

    Explanation:

    Schwann cells are derived from neural crest cells and are responsible for myelination in the peripheral nervous system.
19. Which of the following peripheral nerve fibers is responsible for transmitting sharp, localized pain?
    A. A-alpha fibers
    B. A-delta fibers
    C. C fibers
    D. B fibers

    Correct Answer: B

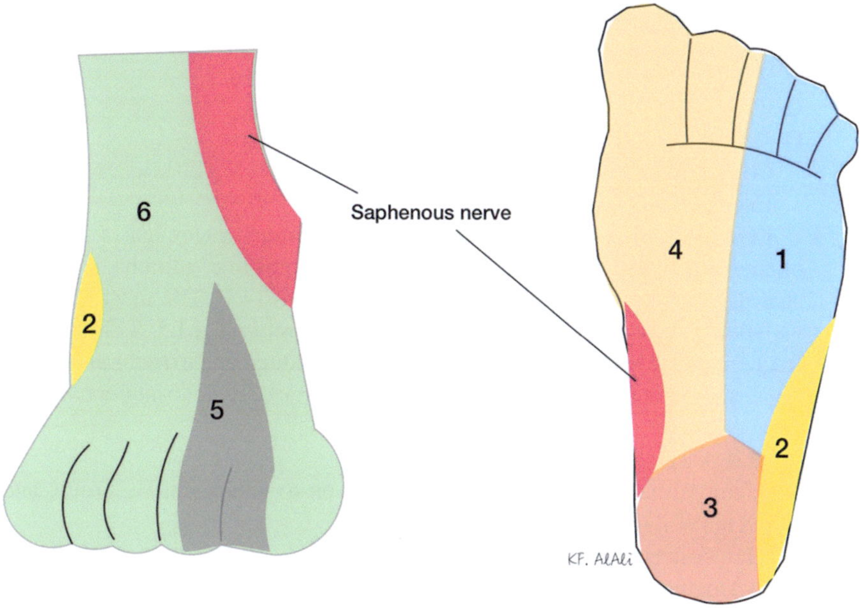

Fig. 16.3 The foot dermatomes

Explanation:

A-delta fibers are thin, myelinated peripheral nerve fibers responsible for transmitting sharp, localized, and fast pain, as well as temperature sensations. They conduct impulses more rapidly than C fibers, which are unmyelinated and associated with dull, aching, and poorly localized pain.

- A-alpha fibers carry motor signals for muscle contraction and proprioception.
- B fibers are preganglionic autonomic fibers and are not involved in somatic pain transmission.

(NB, p. 55)

20. The radial nerve usually bifurcates into the posterior interosseous and superficial sensory at:
    A. Proximal to the elbow joint
    B. At the elbow joint
    C. Distal to the elbow joint
    D. Medial part of the elbow joint

    Correct answer: C.

    Explanation:

    Just distal to the elbow joint, the radial nerve bifurcates into the superficial branch and the posterior interosseous nerve (PIN), in the proximal forearm and at the level of the radial head.

    (MPN. p. 36)

21. The most common lumbar spine level with nerve root anatomical variation is:
    A. L1–L2
    B. L2–L3
    C. L4–L5
    D. L5–S1

    Correct Answer: D. L5–S1

    Explanation:

    Lumbosacral nerve roots can exhibit numerous anatomical variations, often explaining inconsistent neurological symptoms in conditions like herniated discs or lateral stenosis. The incidence is 4–14%. The most common variation is the atypical origin or exit of the nerve roots. The L5–S1 is the most frequently involved level. Variations include intradural and extradural connections, anomalous origins, and conjoined nerve roots, which share a common dural envelope.

    (BS, p. 31)
22. The femoral nerve provides motor innervation to which muscle group, and which nerve roots contribute to its formation?
    A. Hamstrings; L4–L5
    B. Adductors; L2–L3
    C. Quadriceps; L2–L4
    D. Gluteal muscles; L5–S1

    Correct Answer: C

    Explanation:

    The femoral nerve, formed from the L2–L4 nerve roots, is the main motor supply to the quadriceps femoris muscle group, which is responsible for knee extension. It also innervates the iliacus and sartorius muscles, and provides sensory innervation to the anterior thigh and medial leg via the saphenous nerve.

    (EPN, p. 176)
23. Which of the following best describes the anatomical course of the femoral nerve?
    A. It arises from the anterior divisions of L2–L4 and passes through the obturator canal.
    B. It forms within the psoas major, runs lateral to it, and enters the thigh beneath the inguinal ligament.
    C. It arises from the sacral plexus, exits the pelvis via the greater sciatic foramen, and runs posteriorly.
    D. It passes through the adductor canal and supplies the posterior thigh.

    Correct Answer: B

    Explanation:

    The femoral nerve (L2–L4) originates from the posterior divisions of the lumbar plexus. It forms within the psoas major, then travels laterally and passes under the inguinal ligament to reach the anterior thigh.

    (EPN, p. 176)

24. Under the inguinal ligaments, the following structures pass from medial to lateral in the following order:
    A. Femoral artery, femoral vein, femoral nerve
    B. Femoral nerve, femoral vein, femoral artery
    C. Femoral nerve, femoral artery, femoral vein
    D. Femoral vein, femoral artery, femoral nerve

    Correct Answer: D

    Explanation:

    The structures passing under the inguinal ligament follow the order from medial to lateral: Femoral Vein → Femoral Artery → Femoral Nerve (VAN).

    (EPN, p. 176)
25. The axillary nerve innervates which muscle, and where does it originate in the brachial plexus?
    A. Supraspinatus; Upper trunk
    B. Infraspinatus; Lateral cord
    C. Subscapularis; Medial cord
    D. Deltoid; Posterior cord

    Correct Answer: D

    Explanation:

    The axillary nerve arises from the posterior cord of the brachial plexus and contains fibers from C5–C6. It innervates the deltoid and teres minor muscles and provides sensory innervation to the skin over the deltoid region.
26. The long thoracic nerve originates from which spinal nerve roots?
    A. C5–C7
    B. C6–C8
    C. C7–T1
    D. C8–T1

    Correct Answer: A

    Explanation:

    The long thoracic nerve arises from the anterior rami of C5, C6, and C7 spinal nerve roots. It innervates the serratus anterior muscle, which is essential for scapular protraction and stabilization.
27. Which of the following best describes the course of the long thoracic nerve?
    A. Forms anterior to spinal nerve.
    B. It courses between anterior and posterior scalene muscles.
    C. Pass downward behind the proximal brachial plexus.
    D. All of the above are correct.

    Answer: C

    Explanation:

    The long thoracic nerve forms behind the spinal nerves and moves downward behind the proximal brachial plexus. It courses between the anterior and middle scalene muscles. It then passes over the posterolateral part of the first rib and finally reaches the serratus anterior muscle for innervation.

    (EPN, p. 88)

28. The lateral cutaneous nerve of the forearm is a direct continuation of which nerve?
    A. Ulnar nerve
    B. Median nerve
    C. Radial nerve
    D. Musculocutaneous nerve

    Correct Answer: D

    Explanation:

    The lateral cutaneous nerve of the forearm is the terminal sensory branch of the musculocutaneous nerve, which arises from the lateral cord of the brachial plexus (C5–C7).

    (EPN, p. 95)

29. A 28-year-old athlete sustains a shoulder dislocation and later experiences weakness in elbow flexion. Examination reveals intact wrist extension and no involvement of the brachioradialis.

Which nerve is most likely affected?
    A. Radial nerve
    B. Musculocutaneous nerve
    C. Median nerve
    D. Axillary nerve

    Correct Answer: B

    Explanation:

    The musculocutaneous nerve (C5–C6) arises from the lateral cord of the brachial plexus.

    It pierces the coracobrachialis and supplies the biceps brachii and brachialis (elbow flexion). It ends as the lateral antebrachial cutaneous nerve, providing sensation to the lateral forearm (Fig. 16.4).

    (EPN, pp. 95–96)

30. A 35-year-old carpenter presents with weakness in wrist and finger extension but no sensory deficits. Imaging shows compression of a nerve passing through the supinator muscle.

    30a. Which of the following statements best describes the course of this nerve?
    - A. It travels between the two heads of the supinator.
    - B. It passes through the cubital tunnel before entering the supinator muscle.
    - C. It lies deep to the extensor pollicis longus after emerging from the supinator.
    - D. It courses along the median nerve before branching in the distal forearm.

    30b. It innervates which muscle?
    - A. Pronator teres
    - B. Extensor carpi ulnaris
    - C. Flexor digitorum profundus
    - D. Supinator

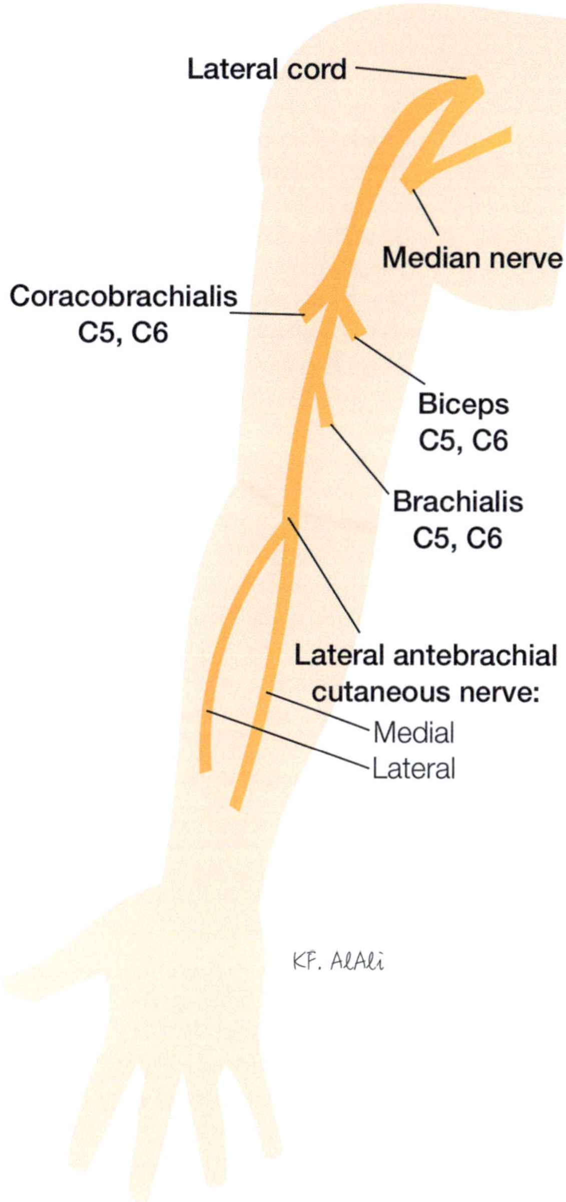

Fig. 16.4 Musculocutaneous nerve course and supply

30c. Through which structure does it pass?
A. Arcade of Struthers
B. Arcade of SpinoGlenoid
C. Arcade of Osborne
D. Arcade of Frohse

30d. One of the following is the sensory area for this nerve:
A. Ventral forearm
B. Tip of the index finger
C. Lateral elbow
D. None of the above

30e This nerve is approached surgically in lateral–dorsal forearm by an incision between two muscles:
A. The brachioradialis and flexor carpi radialis muscles
B. The brachioradialis and extensor carpi radialis longus muscles
C. The pronator teres and flexor carpi radialis muscles
D. The pronator teres and brachioradialis muscles

30f. Which nerve is usually seen during the lateral-dorsal forearm exposure if this nerve?
A. Anterior interosseous nerve
B. The nerve to the carpi radialis longus
C. The nerve to the carpi radialis brevis
D. All of the above

Answers: 30a: A, 30b: B, 30c: D, 30d: D, 30e: B, 30f: C

Explanation:

The nerve is the posterior interosseous nerve (PIN), a branch of the radial nerve. It is a pure motor nerve with no sensory function. It passes deep to the arcade of Frohse, enters the supinator pocket, and travels between the two heads of the supinator muscle. It then moves laterally around the radius into the extensor compartment. Then it runs deep to the extensor digitorum communis and superficial to the abductor pollicis longus, branching into multiple nerves. It supplies the extensor muscles of the forearm.

In the lower forearm, it lies on the interosseous membrane, where it meets the posterior interosseous artery. The PIN is usually approached in the lateral–dorsal forearm with a centered incision between the brachioradialis and extensor carpi radialis longus muscles. Between these two muscles, three nerves will be seen from ventral to dorsal: the superficial radial nerve, the nerve to the carpi radialis brevis, and the PIN.

(EPN, p. 64)

31. All of the following are the contents of the carpal tunnel, EXCEPT:
A. Four tendons of the flexor digitorum superficialis
B. Four tendons of the flexor digitorum profundus
C. One tendon of the flexor pollicis longus
D. One tendon of the flexor pollicis brevis

Correct Answer: D

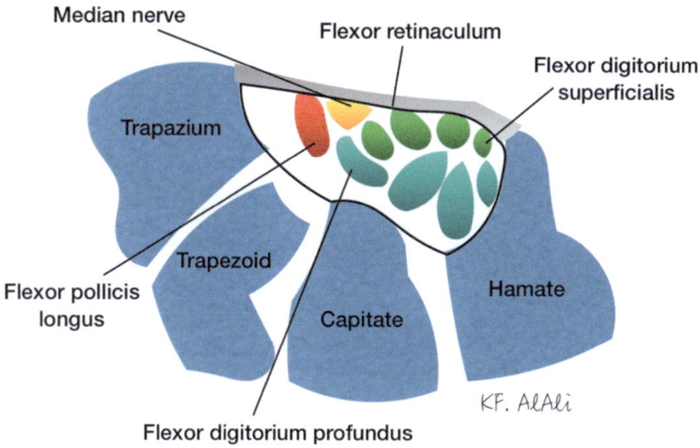

Fig. 16.5 Cross-section through carpal tunnel showing its content

Explanation:

The contents of the carpal tunnel are summarized in the following illustration (Fig. 16.5):

32. The following is the motor action of lumbricals muscle:
    A. Flexing the metacarpophalangeal joints
    B. Extending the proximal interphalangeal joints
    C. Extending the metacarpophalangeal joints
    D. A and B

    Correct Answer: D

    Explanation:

    The lumbricals assist with flexing the metacarpophalangeal joints and extending the proximal interphalangeal joints while the metacarpophalangeal joints are in a hyperextended position and immobilized.

    (MPN, p. 34)
33. Which nerve innervates the majority of the flexor muscles of the forearm?
    A. Median nerve
    B. Ulnar nerve
    C. Radial nerve
    D. Musculocutaneous nerve

    Correct Answer: A

    Explanation:

    The median nerve innervates the majority of the flexor muscles in the forearm, including the pronator teres, flexor carpi radialis, palmaris longus, flexor digitorum superficialis, and the lateral half of flexor digitorum profundus, as well as flexor pollicis longus and pronator quadratus via its anterior interosseous branch. The ulnar nerve innervates only the flexor carpi ulnaris and the medial half of the flexor digitorum profundus, while the radial and musculocutaneous nerves do not innervate forearm flexors.

34. The most outer layer of the peripheral nerve is:
    A. Endoneurium
    B. Axons fibers
    C. Perineurium
    D. Epineurium
    Correct Answer: D
    (Fig. 16.6). (MPN, p. 18)
35. Which of the following is true regarding the sensory innervation of the dorsum of the hand?
    A. The ulnar nerve innervates the entire dorsum of the hand.
    B. The median nerve provides sensory innervation to the back of the thumb.
    C. The radial nerve innervates the dorsum of the thumb and the first two fingers.
    D. The musculocutaneous nerve innervates the dorsum of the hand.
    Correct Answer: C
    (Fig. 16.7)
36. The deep peroneal nerve innervates which muscle?
    A. Gastrocnemius
    B. Tibialis anterior
    C. Flexor digitorum longus
    D. Soleus
    Correct Answer: B

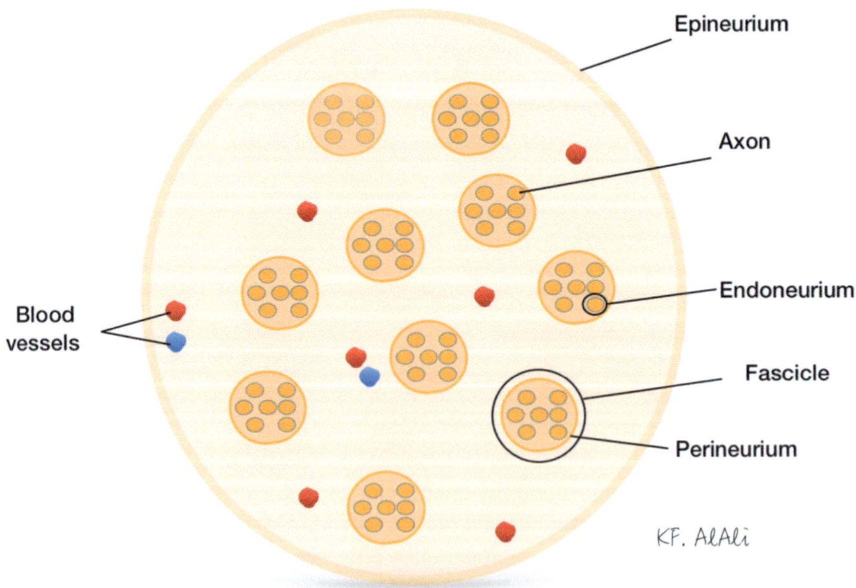

Fig. 16.6 Cross-section of a peripheral nerve showing its layers

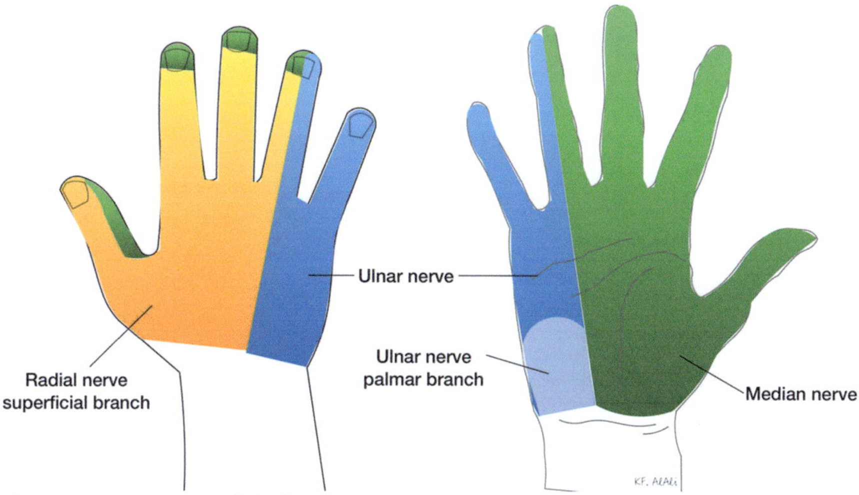

Fig. 16.7 Dermatomes of the hand

Explanation:

The deep peroneal nerve is the major motor branch of common peroneal nerve. It supplies the following: muscles: tibialis anterior, extensor digitorum longus, extensor hallucis longus, and extensor hallucis brevis (Fig. 16.8).

(GB, p. 563)

37. Regarding dorsal root ganglia (DRG):

37a. They contain the cell bodies of which type of neurons?

A. Motor efferents
B. Interneurons
C. Sensory afferents
D. Sympathetic neurons

37b. Which type of neuron does DRG have?

A. Pseudo-unipolar neurons
B. Bipolar neurons
C. Multipolar neurons
D. Interneurons

Correct Answers: 37a: C, 37b: A

Explanation:

Dorsal root ganglia (DRG) are clusters of sensory neuron cell bodies located along the dorsal roots of spinal nerves. They transmit sensory signals, such as pain, temperature, and touch, from the peripheral nervous system to the central nervous system. Each DRG contains pseudo-unipolar neurons, with one branch extending to the periphery and the other to the spinal cord.

(CA, p. 364)

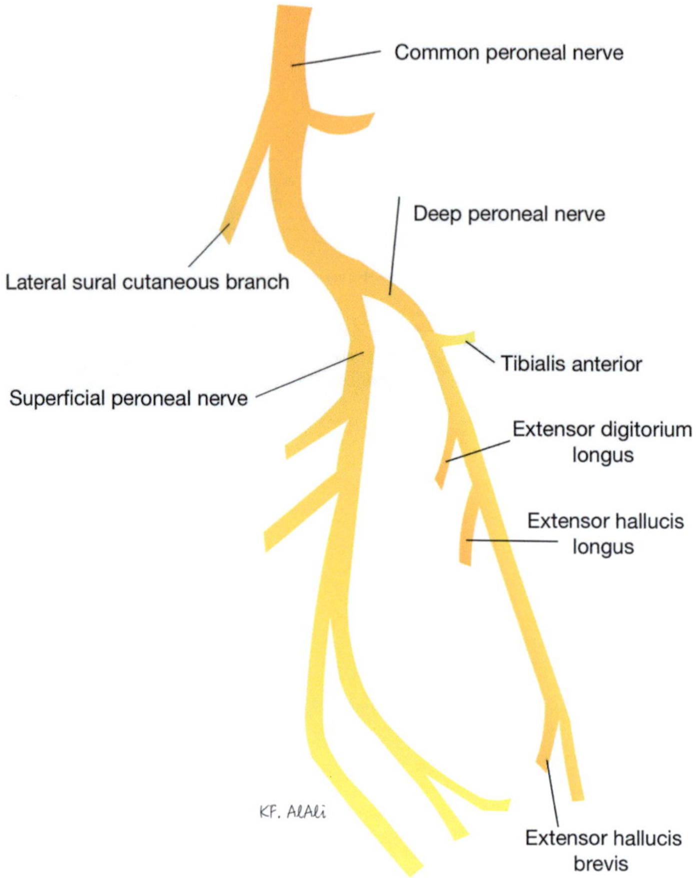

Fig. 16.8 Branches and muscle supply of deep peroneal nerve

38. One of the following muscles from the thenar muscle group is innervated by the ulnar nerve:
    A. Adductor pollicis
    B. Flexor pollicis brevis
    C. Flexor pollicis longus
    D. A and B

    Correct Answer: D

    Explanation:

    Within the thenar muscle group, the adductor pollicis is entirely innervated by the deep branch of the ulnar nerve, while the flexor pollicis brevis has dual innervation—its deep head is innervated by the ulnar nerve, and the superficial head by the median nerve. In contrast, the flexor pollicis longus is not part of the thenar group and is innervated by the anterior interosseous branch of the median nerve. Thus, both adductor pollicis and part of flexor pollicis brevis receive ulnar nerve supply.

    (MPN, p. 32)

39. The sural nerve provides sensory innervation to which region of the body?
    A. Anterior thigh
    B. Plantar surface of the foot
    C. Lateral aspect of the foot
    D. Medial calf
    Correct Answer: C (Fig. 16.3)
40. Which of the following correctly describes the sural nerve's anatomical formation?
    A. It originates at the level of the popliteal fossa.
    B. It is a continuation of the superficial peroneal nerve.
    C. It is solely formed by the tibial nerve.
    D. It is formed by the common peroneal nerve and tibial nerve.
    Correct Answer: D
    Explanation:
    The sural nerve is formed by a medial sural branch from tibial nerve and lateral sural branch of peroneal nerve. Although each branch originates at the level of the popliteal fossa, they merge at the level of two heads of the gastrocnemius muscle.
    (MPN, p. 163)
41. What anatomical feature makes the sural nerve a good donor nerve?
    A. Sural nerve Sensory coverage is overlapped with other sensory nerves.
    B. It has a large diameter and abundant myelination.
    C. It has a constant anatomical location.
    D. It carries inactive motor fibers, making it ideal for functional grafting.
    Correct Answer: A
    Explanation:
    The sural nerve has overlapping sensory innervation, making its damage (e.g., after biopsy or graft) cause usually insignificant numbness along the lateral foot border. Over time, this numb area gradually reduces as neighboring sensory nerves compensate.
    (MPN, p. 163)
42. The sensory innervation of the perineum is provided by which nerve?
    A. Sciatic nerve
    B. Pudendal nerve
    C. Obturator nerve
    D. Femoral nerve
    Correct Answer: B
    Explanation:
    The pudendal nerve, originating from S2–S4, is the primary nerve responsible for sensory innervation of the perineum, including the external genitalia, anal region, and perianal skin. It also carries motor fibers to the external urethral and anal sphincters, making it essential for continence.

43. What anatomical feature of the pudendal nerve helps in differentiating between sciatic nerve palsy and a sacral plexus injury?
    A. It exits the pelvis through the greater sciatic foramen alongside the sciatic nerve.
    B. The pudendal nerve provides motor innervation to the hamstring muscles.
    C. The pudendal nerve is the most distant from the sciatic nerve in the buttock.
    D. All of the above.

    Correct Answer: C

    Explanation:

    The pudendal nerve solely originates from the sacral plexus, S2–S4. It is the farthest nerve in relation to the sciatic nerve in the pelvis, making its deficit in a clinical exam a good indicator for sacral plexus injury and not sciatic nerve injury.

    (EPN, p. 167)
44. To avoid the sciatic nerve in the buttock, where is the safest site to give an intramuscular injection?
    A. Upper outer quadrant
    B. Inferior outer quadrant
    C. Upper inner quadrant
    D. All are safe locations

    Correct Answer: A

    Explanation:

    The sciatic nerve occupies the inner quadrants and courses laterally and inferiorly, avoiding the upper outer quadrant.

    (EPN, p. 167)
45. All of the following are contents of the Guyon's tunnel, EXCEPT:
    A. Deep ulnar nerve
    B. Superficial ulnar nerve
    C. Ulnar artery
    D. Ulnar vein

    Correct Answer: D

    Explanation:

    The contents of Guyon's tunnel are the ulnar nerve with its branches and the ulnar artery. Rarely, there is a small vein in the tunnel.

    (MPN, p. 5)
46. The Guyon's tunnel is formed by two bones, and they are:
    A. Hook of hamate and pisiform
    B. Scaphoid and lunate
    C. Hook of hamate and scaphoid
    D. Trapezoid and pisiform

    Correct Answer: A

    Explanation:

    The Guyon's tunnel is formed between the hook of hamate and the pisiform carpal bones.

    (EPN, p. 57)

47. Which structures form the boundaries of Guyon's tunnel?
    A. Roof: Transverse carpal ligament, Floor: Flexor retinaculum
    B. Roof: Palmar carpal ligament, Floor: Flexor retinaculum
    C. Roof: Flexor retinaculum, Floor: Pisohamate ligament
    D. Roof: Palmar carpal ligament, Floor: Transverse carpal ligament

    Correct Answer: B (Fig. 16.9)

    Explanation:

    The boundaries of Guyon's tunnel are:

    - Roof: Palmar carpal ligament
    - Floor: Flexor retinaculum

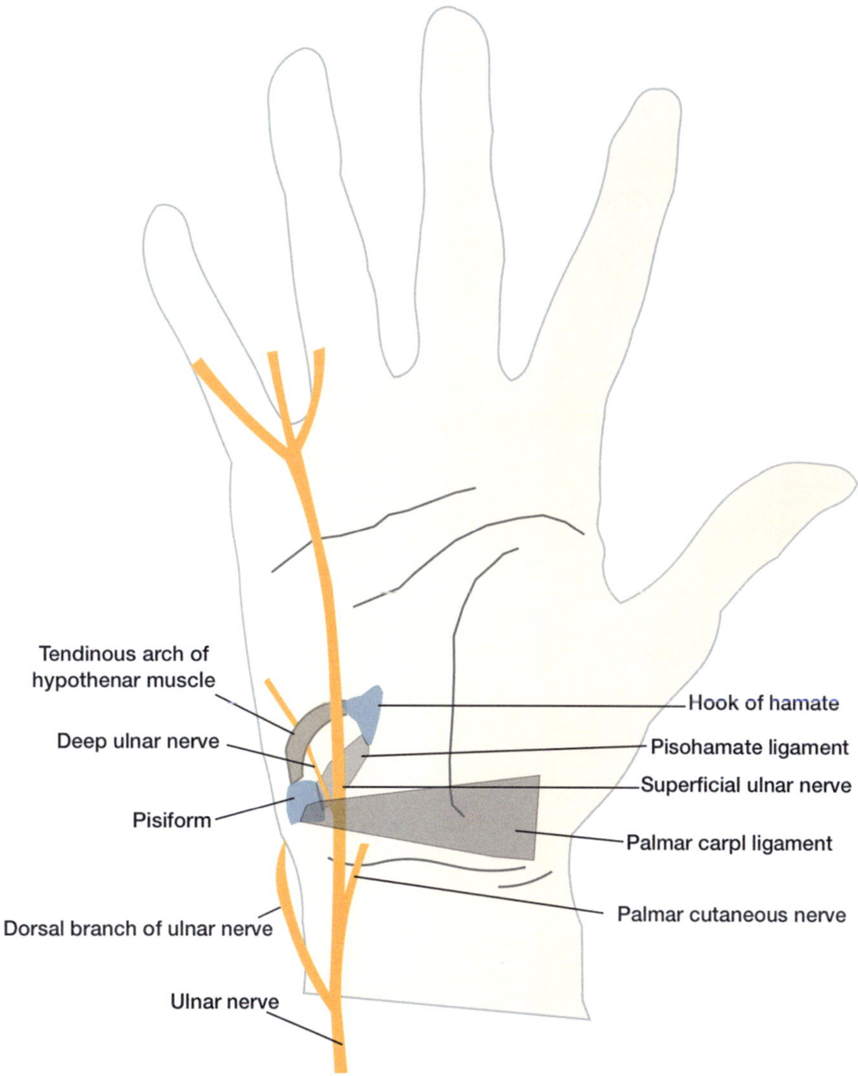

Fig. 16.9 Illustration of Guyon's tunnel borders

- Medial wall: Pisiform
- Lateral wall: Hook of hamate

48. Regarding the course of radial nerve when is just coming off the posterior cord:
    A. The radial nerve originates proximal to the thoracodorsal nerve.
    B. The radial nerve originates proximal to the axillary nerve.
    C. Both A and B are correct.
    D. The radial nerve is the most distal part of the posterior cord.
    Correct Answer: D (Fig. 16.11)
    (MPN, p. 36)
49. Which muscle does the radial nerve pass superficially to as it exits the axilla?
    A. Teres minor
    B. Latissimus dorsi
    C. Pectoralis major
    D. Coracobrachialis
    Correct Answer: B
    Explanation:
    The radial nerve lies superficial to the latissimus dorsi tendon, subscapularis, and teres major as it exits the axilla (Fig. 16.10).

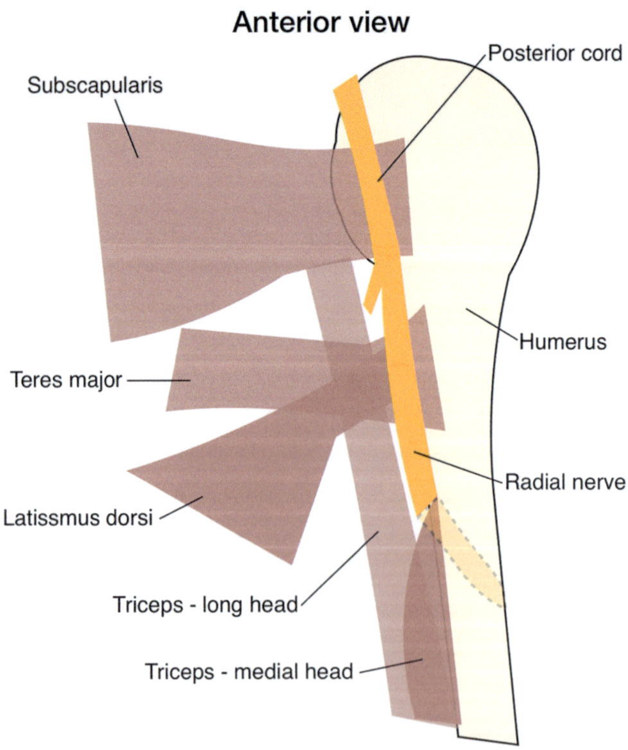

Fig. 16.10 Illustration of median nerve at the axilla. At the distal axilla, the radian nerve pass superficially to three muscles: latissimus dorsi tendon, subscapularis, and teres major

50. The radial nerve provides motor innervation to which of the following muscles?
    A. Biceps brachii
    B. Triceps brachii
    C. Deltoid
    D. Pectoralis major
    Correct Answer: B
51. What is the first innervated muscle by the radial nerve?
    A. Triceps brachii-long head
    B. Triceps brachii-medial head
    C. Triceps brachii-lateral head
    D. All of them have the same innervation
    Answer: A
52. What is the last muscle innervated by the radial nerve?
    A. Extensor pollicis longus
    B. Extensor pollicis brevis
    C. Extensor indicis
    D. Extensor digiti minimi
    Answer: C
    Explanation:
    Radial nerve innervation (4 muscles by radial nerve proper /8 muscles by posterior interosseous nerve)
    - 4 → Radial nerve proper: Triceps , Brachioradialis , ECRL (Extensor Carpi Radialis Longus), ECRB (Extensor Carpi Radialis Brevis)
    - 8 → PIN (Posterior Interosseous Nerve) → (2 / 3 / 3)
      - 2: Supinator, ECU (Extensor Carpi Ulnaris): Key to distinguish proximal radial vs. proximal PIN lesion
      - 3: Extensor digiti group: EDC (Extensor Digitorum Communis), EDM (Extensor Digiti Minimi), EI (Extensor Indicis)
      - 3: Pollicis group: EPL (Extensor Pollicis Longus), EPB (Extensor Pollicis Brevis), AbPL (Abductor Pollicis Longus). (Fig. 16.11)
53. The following is correct about the spiral groove of humerus boundaries:
    A. Inferior border is lateral head of the triceps brachii.
    B. Inferior border is medial head of the triceps brachii.
    C. Inferior border is humeral shaft.
    D. Inferior border is lateral intermuscular septum.
    Correct Answer: B
    Explanation:
    The spiral groove of the humerus is where the radial nerve passes posteriorly from medial to lateral. The boundaries are:
    - Superior: Lateral head of the triceps brachii.
    - Inferior: Medial head of the triceps brachii.
    - Medial: Humeral shaft.
    - Lateral: Lateral intermuscular septum.
    (EPN, p. 61)

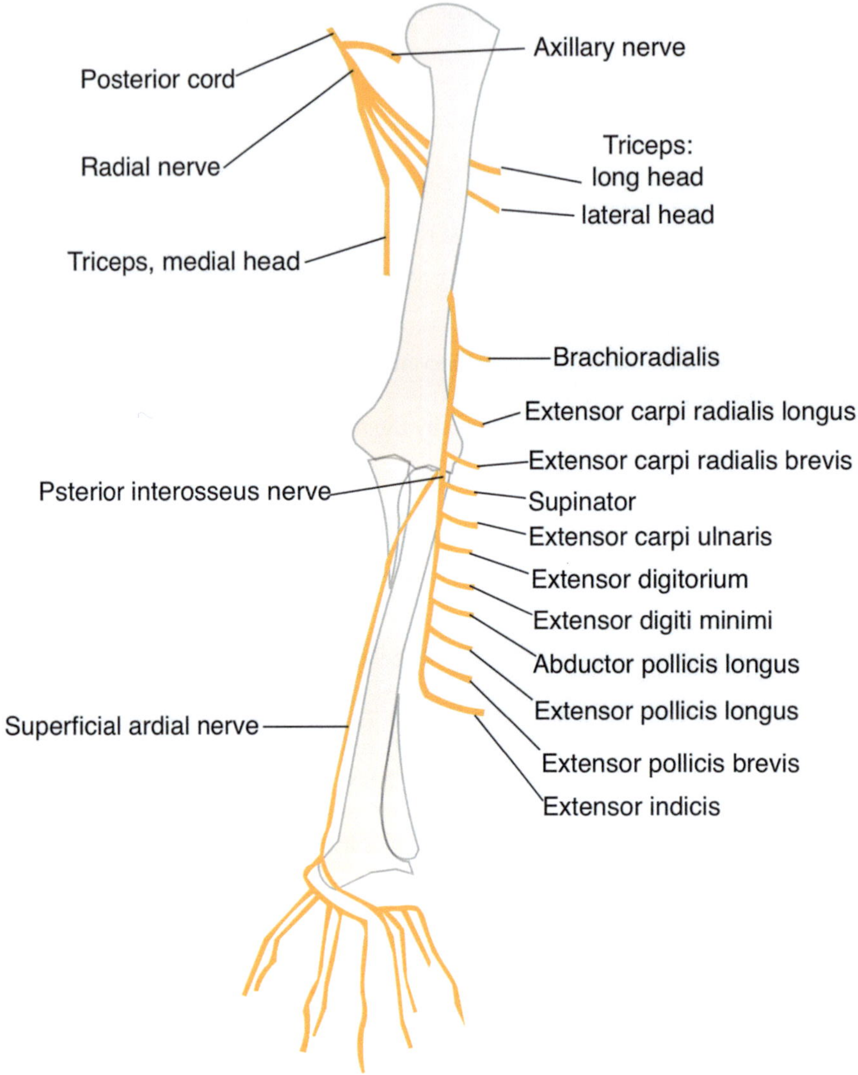

Fig. 16.11 Radial nerve muscles supply

54. One of the following muscles covers the radial nerve after the spiral groove:
    A. Extensor carpi radialis longus
    B. Extensor carpi radialis brevis
    C. Brachialis
    D. A and B

    Correct Answer: D

    Explanation:

    After entering the flexor compartment, the radial nerve runs from the mid-upper arm to the antecubital fossa. It passes beneath three muscles that form an arch over it. These muscles are: brachioradialis, extensor carpi radialis longus and extensor carpi radialis brevis.

(EPN, p. 62)

55. One of the following is correct about the radial nerve tunnel:
    A. Lateral border: brachioradialis
    B. Medial: triceps tendon
    C. Roof: capsule of the radiocapitellar joint
    D. All are correct

    Correct Answer: A

    Explanation:

    The radial tunnel is at the level of the proximal forearm and has approximately 5 cm in length. At this tunnel, the radial nerve is immobile and more superficial, making it prone to injury. The boundaries are:

    Lateral border: brachioradialis, extensor carpi radialis brevis, and extensor carpi radialis longus

    Medial: biceps tendon

    Floor: capsule of the radiocapitellar joint

    Roof: Superficial head of supinator and brachioradialis

    (EPN, p. 62)

56. The following branch of the radial nerve passes through the radial tunnel:
    A. Superficial radial nerve
    B. Posterior interosseous nerve
    C. Main trunk radial nerve
    D. All of the above

    Correct Answer: B

    Explanation:

    The posterior interosseous nerve (PIN), which is the deep motor branch of the radial nerve, passes through the radial tunnel, a potential site of entrapment located in the proximal forearm. The radial tunnel extends from the lateral epicondyle to the proximal edge of the supinator muscle, through which the PIN travels.

    (EPN, p. 62)

57. The fibrous arch of the superficial head of the supinator is known as:
    A. The arcade of Frohse
    B. The arcade of Struthers
    C. The arcade of Osborne
    D. The arcade of Buhler

    Correct Answer: A

    Explanation:

    The arcade of Frohse is a fibrous arch of the superficial supinator, where the posterior interosseous nerve (PIN) can be compressed.

    (EPN, p. 62)

58. The tibial nerve innervates which of the following muscles?
    A. Tibialis anterior
    B. Extensor digitorum longus

C. Peroneus brevis
D. Flexor hallucis longus

Correct Answer: D

Explanation:

The tibial nerve, a branch of the sciatic nerve, innervates the posterior compartment of the leg, including muscles responsible for plantarflexion and toe flexion. One of its key targets is the flexor hallucis longus, which flexes the great toe and assists with push-off during gait.

(EPN, pp. 148–149)

59. Which one of the following is NOT a direct continuation of the tibial nerve?
    A. Saphenous nerve
    B. Lateral plantar nerve
    C. Medial plantar nerve
    D. Posterior tibial nerve

    Correct Answer: A

    Explanation:

    The medial and lateral plantar nerves are terminal branches of the tibial nerve, arising after it passes through the tarsal tunnel. The term posterior tibial nerve is another way of referring to the tibial nerve as it travels through the leg.

    (EPN. P. 148–149)

60. Which branch of the tibial nerve supplies sensation to the heel?
    A. Lateral plantar nerve
    B. Medial plantar nerve
    C. Calcaneal nerve
    D. Sural nerve

    Answer: C

    (see Fig. 16.3)

61. At which level does the tibial nerve usually bifurcate to terminal branches?
    A. Medial malleolus
    B. Ankle joint
    C. Proximal to tarsal tunnel
    D. Distal to tarsal tunnel

    Correct Answer: C

    [74]

62. The tibial nerve receives contributions from which spinal nerve roots?
    A. L2–L3
    B. L4–S1
    C. L2–S1
    D. L4–S3

    Correct Answer: D

    Explanation:

    The tibial nerve is one of the two terminal branches of the sciatic nerve and receives fibers primarily from the L4 to S3 spinal nerve roots. (Fig. 16.12)

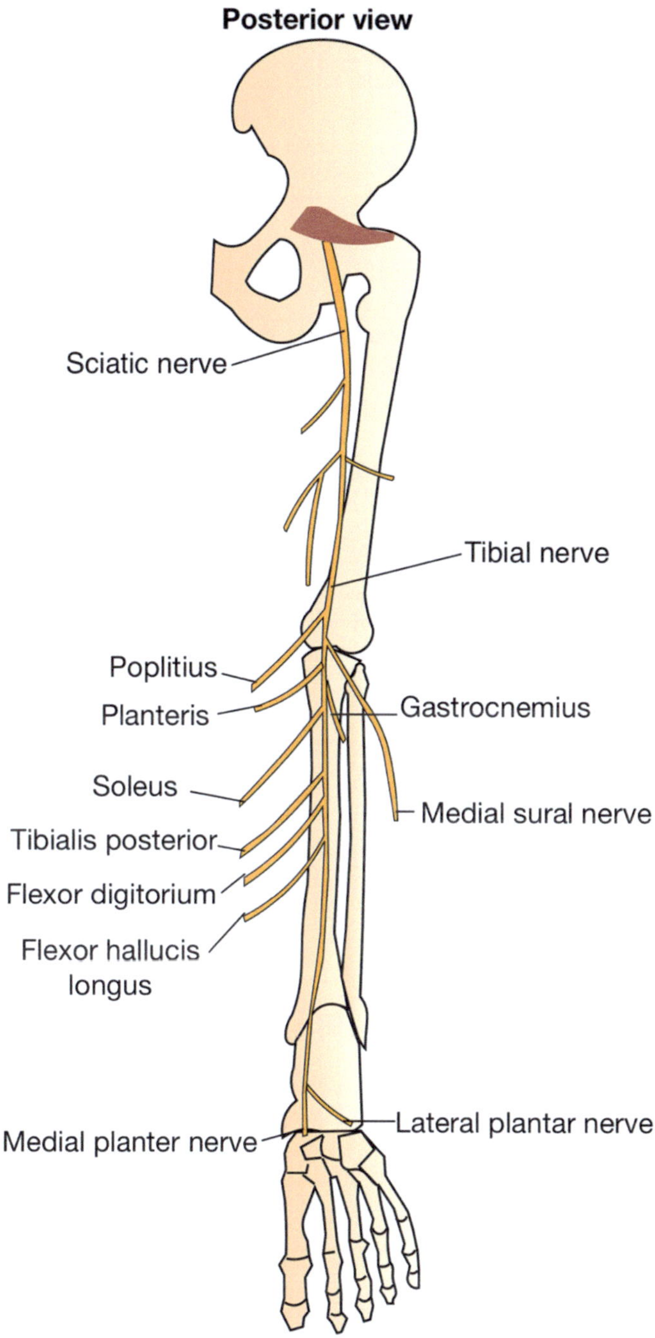

Fig. 16.12 Illustration of tibial nerve muscle supply

63. What anatomical structure lies immediately anterior to the tibial nerve in the tarsal tunnel?
    A. Flexor hallucis longus tendon
    B. Flexor digitorum brevis tendon
    C. Tibialis posterior tendon
    D. Posterior tibial artery
    Correct Answer: D
    Explanation:
    In the tarsal tunnel, the tibial nerve runs posterior to the medial malleolus, along with the posterior tibial artery and vein. Immediately anterior to the tibial nerve is the posterior tibial artery, this relationship is clinically important for both tarsal tunnel syndrome and surgical approaches.
64. The tarsal tunnel roof is:
    A. Medial malleolus
    B. Achilles tendon
    C. Laciniate ligament
    D. Tarsal ligament
    Correct Answer: C
65. All of the following structures pass through tarsal tunnel, EXCEPT:
    A. Flexor hallucis longus tendon
    B. Flexor digitorum brevis tendon
    C. Tibialis posterior tendon
    D. Posterior tibial nerve
    Correct Answer: B
    Explanation:
    The contents of tarsal tunnel from anterior to posterior are Tibialis posterior tendon, Flexor digitorum **longus** tendon, Posterior tibial artery and vein, Tibial nerve and Flexor hallucis longus tendon.
    You can use this mnemonic: **T**he **D**octor **A**nd **N**urse **H**ug (Fig. 16.13). (EPN, p. 143)

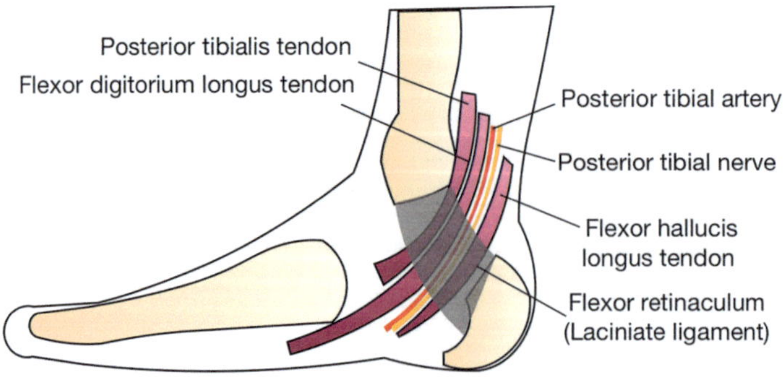

Fig. 16.13 Illustration of tarsal tunnel contents

66. Which muscle does the medial plantar nerve run between as it courses through the foot?
    A. Abductor hallucis and flexor hallucis brevis
    B. Flexor digitorum brevis and quadratus plantae
    C. Abductor hallucis and flexor digitorum brevis
    D. Abductor digiti minimi pedis and flexor digitorum brevis
    Correct Answer: C
67. How does the medial plantar nerve distribute to the toes?
    A. It supplies the first two toes.
    B. It splits into digital nerves for the first three and a half toes.
    C. It supplies all five toes.
    D. It only innervates the big toe.
    Correct Answer: B
    Explanation:
    The posterior tibial nerve bifurcates into medial and lateral plantar nerves. The larger medial plantar travels through the foot's inner region, between the abductor hallucis and flexor digitorum brevis, supplying nerves to the first three-and-a-half toes. Its sensory branches start near the foot's entry point.
    The lateral plantar, after the tarsal tunnel, crosses under the flexor digitorum brevis, dividing into sensory and motor branches between the quadratus plantae and abductor digiti minimi pedis, similar to the ulnar nerve.
    (EPN, p. 144)
68. Which nerve is responsible for the motor supply to the adductor magnus muscle?
    A. Femoral nerve
    B. Tibial nerve
    C. Obturator nerve
    D. B and C
    Correct Answer: D
    Explanation:
    The adductor magnus is innervated by both the tibial nerve and the posterior division of the obturator nerve.
    (EPN, p. 179)
69. A patient comes to your clinic with recent onset of weakness in hip adduction after undergoing a procedure for an inguinal hernia. They mention the surgeon spoke about unusual anatomy. Which anatomical variation might explain this weakness?
    A. An additional ilioinguinal nerve
    B. An accessory obturator nerve
    C. An aberrant femoral nerve course
    D. A duplicated sciatic nerve
    Correct Answer: B.
    Explanation:
    If present, an accessory obturator nerve would contribute to the innervation of muscles like the pectineus, which is usually innervated by the femoral

nerve. It does not pass through the obturator canal. It passes over the superior pubic ramus. If injured during surgery, it could lead to weakness in hip adduction (pectineus muscle weakness).

(EPN, p. 179)

70. After leaving the psoas major, the obturator nerve runs:
    A. Over the iliac crest
    B. Between the psoas and the iliac vessels
    C. Through the greater sciatic foramen
    D. Lateral to the femoral artery

    Correct Answer: B

    Explanation:

    The obturator nerve arises from L2–L4 within the psoas major. Then, it courses inferomedially between the psoas and iliac vessels toward the pelvis. It exits via the obturator canal, splitting into anterior and posterior divisions. Both divisions pierce the obturator externus. The anterior division runs over adductor brevis, under adductor longus, and gives a cutaneous branch to the medial thigh. The posterior division passes deep to the pectineus, supplying the adductor magnus.

    An accessory obturator nerve (L3–L4) is found in one-third of cases. It bypasses the obturator canal to innervate the pectineus, which is usually supplied by the femoral nerve.

    (EPN, p. 179)

71. In the lateral arm, the radial nerve lies between:
    A. Brachialis and brachioradialis muscles
    B. Biceps and brachioradialis muscles
    C. Biceps and brachialis muscles
    D. Two head of biceps muscles

    Correct Answer: A

    Explanation:

    In the lateral arm, the radial nerve travels from the posterior compartment (after passing through the radial groove of the humerus) to the anterior compartment by piercing the lateral intermuscular septum. It then courses between the brachialis (medially) and brachioradialis (laterally) as it descends toward the elbow, where it divides into the superficial radial nerve and the posterior interosseous nerve.

    (MPN, p. 36)

72. Which nerve provides sensory innervation to the inferior outer quadrant of the gluteal region?
    A. Sciatic nerve
    B. Superior cluneal nerves
    C. Inferior cluneal nerve
    D. Iliohypogastric nerve

    Correct Answer: C

Explanation:

The inferior cluneal nerves are cutaneous branches of the posterior femoral cutaneous nerve (S1–S3). They provide sensory innervation to the inferior aspect of the gluteal region, particularly the lower and lateral (inferolateral) quadrant of the buttock.

(EPN, p. 203)

73. Iliohypogastric nerve supply the following muscle(s):
    A. Internal and transverse abdominal muscles
    B. External oblique muscle
    C. Cremaster muscle
    D. All of the above

    Correct Answer: A

    Explanation:

    The iliohypogastric nerve, arising from L1, provides motor innervation primarily to the internal oblique and transversus abdominis muscles, and sensory innervation to the skin over the hypogastric and gluteal regions.

    (MPN, p. 44)

74. A 40-year-old office worker presents with weakness in pinching objects between his thumb and index finger. There is no sensory loss, and wrist flexion remains normal.

    74a. Which of the following muscles is most likely affected?
    - A. Flexor carpi radialis
    - B. Flexor digitorum profundus (index and middle fingers)
    - C. Flexor pollicis brevis
    - D. Flexor carpi ulnaris

    74b. The nerve affected in this case also innervates one of the following muscles:
    - A. Pronator teres
    - B. Flexor carpi radialis
    - C. Flexor pollicis longus
    - D. Flexor digitorum superficialis

    Correct Answers: 74a: B, 74b:C

    Explanation:

    The anterior interosseous nerve innervates flexor digitorum profundus I and II, flexor pollicis longus, and pronator quadratus.

    (MPN, p. 5)

75. Which of the following is NOT innervated by the median nerve at the elbow?
    A. Pronator teres
    B. Flexor carpi ulnaris
    C. Palmaris longus
    D. Flexor digitorum superficialis

    Correct Answer: B

    Explanation

    The median nerve does not innervate the flexor carpi ulnaris, which is supplied by the ulnar nerve.

    (MPN, p. 28)

76. The thenar branch of median nerve innervate all of the following, EXCEPT:
    A. Abductor pollicis brevis
    B. Flexor pollicis brevis
    C. Flexor pollicis longus
    D. Opponens pollicis

    Correct Answer: C

    Explanation:

    The thenar branch of the median nerve, or recurrent branch, supplies the following muscles (LOAF):

    L: lateral two lumbricals

    O: opponens pollicis

    A: abductor pollicis brevis

    F: flexor pollicis brevis (superficial head)

    (MPN, p. 28)
77. One of the following is a distinctive feature of the pronator quadratus muscle:
    A. It is a weak forearm pronator.
    B. It has a distal attachment on the medial surface of the radius.
    C. It originates from the lateral epicondyle of the humerus.
    D. It has weak forearm supination action.

    Correct Answer: A

    Explanation:

    The pronator quadratus muscle is a weak forearm supinator, innervated by the anterior interosseous nerve. It is a deep distal forearm muscle and originates from the medial, anterior ulna and inserts on the lateral, anterior radius.

    (EPN, p. 12)
78. The anterior interosseous nerve supplies which muscles?
    A. Supinator
    B. Flexor pollicis longus
    C. Adductor pollicis
    D. Medial half of Flexor digitorum profundus

    Correct Answer: B (Fig. 16.14)

    (EPN, p. 1)
79. Where does the palmar cutaneous branch of the median nerve typically arise?
    A. Proximal to the carpal tunnel
    B. Within the carpal tunnel
    C. At the level of the wrist joint
    D. Distal to the carpal tunnel

    Correct Answer: A

    Explanation

    The palmar cutaneous branch of the median nerve arises just proximal to the carpal tunnel approximately 5 cm from the wrist crease. It crosses the wrist, running superficial to the flexor retinaculum. It provides sensory innervation to the thenar eminence and the proximal radial palm.

    (MPN, p. 26)

80. One of the following is correct about median nerve:
    A. The lateral cord providing mostly motor axons from C6 and C7.
    B. It is deep to the brachial artery in the arm.
    C. In the forearm it passes superficial to the flexor digitorum superficialis, but deep to the underlying flexor digitorum profundus.
    D. It passes under the bicipital aponeurosis.

    Correct Answer: D

    Explanation:

    The median nerve passes under the bicipital aponeurosis (lacertus fibrosus) in the cubital fossa as it enters the forearm. This anatomical relationship is important clinically, as the aponeurosis can be a site of compression of the median nerve (Lacertus syndrome, also known as bicipital aponeurosis syndrome).

    (MPN, p. 26)

81. Regarding the medial cord contribution to the median nerve, which statement is CORRECT?
    A. It provides mostly motor axons to the median nerve.
    B. It carries fibers primarily from C5 and C6 nerve roots.
    C. It does not contribute to any sensory function of the median nerve.
    D. It forms the entire median nerve independently without input from the lateral cord.

    Correct Answer: A

    Explanation:

    The medial cord contributes to the median nerve, mainly supplying motor fibers to intrinsic hand muscles. It carries fibers from C8 to T1. The lateral cord (C5–C7) also contributes to the median nerve, mainly sensory axons. The median nerve contains both motor and sensory fibers, and its formation requires input from both cords of the brachial plexus.

    (EPN, p. 1)

82. Where might the medial and lateral cord components of the median nerve fuse in some individuals?
    A. Always in the axilla
    B. Below the clavicle
    C. Along the upper arm
    D. Just before the axilla

    Correct Answer: C

    The medial and lateral cords fuse to form median nerve anywhere along the upper arm and sometimes as low as the elbow (Fig. 16.14).

    (EPN, p. 1)

83. The median nerve enters the antecubital fossa:
    A. Medial to the biceps brachi
    B. Lateral the biceps brachi
    C. Over medial the biceps brachi
    D. Underneath the biceps brachi

    Correct Answer: A

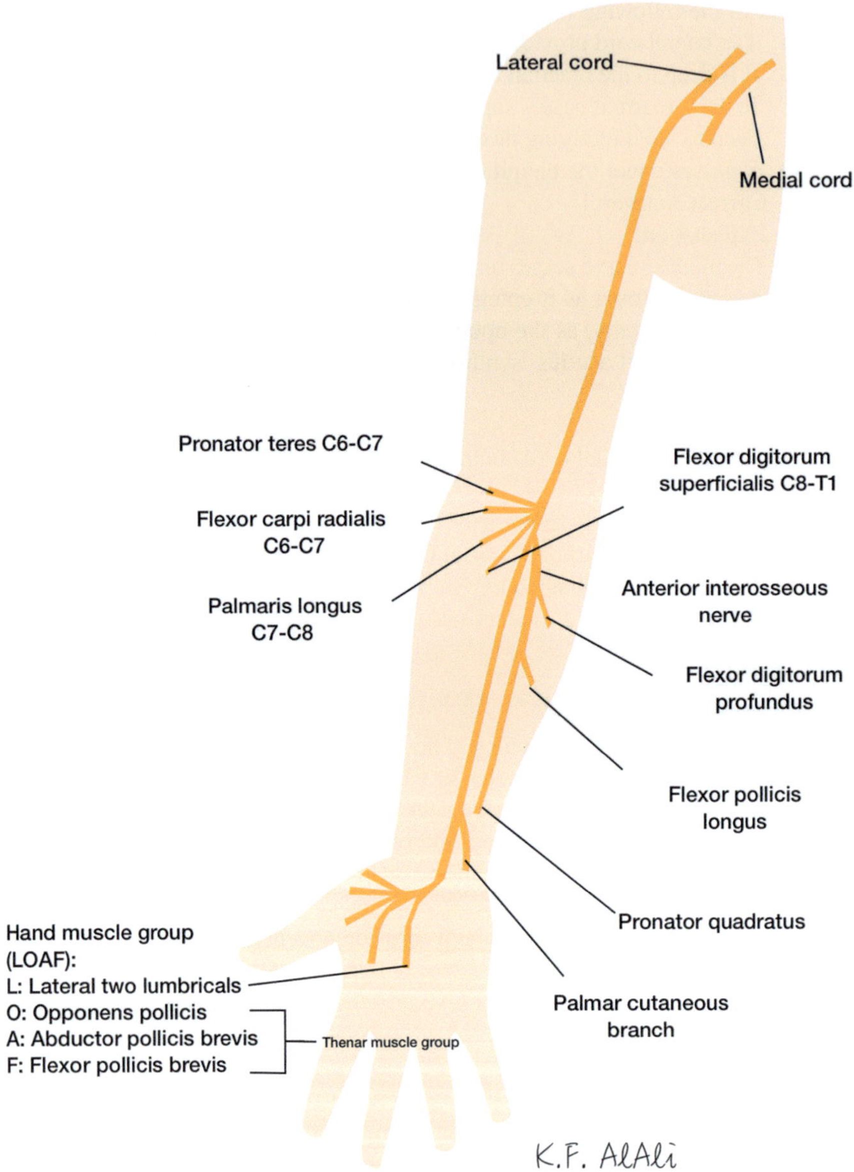

Fig. 16.14 Median nerve course and muscles supply

Explanation:

As the median nerve enters the antecubital fossa, it lies medial to the tendon of the biceps brachii muscle and brachial artery. This anatomical arrangement is important during venipuncture, nerve blocks, and in recognizing compression syndromes at the elbow.

(EPN, p. 2)

84. One of the following is CORRECT about lacertus fibrosis:
    A. It is a fibrous expansion of the biceps brachii tendon.
    B. It directly inserts into the radial tuberosity.
    C. It originates from the coracobrachialis muscle.
    D. It primarily functions as an elbow extensor.

    Correct Answer: A

    Explanation:

    The lacertus fibrosus (bicipital aponeurosis) is a fibrous extension of the biceps brachii tendon that extends medially, blending with the antebrachial fascia. It covers brachial artery, median nerve, and underlying muscles.

    (EPN, p. 2)
85. The following three structures cover the median nerve in the antecubital fossa:
    A. Bicipital aponeurosis, brachialis, and flexor digitorum superficialis
    B. Bicipital aponeurosis, flexor carpi ulnaris, and flexor digitorum superficialis
    C. Bicipital aponeurosis, pronator teres, and flexor digitorum superficialis
    D. Bicipital aponeurosis, flexor digitorum superficialis, and extensor carpi radialis longus

    Correct Answer: C

    (EPN, p. 3)
86. Which structure does the median nerve pass under first in the antecubital fossa?
    A. Humeral head of pronator teres
    B. Flexor digitorum superficialis
    C. Brachioradialis muscle
    D. Bicipital aponeurosis

    Correct Answer: D

    Explanation:

    As the median nerve enters the antecubital fossa, it first passes under the bicipital aponeurosis (also called the lacertus fibrosus)

    (EPN, p. 2)
87. The greater occipital nerve originates from the dorsal ramus of:
    A. C1
    B. C2
    C. C1–C2
    D. C3

    Correct Answer: B

    (EPN, p. 113)
88. Which of the following structures is innervated by the greater occipital nerve?
    A. External ear
    B. Lower eyelid
    C. Posterior scalp
    D. Skin over the mastoid process.

    Correct Answer: C

Explanation:

The greater occipital nerve is the dorsal ramus of the second cervical spinal nerve (C2). It emerges between the first and second cervical vertebrae, travels superiorly, and pierces the semispinalis capitis and trapezius muscles to provide sensory innervation to the posterior scalp, especially the occipital region.

(ABN, p. 93)

89. Which of the following structures is innervated by the lesser occipital nerve?
    A. External ear
    B. Lower eyelid
    C. Lower scalp
    D. Skin over the mastoid process

    Correct Answer: D

    (ABN, p. 93)
90. Injury to the posterior cord of the brachial plexus would most likely affect which of the following functions?
    A. Wrist flexion
    B. Finger flexion
    C. Shoulder abduction
    D. Thumb opposition

    Correct Answer: C

    Explanation:

    The posterior cord gives two terminal branches: the axillary nerve and the radial nerve. The axillary nerve supplies the deltoid muscle which abduct the shoulder.
91. The lumbar plexus is form by:
    A. Anterior branches of spinal nerve L1–L4
    B. Posterior branches of spinal nerve L1–L4
    C. Anterior branches of spinal nerve L2–L5
    D. Posterior branches of spinal nerve L2–L5

    Correct Answer: A

    (MPN, p.10)
92. The radial nerve pierces the following structure in the arm?
    A. Lateral intermuscular septum
    B. Medial intermuscular septum
    C. Triceps muscle
    D. Biceps muscle

    Correct Answer: A

    (EPN, p. 61)
93. Regarding the thoracodorsal nerve

    93a. It innervates which muscle?
    A. Trapezius
    B. Rhomboids
    C. Serratus anterior
    D. Latissimus dorsi

    93b. It originates from:
    A. Lateral cord
    B. Medial cord

C. Posterior cord
D. A and B

93c. It arises between:
A. Upper and lower subscapular nerves
B. Medial and lateral pectoral nerves
C. Radial and musculocutaneous nerves
D. Subclavius and suprascapular nerves

Correct Answers: 93a: D, 93b: C., 93c: A.

Explanation:

The thoracodorsal nerve, a minor branch of the posterior cord, emerges between the upper and lower subscapular nerves. It supplies the latissimus dorsi muscle. To evaluate its function, the patient performs arm adduction while keeping the elbow flexed at 90°.

(EPN, p. 108)

94. The infrapatellar nerve branches from
A. Femoral nerve
B. Tibial nerve
C. Common peroneal nerve
D. Saphenous nerve

Correct Answer: D.

(EPN. P. 189)

95. The typical anatomical course of the infrapatellar branch of the saphenous nerve is:
A. It has always a horizontal course to the knee.
B. It has always a vertical course to the knee.
C. It runs lateral to the patellar tendon.
D. It has variable anatomical course.

Correct Answer: D

Explanation:

The infrapatellar branch of the saphenous nerve is at risk from knee surgeries. It has a variable anatomical course, and there is no definitive safety zone when doing knee surgeries. Its location is best identified by ultrasound.

[75]

96. One of the following is correct about the suprascapular notch, EXCEPT:
A. The superior border is the superior border of the scapula.
B. The lateral border is the base of the coracoid process.
C. The superior transverse scapular ligament forms the base.
D. It contains the suprascapular vein.

Correct Answer: C

Explanation:

The superior transverse scapular ligament (suprascapular ligament) forms the roof to convert the notch into a foramen. The suprascapular nerve passes through the foramen where the suprascapular vein and artery pass over the superior transverse scapular ligament.

(TS, p. 50)

97. Before entering the suprascapular notch, the suprascapular nerve passes between:
    A. Inferior belly of the omohyoid and the trapezius muscle
    B. Teres minor and infraspinatus muscles
    C. Subclavius and sternocleidomastoid muscle
    D. Latissimus dorsi and rhomboid major
    Correct Answer: A
    (EPN, P, 92)
98. During anterior exposure of the suprascapular nerve, the best way to identify it is by:
    A. Tracing it from the posterior cord of the brachial plexus
    B. Locating it as it passes superior to the transverse scapular ligament
    C. Following it as it converges with the inferior belly of the omohyoid at scapula
    D. Locating it between the infraspinatus muscles and supraspinatus
    Correct Answer: C (Fig. 16.15)
    (EPN, p. 92)
99. Which nerve is at risk of injury during a pelvic fracture, leading to weakness in adduction of the thigh?
    A. Femoral nerve
    B. Sciatic nerve
    C. Obturator nerve
    D. Pudendal nerve
    Correct Answer: C

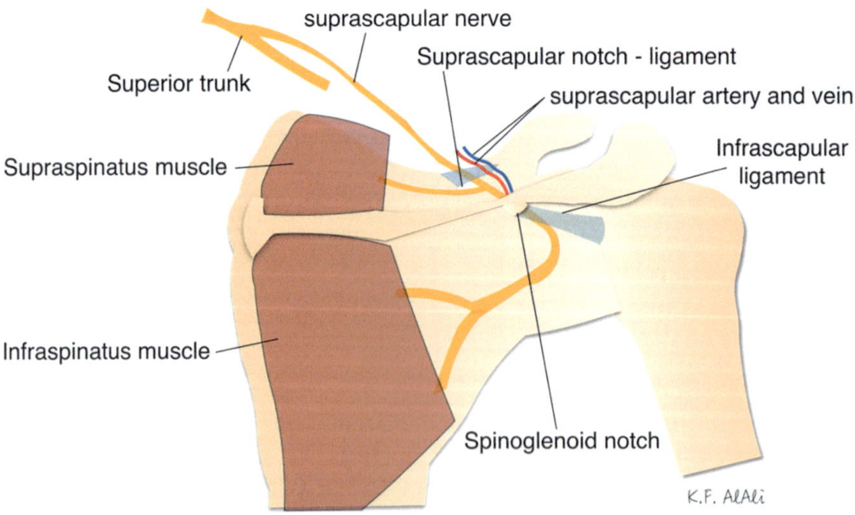

Fig. 16.15 Posterior view of scapula showing the suprascapular nerve with its branches

Explanation:

The obturator nerve, posterior division, supplies the adductor magnus muscle.

(EPN, p. 179)

100. The sensation of the posterior thigh is primarily supplied by which nerve?
    A. Posterior femoral cutaneous nerve
    B. Sciatic nerve
    C. Lateral femoral cutaneous nerve
    D. Femoral nerve

    Correct Answer: A

101. One of the following is CORRECT about the posterior femoral cutaneous nerve:
    A. It exits the pelvis via the greater sciatic foramen.
    B. It provides motor innervation to the hamstring muscles.
    C. It originates from the lumbar plexus.
    D. It runs lateral to the sciatic nerve throughout its course.

    Correct Answer: A

    Explanation:

    The posterior femoral cutaneous nerve is a sensory nerve originating from the sacral plexus (S1–S3). It exits the pelvis via the greater sciatic foramen, traveling inferior to the piriformis muscle posteriorly first to the sciatic nerve, then become medial. It descends in the posterior thigh, providing cutaneous innervation to the posterior thigh, inferior gluteal region, and popliteal fossa. It also gives rise to the perineal branch, supplying part of the perineum.

102. The intercostobrachial nerve, provides sensation to which area?
    A. Lateral forearm
    B. Posterior shoulder
    C. Dorsum of the hand
    D. Upper medial arm

    Correct Answer: D

    Explanation:

    The intercostobrachial nerve refers to the lateral cutaneous branch of the second intercostal nerve. It originates anterior to the long thoracic nerve and supplies sensory innervation to the axillary skin and a variable area on the medial upper arm. It is often cut during axillary lymph node dissection.

    (MPN, p. 1)

103. The subscapularis muscle is innervated by which nerve, and what is its primary action?
    A. Axillary nerve; arm abduction
    B. Upper and lower subscapular nerves; arm internal rotation
    C. Radial nerve; arm extension
    D. Suprascapular nerve; arm external rotation

    Correct Answer: B

Explanation:

The upper subscapular nerve innervates the subscapularis muscle, while the lower subscapular nerve supplies the distal part of the subscapularis.

The subscapularis muscle is involved in arm internal rotation.

(MPN, p. 4)

104. The sensory innervation to the posterior aspect of the external ear is provided by which nerve?
   A. Auriculotemporal nerve
   B. Facial nerve
   C. Greater auricular nerve
   D. V1 branch of trigeminal nerve

   Correct Answer: C

   (EPN, p. 117)

105. The anteriolateral boundary of the greater sciatic foramen is:
   A. Greater sciatic notch of the ilium
   B. Sacrotuberous ligament
   C. Sacrospinous ligament and the ischial spine
   D. Anterior sacroiliac ligament

   Correct Answer: A

   Explanation:

   The greater sciatic foramen is enclosed by several structures. Superiorly, it is bordered by the anterior sacroiliac ligament. Posteromedially, the sacrotuberous ligament forms its boundary. Anterolaterally, it is framed by the greater sciatic notch of the ilium. Finally, inferiorly, it is limited by the sacrospinous ligament and the ischial spine.

   (CA, p. 324)

106. The lateral and medial cords contribute to an "M" like branches, the medial limb of the "M" is
   A. Musculocutaneous nerve
   B. Median nerve
   C. Radial nerve
   D. Ulnar nerve

   Correct Answer: D

   Explanation:

   The musculocutaneous nerve forms the lateral limb of the "M" shape, while the ulnar nerve forms the medial limb. The median nerve is created at the center where the lateral and medial cords converge in a V-shaped junction.

   (EPN, p. 36)

107. In exposure for the median nerve in the proximal forearm, the muscle that is usually the median nerve hidden in its lateral border (picked up with forceps in the image Fig. 16.16).
   A. Brachioradialis
   B. Flexor carpi radialis
   C. Pronator teres
   D. None of the above

   Correct Answer: B

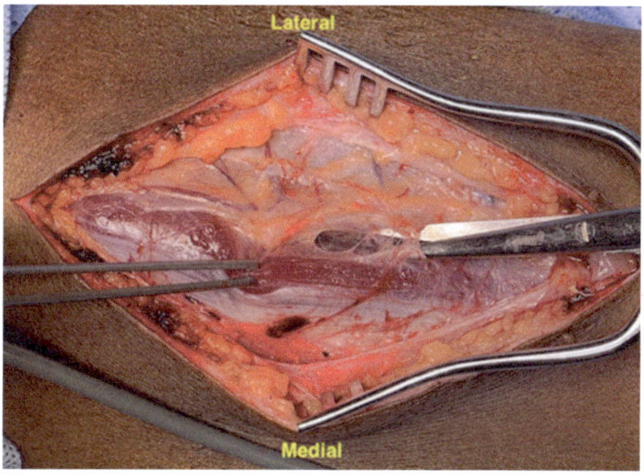

Fig. 16.16 Case 107 diagram

Explanation:

In the forearm, the median nerve courses between the humeral and ulnar heads of the pronator teres before traveling deep to the flexor digitorum superficialis. Flexor carpi radialis lies superficially and laterally to the median nerve, often covering it during surgical dissection.

(EPN, p. 5)

108. The first ulnar innervated muscle is:
    A. Flexor digitorum superfecialis
    B. Flexor digitorum profundus
    C. Flexor carpi ulnaris
    D. Pronotor teres

    Correct Answer: C
    (MPN, p. 31)
109. The deep branch of the ulnar nerve supplies which of the following muscles?
    A. Brachioradialis
    B. Adductor pollicis
    C. Flexor pollicis longus
    D. Extensor carpi ulnaris

    Correct Answer: B (Fig. 16.17)
    (EPN, p. 36)
110. In 50% of patients, the ulnar nerve, after piercing the medial intermuscular septum, passes underneath a structure called?
    A. Intermuscular canal
    B. Arcade of Froshe
    C. Arcade of Struthers.
    D. Unnamed ligament between triceps and biceps

    Correct Answer: B
    (EPN, p. 30)

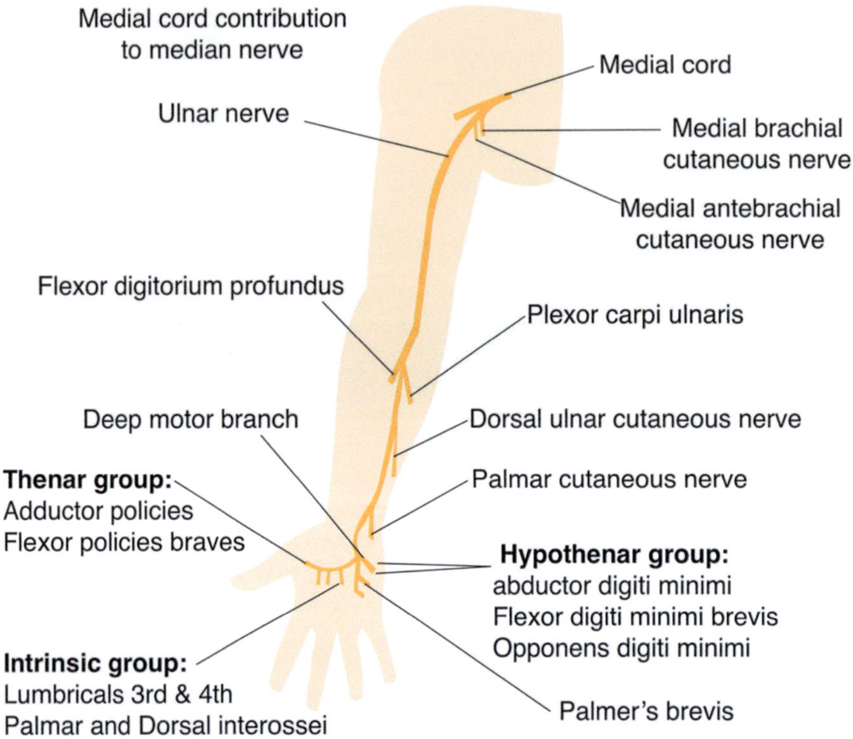

Fig. 16.17 Ulnar nerve branches and muscle supply

111. Which of the following is TRUE about the arcade of Struthers?
   A. It is an extension of the lateral intermuscular septum.
   B. It attaches to the lateral head of the triceps.
   C. It is located about two-thirds down the arm.
   D. It forms a tunnel for the ulnar and median nerves.
   Correct Answer: C
   Explanation:
   In approximately 50% of individuals, the ulnar nerve passes underneath an extension of the intermuscular septum, forming an arch-like structure that connects to the medial head of the triceps. This short fibrous band, located about two-thirds down the arm, is known as the arcade of Struthers.
   (EPN, p. 30)
112. Which statement correctly differentiates the arcade of Struthers from the ligament of Struthers?
   A. Arcade of Struthers compresses the median nerve; ligament of Struthers affects the ulnar nerve.
   B. Arcade of Struthers forms a bony tunnel, while ligament of Struthers is purely fibrous.

Table 16.1 The differences between arcade and ligament of Struthers

Feature	Arcade of Struthers	Ligament of Struthers
Type	Fibrous band (extension of intermuscular septum the medial head of the triceps)	Fibrous or bony band (remnant of supracondylar process)
Location	About two-thirds down the arm, near the medial head of the triceps	Near the distal humerus, extending from the supracondylar process to the medial epicondyle
Prevalence	Present in ~50% of individuals	Found in ~1% of the population
Structures involved	Ulnar nerve passes through it	Median nerve and brachial artery may pass beneath it
Clinical relevance	Can cause ulnar nerve compression, leading to weakness and numbness in the hand	Can cause median nerve compression, mimicking pronator teres syndrome

C. Arcade of Struthers is at the distal humerus; ligament of Struthers is at mid-arm.
D. Arcade of Struthers is near the medial triceps; ligament of Struthers is a remnant of the supracondylar process.

Correct Answer: D

Explanation:

The following table summarizes the differences (Table 16.1):

113. In the elbow, the ulnar nerve enters a groove which is called:
A. Olecrano-epicobdylar groove
B. Medial epicondyle groove
C. Postcondylar groove
D. The groove has no name

Correct Answer: C

Explanation:

After passing from medial head of the triceps in the lower arm, the ulnar nerve enters the postcondylar groove—a curved bony channel situated between the medial epicondyle of the humerus (anterior and medial) and the olecranon of the ulna (posterior and lateral). In this groove, the ulnar nerve is highly susceptible to external trauma.

(EPN, p. 31)

114. Regarding the cubital tunnel:

114a. Where is the cubital tunnel located?
A. Proximal to postcondylar groove
B. Distal to postcondylar groove
C. Medial to postcondylar groove
D. Lateral to postcondylar groove

114b. Which statement correctly describes the segments of the cubital tunnel?
A. The first segment lies beneath an aponeurosis bridging the medial epicondyle and olecranon.
B. The second segment is where the ulnar nerve passes under the Osborne ligament.

C. The first segment is where the ulnar nerve enters the postcondylar groove.
D. The second segment lies between the heads of the pronator teres.

142c. What is the name of the aponeurosis in the first segment?
A. Arcade of Osborne
B. Osborne ligament
C. Osborne band
D. All of the above are correct.

Correct Answers: 142a: B, 142b: A, 142c: D

Explanation:

The cubital tunnel is located just beyond the postcondylar groove. It has two segments:

Proximal segment: The ulnar nerve passes beneath an aponeurosis that connects the proximal tendons of the flexor carpi ulnaris (FCU). This aponeurosis may extend between the medial epicondyle and olecranon, sometimes covering the postcondylar groove.

Distal segment: The nerve continues between and under the two heads of the FCU. In about 75% of individuals, a thickened aponeurosis, known as the **Osborne band (also known as Osborn ligament, arcade of Osborn, Osborne fascia, or the cubital tunnel retinaculum)**, may further enclose the nerve (Fig. 16.18).

(EPN, p. 32)

115. In the forearm, the ulnar nerve passes underneath flexor carpi ulnaris muscle but above the following muscle:
A. Flexor digitorum profundus
B. Flexor pollicis longus

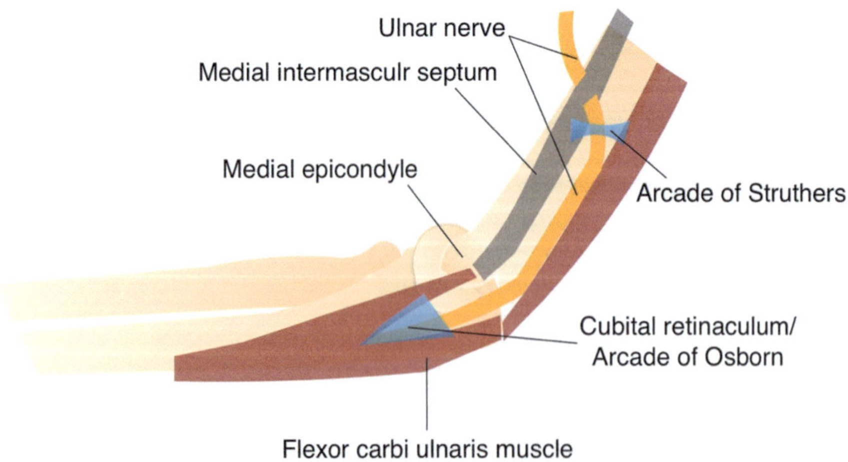

Fig. 16.18 Medial elbow showing areas of possible entrapment of ulnar nerve causing cubital tunnel syndrome

C. Pronator teres
D. Brachioradialis

Correct Answer: A

Explanation:

In the forearm, the ulnar nerve enters by passing between the two heads of the flexor carpi ulnaris, and then travels deep to that muscle, but superficial (above) the flexor digitorum profundus (FDP) muscle. It continues this course as it descends toward the wrist.

(EPN, p. 35)

116. In the distal forearm, the ulnar nerve lies between which two tendons?
A. Flexor carpi radialis tendon medially and the palmaris longus tendon laterally
B. Flexor pollicis longus tendon medially and the brachioradialis tendon laterally
C. Pronator teres tendon medially and the flexor digitorum profundus tendon laterally
D. Flexor carpi ulnaris tendon medially and the flexor digitorum superficialis tendon laterally

Correct Answer: D

(EPN, p. 35)

117. Which statement is TRUE regarding the sensory branches of the ulnar nerve in the forearm?
A. The palmar ulnar cutaneous nerve arises 5–10 cm proximal to the wrist and supplies the dorsum of the hand.
B. The dorsal ulnar cutaneous nerve arises from the dorsomedial aspect of the ulnar nerve and supplies the hypothenar eminence.
C. The palmar ulnar cutaneous nerve enters the subcutaneous space near the distal wrist crease.
D. Both the dorsal and palmar ulnar cutaneous nerves branch from the ulnar nerve just before it enters Guyon's canal.

Correct Answer: C

Explanation:

Palmar ulnar cutaneous nerve arises 5–10 cm proximal to the wrist crease and supply palmar part of ulnar supply to the hypothenar eminence and proximal ulnar aspect of the palm.

(EPN, p. 35) (MPN, p. 31)

118. The first branch from the medial cord of the brachial plexus is:
A. Medial pectoral nerve
B. Medial brachial cutaneous nerve
C. Ulnar nerve
D. Lower subscapular nerve

Correct Answer: A (Fig. 16.1)

119. The lateral sural nerve is a branch of:
   A. Sciatic nerve
   B. Tibial nerve
   C. Common peroneal nerve
   D. Deep peroneal nerve
   Correct Answer: C (Fig. 16.8)
   (EPN, p. 142)
120. The femoral nerve passes between the following muscles:
   A. Iliacus and psoas major muscles
   B. Psoas major and psoas minor muscles
   C. Iliacus and quadratus lumborum muscles
   D. Psoas major and quadratus lumborum muscles
   Correct Answer: A
   Explanation:
   The femoral nerve arises from the lumbar plexus (L2–L4) and descends between the iliacus and psoas major muscles in the pelvis.
   (EPN, p. 176)
121. The median nerve passes between which two muscles in the forearm before entering the carpal tunnel?
   A. Flexor carpi radialis and palmaris longus
   B. Flexor digitorum profundus and flexor digitorum superficialis
   C. Pronator teres and flexor carpi ulnaris
   D. Brachioradialis and extensor carpi radialis longus
   Correct Answer: A
   Explanation:
   In the distal forearm, the median nerve lies between the palmaris longus tendon medially and the flexor carpi radialis tendon laterally, just before passing into the carpal tunnel.
   (MPN, p. 6)
122. The radial nerve travels in the spiral groove of the humerus along with which vascular structure?
   A. Ulnar artery
   B. Brachial artery
   C. Deep brachial artery
   D. Median artery
   Correct Answer: C
   (EPN, p. 59)
123. After leaving the brachial plexus, the axillary nerve passes through which anatomical space to reach the deltoid muscle?
   A. Triangular space
   B. Triangular interval
   C. Subclavian triangle
   D. Quadrangular space
   Correct Answer: D

124. Axillary nerve passes into quadrangular space along with which structure?
   A. Anterior circumflex humeral artery
   B. Posterior circumflex humeral artery
   C. Medial circumflex humeral artery
   D. All of the above

   Correct Answer: B

   Explanation:

   The posterior circumflex humeral artery travels posteromedially with the axillary nerve. They both exit the axilla through the quadrangular space (Fig. 16.19).

   (EPN, p. 100)

125. The musculocutaneous nerve pierces which muscle as it enters the forearm?
   A. Brachialis
   B. Biceps brachii
   C. Coracobrachialis
   D. Pronator teres

   Correct Answer: C

   (EPN, p. 95)

126. The sciatic nerve typically exits the pelvis through the greater sciatic foramen, passing below which muscle?
   A. Piriformis
   B. Gluteus maximus

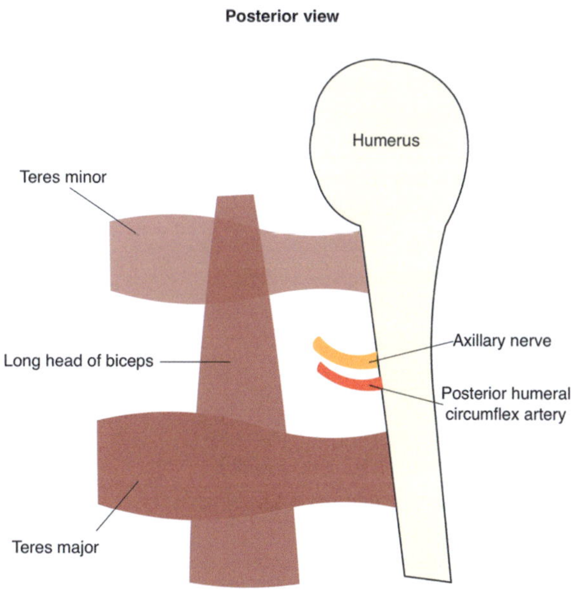

Fig. 16.19 Axillary nerve pathway

C. Obturator internus
D. Quadratus femoris
Correct Answer: A
(EPN, p. 139)

127. After passing underneath the piriformis muscle, the sciatic nerve becomes underneath which muscle?
A. Obturator internus
B. Gluteus maximus
C. Quadratus femoris
D. Gluteus medius
Correct Answer: B
(EPN, p. 139)

128. In the posterior thigh, the sciatic nerve passes between which two muscles?
A. Semitendinosus and semimembranosus muscles
B. Semitendinosus and adductor magnus muscles
C. Semitendinosus and long head of biceps femoris muscles
D. Adductor magnus muscles and long head of biceps femoris muscles
Correct Answer: C
(EPN, p. 139)

129. The femoral triangle is bordered by all of the following structures EXCEPT:
A. Inguinal ligament
B. Sartorius muscle
C. Adductor longus muscle
D. Adductor magnus muscle
Correct Answer: D (Fig. 16.20)
(EPN, p. 176)

130. The superior gluteal nerve passes through the greater sciatic foramen and supplies which muscle directly as it passes superior to the piriformis:
A. Gluteus maximus
B. Gluteus medius
C. Quadratus femoris
D. Gemellus superior
Correct Answer: B
Explanation:
The superior gluteal nerve arises from L4, L5, and S1. It exits the greater sciatic foramen above the piriformis and supplies the gluteus medius, gluteus minimus, and tensor fascia latae, which work together to abduct the hip.
(EPN, p. 199)

131. The inferior gluteal nerve exits the pelvis through the greater sciatic foramen to innervate which muscle?
A. Gluteus medius
B. Gluteus minimus
C. Piriformis
D. Gluteus maximus
Correct Answer: D

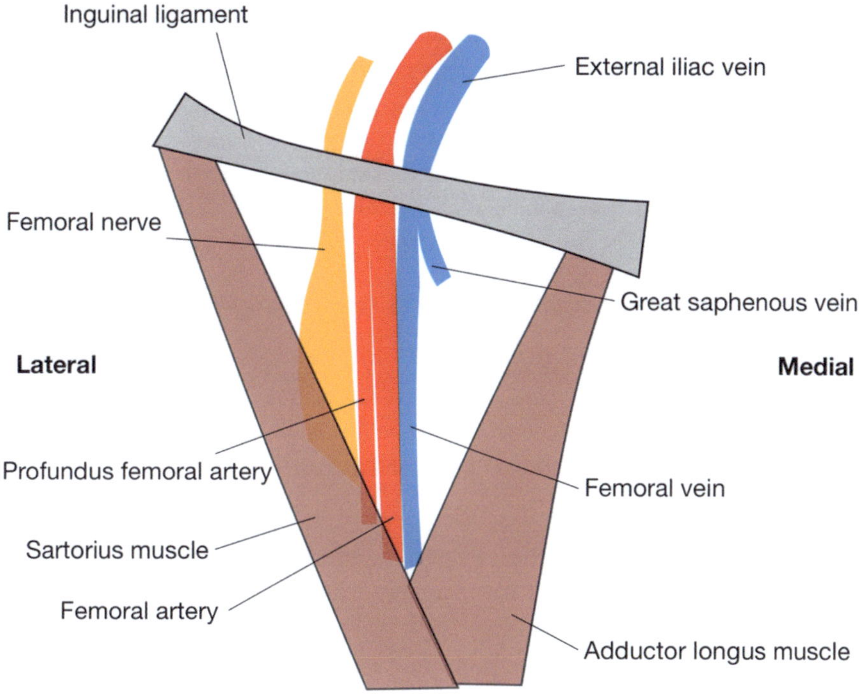

Fig. 16.20 Femoral triangle borders and contents

Explanation:

The inferior gluteal nerve arises from L5, S1, and S2. It exits the greater sciatic foramen and supplies gluteus maximus.

(EPN, p. 199)

132. The deep peroneal nerve innervates which muscles in the anterior compartment of the leg before it crosses the ankle joint?
   A. Tibialis anterior and extensor digitorum longus
   B. Soleus and gastrocnemius
   C. Peroneus longus and peroneus brevis
   D. Tibialis posterior and flexor hallucis longus
   Correct Answer: A
   (EPN, p. 151)
133. The first muscle which is innervated by musculocutaneous nerve is:
   A. Biceps brachii
   B. Coracobrachialis
   C. Brachialis
   D. Brachioradialis
   Correct Answer: B (MPN, p. 24)

134. Which statement correctly describes the course of the superficial peroneal nerve?
    A. It arises from the tibial nerve and runs deep to the gastrocnemius.
    B. It pierces the crural fascia in the lower third of the leg to become subcutaneous.
    C. It remains deep throughout the leg and only supplies the peroneus muscles.
    D. It passes posterior to the lateral malleolus before entering the foot.

    Correct Answer: B

    (EPN, p. 146)
135. The superficial peroneal nerve provides sensory innervation to which of the following areas?
    A. The lateral side of the little toe
    B. The plantar surface of the foot
    C. The dorsum of the foot except for the first web space
    D. The medial malleolus and medial foot

    Correct Answer: C

    (EPN, p. 146)
136. Which muscles are innervated by the superficial peroneal nerve?
    A. Tibialis anterior and extensor digitorum longus
    B. Peroneus longus and extensor hallucis longus
    C. Peroneus brevis and soleus
    D. Peroneus longus and peroneus brevis

    Correct Answer: D (Fig. 16.21)
137. In the supraclavicular approach, the accessory nerve can be identified at the:
    A. Anterior surface of the trapezius at its medial border
    B. Anterior surface of the trapezius at its lateral border
    C. Posterior surface of the trapezius at its medial border
    D. Posterior surface of the trapezius at its lateral border

    Correct Answer: A

    Explanation:

    The accessory nerve courses superficially in the posterior triangle of the neck. It lies at the anterior surface of the trapezius. It runs deep to the sternocleidomastoid (SCM) and then emerges to supply the trapezius muscle from its medial border.

    (SSW, p. 2154)
138. The key in infraclavicular exploration of the brachial plexus is to identify:
    A. The lateral cord
    B. The medial cord
    C. Median nerve
    D. Ulnar nerve

    Correct Answer: C

    Explanation:

    The key neural structure to be identified here is the median nerve, which is characterized by a Y-shape at its takeoff from both the lateral and medial

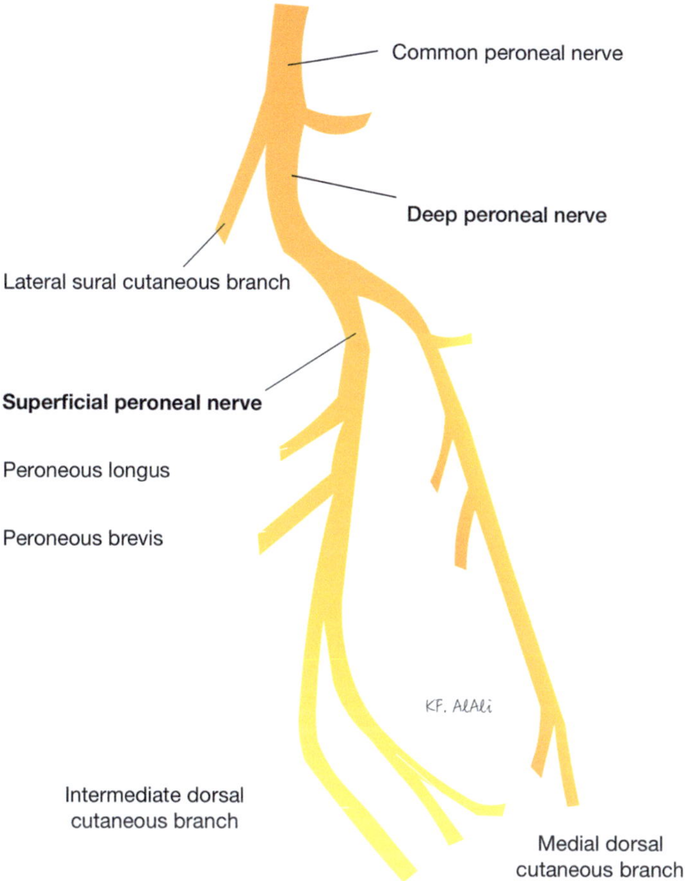

Fig. 16.21 Superficial peroneal nerve supplied muscles and branches

cords. The lateral cord is the first neural structure seen typically during the infraclavicular exposure.

(SSW, p. 2155)

139. During the exposure of the superficial radial nerve at the forearm, the nerve will be found between:
   A. Tendons of the extensor carpi radialis longus and the brachioradialis muscles
   B. Tendons of the flexor carpi ulnaris and palmaris longus
   C. Extensor digitorum and extensor carpi ulnaris muscles
   D. Pronator teres and flexor digitorum superficialis

   Correct Answer: A

   (OPN, p. 130)

140. In most individuals, the superficial radial nerve pierces the fascia approximately how far proximal to Lister's tubercle?
    A. 2 cm
    B. 5 cm
    C. 9 cm
    D. 15 cm

    Correct Answer: C

    (PNN, p. 1099)

141. After emerging subcutaneously, the superficial radial nerve typically divides into how many main branches?
    A. One
    B. Two
    C. Three
    D. Four

    Correct Answer: B

    (PNN, p. 1099)

142. The distal superficial radial nerve branches were found in which specific anatomical triangle?
    A. Guyon's canal triangle
    B. Cubital fossa triangle
    C. Anatomical snuffbox
    D. Isosceles triangle

    Correct Answer: D

    Explanation:

    All of the branches of the superficial radial nerve were found in the radial half of an isosceles triangle. The triangle is formed by the radial styloid, Lister's tubercle, and the exit of the superficial radial nerve.

    (PNN, p. 1106)

143. The extensor indicis proprius muscle is supplied by
    A. Posterior interosseous nerve
    B. Anterior interosseous nerve
    C. Radial main trunk
    D. Superficial radial nerve

    Correct Answer: A

    Explanation:

    The posterior interosseous nerve supplies the extensor muscles of the fingers, including the extensor indicis proprius muscle, which extends the index finger.

    (EPN, p. 71)

144. Why does the common peroneal nerve have another name, fibular nerve?
   A. Because it anatomically aligns with the fibular artery
   B. Due to its embryological origin, the lumbar plexus, which historically used "fibular" terminology
   C. To reflect the updated anatomical terminology that emphasizes its close association with the fibula
   D. To avoid confusion with the perineal pelvic region

   Correct Answer: D

   Explanation:

   The peroneal nerve was renamed the fibular nerve in 1998, in an effort to avoid confusion with the perineal pelvic region, but the name change has not been commonly accepted, and both terms are used.

   (PNN, p. 2303)

Peripheral Nerve Injuries and Nerve Physiology

17

1. The axoplasmic transport mechanism that moves materials from the nerve terminal toward the cell body is known as:
   A. Fast anterograde transport
   B. Slow anterograde transport
   C. Fast retrograde transport
   D. Slow retrograde transport

   Correct Answer: C

   Explanation:

   Fast axonal retrograde transport moves materials from the axon terminal back to the soma at a speed of 200–400 mm/day. This process is crucial for membrane recycling, signaling, and cellular maintenance. It is driven by the motor protein dynein, which transports endocytosed vesicles, signaling molecules, and degraded proteins toward the cell body.

   (NB, p. 27)
2. Which of the following best describes the role of internodal segments in saltatory conduction within peripheral myelinated nerves?
   A. Sites of action potential generation
   B. Areas rich in voltage-gated potassium channels
   C. Regions where neurotransmitter synthesis occurs
   D. Segments that prevent ion leakage, increasing conduction velocity

   Correct Answer: D

   (FCN, p. 86)
3. Regarding Wallerian degeneration:

   3a. It occurs at:
   A. Proximal stump
   B. Distal stump
   C. Both proximal and distal stumps
   D. It occurs only in motor nerve

K. F. AlAli, H. T. Hashim, *Spine Surgery and Peripheral Nerve Surgery*,
https://doi.org/10.1007/978-3-031-98543-0_17

3b. It starts within:
  A. 6 h post injury
  B. 12 h post injury
  C. 24 h post injury
  D. 48 h post injury

3c. The first step starts with:
  A. Myeline degeneration
  B. Schwan cell proliferation
  C. Formation of bands of Bungner
  D. Axon regeneration

3d. What is the primary role of Bands of Bungner in nerve regeneration?
  A. Axonal growth cones extending to muscles
  B. Schwann cell columns guiding axons
  C. Fibrotic bands blocking regeneration
  D. Synaptic junctions with muscles

Correct Answers: 3a: B, 3b: C, 3c: A, 3c: B

Explanation:

Wallerian degeneration is the process that happen after the injury within 24 h in the distal stump. The proximal stump stays connected to the neuron's nucleus, so it does not undergo this degeneration in the same way The distal stump, however, experiences a cascade of cellular and molecular events due to the loss of axoplasmic transport. It stars with myelin degeneration, followed by Schwann cell proliferation, clearance of axonal debris, and formation of bands of Büngner to guide axonal regeneration, culminating in potential remyelination and functional recovery over weeks to months (Fig. 17.1).

(FCB, p. 114)

4. What is the key molecular event in Schwann cells that promotes peripheral nerve regeneration after injury?
   A. Upregulation of myelin genes
   B. Downregulation of c-Jun transcription factor
   C. Formation of glial scar tissue
   D. Dedifferentiation and upregulation of repair-supportive features

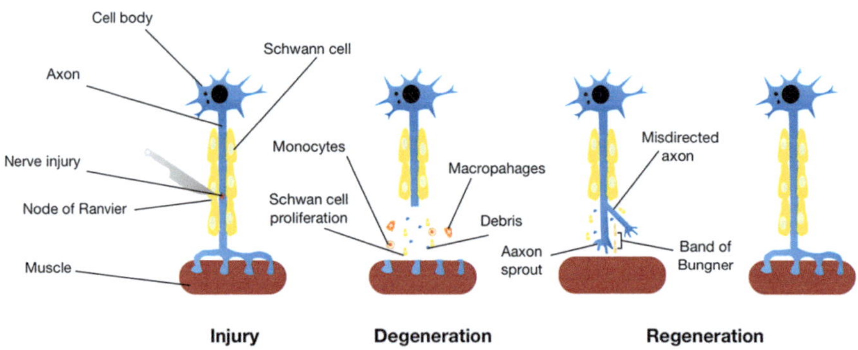

Fig. 17.1 Process of Wallerian degeneration and nerve regeneration after an injury

Correct Answer: D

Explanation:

After nerve injury, Schwann cells dedifferentiate, downregulate myelin genes, and activate repair-supportive features, including trophic factor production and innate immune response activation.

(FCB, p. 118)

5. How soon after a clean cut injury do axons begin to sprout from the proximal stump in the PNS?
   A. Within a few h
   B. After 24 h
   C. After 1 week
   D. After 3 weeks

   Correct Answer: A

   Explanation:

   Following a clean cut, axons begin to sprout from the proximal stump within a few h, driven by growth cones. In crush injuries, sprouting may be delayed up to a week due to axonal dieback, but a clean cut allows for a faster response.

   (FCB, p. 119)

6. A lesion of the superior gluteal nerve would result in which of the following gait abnormalities?
   A. Steppage gait
   B. Trendelenburg gait
   C. Waddling gait
   D. Spastic gait

   Correct Answer: B

   Explanation:

   Superior gluteal nerve injury results in Trendelenburg gait due to weakened hip abductors (gluteus medius muscle).

   [76]

7. All of the following is correct regarding end-to-end nerve repair, EXCEPT:
   A. Achieve continuity of the nerve stumps without tension.
   B. Proper alignment of the fascicles
   C. Use of multiple absorbable stitches
   D. Aligning the longitudinal blood vessels in the epineurium

   Correct Answer: C

   Explanation:

   The main objective of nerve repair is to reconnect nerve ends without tension, ensuring proper fascicular alignment. Fascicle positioning is confirmed by aligning longitudinal blood vessels within the epineurium. Under magnification, coaptation is performed with fine nylon sutures (8–0 or 9–0). It is advisable to use a minimal number of sutures (usually four) to reduce the scarring process.

   (MPN, p. 75)

8. A 32-year-old patient develops foot drop after an extensive hip surgery. Nerve conduction studies show prolonged latency but normal amplitude in the common peroneal nerve. What is the most likely mechanism of injury?
   A. Neuropraxia
   B. Axonotmesis
   C. Wallerian degeneration
   D. Neurotmesis

   Correct Answer: A

   Explanation:

   Neuropraxia caused by loss of myelination with intact axons. Amplitude in a nerve conduction study measures the number of axons; therefore, it is normal in neuropraxia. Neuropraxia is characterized by conduction block causing prolonged latency in conduction study.

   (MPN, p. 19)
9. A 45-year-old woman develops numbness and weakness in her hand after a complex wrist fracture. Nerve conduction studies suggest damage to the median nerve. Upon surgical exploration, the nerve is found to be contused but not transected. What is the next best step in surgical management?
   A. Nerve grafting
   B. End-to-end repair
   C. Neurolysis
   D. Nerve transfer

   Correct Answer: C

   Explanation:

   Neurolysis is appropriate in cases of contusion without transection, allowing the nerve to recover without tension or grafting. Even if nerve repair is required, neurolysis is crucial to free the nerve from tension and enhance its vascularity.

   (MPN, p. 75)
10. All of the following is NOT a type of end-to-end nerve repair:
    A. Epineural repair
    B. Grouped fascicular repair
    C. Fascicular repair
    D. Grafting repair

    Correct Answer: D

    Explanation:

    End-to-end nerve repair is a microsurgical technique used to reconnect injured nerve ends to restore function. It is typically performed when a nerve is cleanly transected and there is no significant gap between the stumps. Grafting is used to reconnect stumps if there is a gap between them by using a nerve graft.

    (MPN, p. 76)

11. A young athlete sustains a penetrating injury to the forearm that severs the median nerve. After 12 months, no signs of functional recovery are observed. Which of the following would most likely be the recommended surgical procedure?
    A. Nerve grafting
    B. Tendon transfer
    C. Nerve transfer
    D. End-to-end repair

    Correct Answer: C

    Explanation:

    After prolonged nerve injury (typically more than 12 months) without recovery, nerve transfers may be the best option to restore motor function, especially when reinnervation time is a concern.

    [77]
12. The following are indications for nerve transfer, EXCEPT:
    A. Root avulsions
    B. Distal lesions
    C. Poor surgical bed for graft
    D. Insufficient autologous graft available

    Correct Answer: B

    Explanation:

    Nerve transfer is indicated when direct nerve repair is not feasible due to a large gap, excessive tension, or prolonged denervation. It is commonly used in proximal nerve injuries, brachial plexus avulsions, chronic nerve damage (>12–18 months), severe crush injuries, or failed primary repairs.

    [77]
13. Which Sunderland degree of nerve injury corresponds to Seddon's neurapraxia?
    A. First degree
    B. Second degree
    C. Third degree
    D. Fourth degree

    Correct Answer: A

    Explanation:

    Sunderland's first-degree injury is a conduction block with no structural damage (like Seddon's neurapraxia), affecting only nerve function temporarily.

    (MPN, p. 19)

14. A 35-year-old carpenter accidentally strikes his wrist with a hammer, causing weakness in finger flexion and numbness in the median nerve distribution. Imaging shows no nerve transection, but electromyography (EMG) after two weeks reveals Wallerian degeneration distal to the injury site. Strength and sensation gradually improve over three months without surgery.
    What is the Sunderland classification of this nerve injury?
    A. First degree
    B. Second degree
    C. Third degree
    D. Fourth degree
    Correct Answer: B
    Explanation:
    A second-degree injury (axonotmesis) involves axonal disruption with intact endoneurium, perineurium, and epineurium. Wallerian degeneration occurs, but spontaneous recovery is possible due to preserved connective tissue, matching the gradual recovery in this case.
    (MPN, P. 19)
15. A patient presents with a peripheral nerve injury where the axon, endoneurium, and perineurium are disrupted, but the epineurium remains intact. What is the Sunderland classification for this injury?
    A. Second degree
    B. Third degree
    C. Fourth degree
    D. Fifth degree
    Correct Answer: C
    Explanation:
    A fourth-degree injury involves disruption of the axon, endoneurium, and perineurium, with only the epineurium intact. This severe injury disrupts the nerve's continuity, often leading to neuroma formation and requiring surgical repair.
    (MPN, p. 19)
16. In peripheral nerve injury, axonotmesis in Seddon classification is equivalent to which Sunderland grade:
    A. II
    B. III
    C. IV
    D. All of the above
    Correct Answer: D
    (MPN, p. 19)
17. A 40-year-old motorcyclist sustains a deep laceration to the upper arm in a crash, severing the ulnar nerve completely. Surgical exploration reveals a gap between the nerve ends, with no continuity of any nerve layers. After nerve repair, recovery is incomplete despite months of rehabilitation.

How would this injury be classified using Sunderland's system?

A. Third degree
B. Fourth degree
C. Fifth degree
D. Second degree

Correct Answer: C

Explanation:

A fifth-degree injury (neurotmesis in Seddon) involves complete transection of the nerve, including the axon and all connective tissue layers (endoneurium, perineurium, epineurium). The gap and lack of continuity confirm this severity, often resulting in incomplete recovery even with surgery.

(MPN, p. 19)

The Seddon and Sunderland nerve injury classification are summarized:

Seddon's Classification:

- Neurapraxia: Mildest, no structural damage
- Axonotmesis: Axon damage with intact connective tissue, allowing regeneration
- Neurotmesis: Complete disruption, no spontaneous recovery
- Sunderland's Classification:
- 1st Degree: Matches neurapraxia
- 2nd Degree: Matches axonotmesis with intact endoneurium
- 3rd Degree: Adds endoneurial damage, complicating regeneration
- 4th Degree: Perineurial damage, often leading to neuroma
- 5th Degree: Complete transection, equivalent to severe neurotmesis
- Overlap and Differences:
- Seddon's axonotmesis corresponds to Sunderland's second and third degrees
- Seddon's neurotmesis covers Sunderland's fourth and fifth degrees
- Sunderland's system provides finer granularity by distinguishing damage to specific nerve layers, aiding in surgical decision-making

18. Which of the following statements about the axon hillock is TRUE regarding action potential initiation in peripheral nerves?

A. It has the highest concentration of voltage-gated sodium channels.
B. It is the site of neurotransmitter release.
C. It contains Nissl bodies for protein synthesis.
D. It is insulated by myelin sheath.

Correct Answer: A

Explanation:

The axon hillock is the specialized region of a neuron where the axon originates from the cell body and is crucial for the initiation of an action potential. It contains a high density of voltage-gated sodium channels, making it the most excitable part of the neuron.

19. In the context of peripheral nerve excitability, the term "accommodation" refers to:
    A. Decreased threshold due to rapid stimuli
    B. The ability of a nerve to regenerate after injury
    C. The summation of excitatory postsynaptic potentials
    D. Increased threshold due to prolonged depolarization

    Correct Answer: D

    Explanation:

    Peripheral nerve accommodation occurs when a gradually increasing stimulus fails to trigger an action potential. This happens because sodium channel inactivation and potassium channel activation counteract depolarization, preventing the nerve from reaching the threshold. This process helps regulate nerve excitability, preventing overstimulation and contributing to sensory adaptation and motor control.

    [78]
20. Regarding axillary nerve injury:

    20a. What is the typical scenario for axillary nerve injury?
    A. Fracture of the clavicle
    B. Fracture of the surgical neck of the humerus
    C. Compression in the axilla during crutch use
    D. Anterior shoulder dislocation

    20b. What is the typical associated injury?
    A. The anterior circumflex artery injury
    B. The posterior circumflex artery injury
    C. Axillary artery injury
    D. All of the above

    20c. During the surgical exposure, the injured axillary proximal stump is usually found:
    A. Above the coracoid process
    B. Below the coracoid process
    C. Lateral to surgical neck of humerus
    D. 2–3 cm medial to surgical neck of humerus

    Correct Answers: 20a: D, 20b: B, 20c: B

    Explanation:

    Axillary nerve injuries typically results from anterior shoulder dislocations. This can lead to injury to the posterior circumflex humeral artery causing pseudoaneurysm. During surgical exposure, the proximal stump is typically located below the coracoid process, while the distal stump might be entrapped in fibrotic tissue and may require a separate posterior incision for access. Surgical repair often involves nerve grafting.

    (PNG, p. 247)

21. Which of the following findings best differentiates medial cord injury from proximal ulnar nerve injury?
    A. Sensory loss only in the medial hand and little finger
    B. Weakness in flexor carpi ulnaris and medial flexor digitorum profundus without median nerve involvement
    C. Sensory loss in the medial forearm and upper arm
    D. Normal sensation in the medial forearm with intrinsic hand muscle weakness

    Correct Answer: C

    Explanation:

    A medial cord injury affects the ulnar nerve, median nerve, and medial cutaneous nerves, causing sensory loss in the medial forearm and upper arm plus the hand. A proximal ulnar nerve injury only impacts the medial hand sensation and ulnar-supplied muscles. Option C highlights the medial cord's unique sensory territory (forearm and upper arm), distinguishing it from ulnar nerve injury.

    (EPN, p. 28)

22. In peripheral nerve regeneration:

    22a. which cells form the regeneration tube guiding axonal regrowth?
    A. Oligodendrocytes
    B. Schwann cells
    C. Astrocytes
    D. Microglia

    22b. What factor do these cells secrete to facilitate this process?
    A. Nogo protein
    B. Glial fibrillary acidic protein (GFAP)
    C. Nerve Growth Factor (NGF)
    D. Brain-derived neurotrophic factor (BDNF)

    Answers: 22a: B, 22b: C

23. The following nerve can be injured during cubital tunnel release.
    A. Main trunk medial antecubital cutaneous
    B. Anterior branch of medial antecubital cutaneous nerve
    C. Posterior branch of medial antecubital cutaneous nerve
    D. All of the above

    Explanation Answer: C

    Explanation:

    The posterior branch of the medial antebrachial cutaneous nerve (MACN) is most commonly injured during cubital tunnel release due to its closeness to the medial epicondyle and surgical site. While the main MACN trunk (A) and anterior branch (B) could be at risk with a wider incision.

    (EPN, p. 28)

24. During the repair of a median nerve laceration at the forearm level, the surgeon uses an operating microscope to perform the repair. Which of the following steps is critical to ensure precise fascicular alignment?
    A. Use a running suture technique to avoid gapping.
    B. Perform a group fascicular repair with minimal sutures.
    C. Use fibrin glue alone without sutures to reduce manipulation.
    D. Ensure precise alignment of the epineurium only.

    Correct Answer: B

    Explanation:

    In cases where fascicular alignment is important (e.g., major mixed nerves), group fascicular repair using a few fine sutures ensures better alignment and functional recovery. Excessive sutures or manipulation increases the risk of fibrosis and poor outcomes.

    (MPN, p.75)
25. Which of the following statements best describes the appropriate management of a high-energy traumatic nerve injury caused by a laceration from a sharp object?
    A. Delayed surgical exploration after 3 weeks
    B. Delayed surgical exploration after 3 months
    C. Immediate surgical exploration and repair
    D. Immobilization and observation for spontaneous recovery

    Correct Answer: C

    Explanation:

    Sharp lacerations of nerves typically require immediate surgical exploration and repair to prevent further damage and optimize recovery.

    (MPN, p. 20)
26. In blunt laceration of a peripheral nerve, what is the most appropriate timing for surgical exploration?
    A. Immediate
    B. 3 weeks
    C. 3 months
    D. 12 months

    Correct Answer: B

    Explanation:

    In cases of blunt lacerations, contaminated wounds, or extensive soft-tissue loss, a delayed nerve repair (3 weeks) is recommended. This waiting period allows the swollen and bruised nerve ends to heal, clearly defining the boundary between healthy and damaged tissue. This improves the chances of successful reconstruction, either through end-to-end repair or, more commonly, nerve grafting for better functional recovery.

    (MPN, p. 20)

27. In a closed nerve injury due to a crush mechanism, what is the most appropriate timing for surgical exploration if there is no clinical or electrical evidence of recovery?
    A. Immediate
    B. 3 weeks
    C. 3 months
    D. 6 months

    Correct Answer: C

    Explanation:

    Closed nerve injuries such as crush injuries are often observed for spontaneous recovery, but if there is no improvement after 3–6 months, surgical exploration is recommended.

    (MPN, p. 22)

    A 19-year-old suffers a gunshot wound to the thigh, resulting in sciatic nerve palsy. What is the appropriate initial surgical exploration timing if there is no recovery?
    A. Immediate
    B. 3 weeks
    C. 3 months
    D. 6 months

    Correct Answer: C

    Explanation:

    Gunshot wounds are classified as closed injuries with preserved continuity. Surgery is delayed 3–4 months to allow potential spontaneous recovery (e.g., axonotmesis), as most lesions are not transections but heat/shock wave damage. Exploration occurred due to lack of recovery.

    Summary: The **"Rule of Three"** guides surgical timing in traumatic peripheral nerve injuries.

    It recommends immediate repair (within 3 days) for clean, sharp injuries, early intervention (within 3 weeks) for blunt or contusion injuries, and delayed surgery (at 3 months) for closed injuries to allow nerve degeneration and clearer surgical planning.

    [79]
28. A 30-year-old undergoes exploration of a median nerve injury 3 months after a crush trauma, revealing a neuroma in continuity. Intraoperative nerve action potential (NAP) testing shows no recordable signal across the lesion. What should the surgeon do next?
    A. Perform neurolysis as prognosis is poor
    B. Resect neuroma and graft
    C. Suture stumps directly
    D. Delay surgery to allow further regeneration

    Correct Answer: B

Explanation:

In case of neuroma in continuity with no NAP indicates scar tissue blocking regeneration (neurotmesis), resection of the scar and grafting with autologous nerve tissue is required, as healthy axons are not present to support spontaneous recovery.

[79]

29. What is the primary purpose of performing an intraoperative Nerve Action Potential (NAP) test during peripheral nerve surgery?
    A. To measure muscle contraction strength distal to the lesion
    B. To determine the thickness of the epineurium
    C. To evaluate blood flow to the nerve
    D. To assess the presence of viable axons

    Correct Answer: D

    Explanation:

    NAP testing evaluates whether functioning axons traverse a lesion (e.g., neuroma in continuity), guiding whether to preserve or resect the nerve segment.

    [79]
30. In NAP testing for a median nerve injury, how are the electrodes positioned relative to the lesion site?
    A. Stimulating electrode distal and recording electrode proximal to the lesion
    B. Both electrodes placed proximal to the lesion
    C. Stimulating electrode proximal and recording electrode distal to the lesion
    D. Both electrodes placed distal to the lesion

    Correct Answer: C

    Explanation:

    Placing the stimulating electrode proximal to the lesion and the recording electrode distal to it, allowing detection of action potentials crossing the injured segment.

    [79]
31. A surgeon is performing NAP testing on a sciatic nerve injury 3 months post-trauma. After isolating the nerve and placing the proximal stimulating electrode and distal recording electrode around a neuroma in continuity, what is the next step?
    A. Apply a supramaximal stimulus and observe for a recordable NAP
    B. Measure the nerve diameter with a caliper
    C. Suture the nerve ends to stabilize the electrodes
    D. Irrigate the nerve with saline to improve conduction

    Correct Answer: A

    Explanation:

    After positioning the electrodes, the surgeon applies a supramaximal stimulus and checks for a recordable NAP to assess axonal function.

    [79]

32. A patient with a mid-level ulnar nerve injury following an industrial accident is scheduled for repair. The surgeon decides to perform an end-to-end epineurial repair. Which of the following is the correct first step?
    A. Mobilization of the nerve ends to reduce tension
    B. Direct suturing of the nerve ends without mobilization
    C. Suturing of individual fascicles
    D. Nerve graft placement without tension

    Correct Answer: A

    Explanation:

    Nerve stumps must be mobilized to reduce tension before repair. The tension at the repair site impedes recovery by restrict blood supply. It is also used to reduce the length of the graft. The shorter the graft the better for functional recovery.

    (PNG, p. 196)
33. A 45-year-old male presents with weakness in his right hand and numbness in his ring and little fingers after a fall. As part of nerve conduction study, on stimulation of the median nerve at the elbow produces a larger compound muscle action potential (CMAP) at the abductor digiti minimi compared to wrist stimulation. This suggests:
    A. Double crush syndrome affecting both the median and ulnar nerves
    B. Martin–Gruber anastomosis
    C. C8-T1 radiculopathy
    D. Pronator teres syndrome with median-to-ulnar crossover

    Correct Answer: B

    Explanation:

    In Martin–Gruber anastomosis, median nerve fibers cross to the ulnar nerve in the forearm, innervating ulnar-supplied muscles (e.g., ADM). Elbow stimulation activates these fibers, increasing CMAP amplitude compared to wrist stimulation, where only the median nerve's usual path is tested.

    (MPN, p. 30)
34. The most appropriate treatment for a patient with a neuroma in continuity with persistent pain and no functional recovery after 6 months is:
    A. Observation and pain management
    B. Neurolysis
    C. Nerve grafting
    D. Nerve transfer

    Correct Answer: C

    Explanation:

    Neuroma in continuity is treated as blunt nerve injury. If there is no meaningful functional recovery after 3 months, surgical exploration is indicated. In this case, there was no functional recovery at all making nerve grafting is the most appropriate surgical approach.

    [79]

35. In a traumatic brachial plexus injury with complete avulsion of the C5 and C6 roots, the surgeon opts for a nerve transfer procedure. Which of the following nerves is typically transferred to restore elbow flexion in this scenario?
    A. Lateral pectoral nerve to musculocutaneous nerve
    B. Intercostal nerves to musculocutaneous nerve
    C. Spinal accessory nerve to axillary nerve
    D. Median nerve to radial nerve

    Correct Answer: B

    Explanation:

    In brachial plexus injuries involving C5 and C6 root avulsion, intercostal nerves or medial pectoral nerve are often transferred to the musculocutaneous nerve to restore elbow flexion, as they provide motor function and are expendable in this context.

    (MPN, p. 160)
36. All of the following is characteristics of an ideal nerve transfer donor**,** EXCEPT**:**
    A. Pure motor or sensory nerve
    B. Adjacent to the recipient nerve
    C. Donor fascicle muscle groups must have at least grade 4/5 MRC power
    D. Donor from muscle different muscle compartment than the recipient

    Correct Answer: D

    Explanation:

    An **ideal donor nerve for transfer** should have specific characteristics to maximize functional recovery. It should be **pure** (motor or sensory) to match the target function, **adjacent** to minimize dissection, and **expendable**, meaning its loss would not cause significant functional deficits. The donor must be **uninjured** with at least **grade 4/5 strength** to ensure effectiveness, and **remote** from the injury zone to allow easier dissection. Ideally, it should also be **proximate** to the target motor point to speed up reinnervation, have an **adequate size match** to prevent diameter mismatch, and be **educatable**, meaning it should ideally supply a muscle in the same functional group to ease motor relearning and reduce unwanted movements.

    (SSW, p. 2154)
37. All of the following are commonly used nerve transfer for brachial plexus injury, EXCEPT:
    A. Spinal accessory nerve to suprascapular nerve
    B. Medial pectoral nerve to axillary nerve
    C. Dorsal scapular nerve to median nerve
    D. Anterior interosseus nerve to ulnar nerve

    Correct Answer: C

    Explanation:

    Common donor nerves for median nerve transfer are sensory intercostals, contralateral C7, ulnar nerve fascicle and brachialis branch of musculocutaneous nerve.

    (SSW, p. 2153)

38. All of the following are possible donor nerves for transfer for radial nerve injury, EXCEPT:
    A. Motor intercostals
    B. Contralateral C7
    C. Dorsal scapular nerve
    D. Spinal accessory
    Correct Answer: D
    (SSW, p, 2153)
39. The most common cause of iatrogenic injury to the spinal accessory nerve is:
    A. Cervical lymph node biopsy at the anterior triangle
    B. Cervical lymph node biopsy at the posterior triangle
    C. Posterior shoulder surgery
    D. Anterior shoulder surgery
    Correct Answer: B
    Explanation:
    Spinal accessory nerve injury occurs in approximately **3%–8%** of cases following **diagnostic lymph node biopsy** in the **posterior triangle of the neck**. In addition to surgical causes, the nerve can also be damaged by minor trauma, such as whiplash or injuries sustained during wrestling. These injuries often involve stretching or traction, which can disrupt the nerve's microvascular supply, leading to ischemia and subsequent axonal degeneration.
    (SSW, p. 2222)
40. During surgical decompression of the common peroneal nerve at the fibular head, which of the following anatomical structures is most critical to preserve to avoid inadvertent injury during the procedure?
    A. Lateral sural cutaneous nerve
    B. Superficial peroneal nerve
    C. Tibial nerve
    D. Popliteal artery
    Correct Answer: A
    Explanation:
    The lateral sural cutaneous nerve branches from the common peroneal nerve and provides sensory innervation to the lateral calf. It is located superficially in the area of the fibular head and should be preserved during peroneal nerve decompression specially during the proximal decompression of the common peroneal nerve.
    [80]
41. Distal sural nerve can be injured during the following procedure:
    A. Open reduction and internal fixation of a tibial shaft fracture
    B. Fasciotomy for anterior compartment syndrome
    C. Medial malleolus fracture fixation
    D. Repair of the Achilles tendon
    Correct Answer: D

Explanation:

Distal sural nerve branches injury is uncommon and may occur following a lateral ankle sprain or as an iatrogenic complication during procedures involving the Achilles tendon or lateral ankle region.

[80]

42. A 34-year-old man sustains a high-energy trauma resulting in sciatic nerve injury with loss of motor function and partial sensory recovery. He undergoes surgical repair. Which factor is most likely to negatively impact his motor recovery?
    A. Delay in surgical intervention of 4 weeks
    B. The nerve injury occurring at the thigh level
    C. Immediate intraoperative neurolysis
    D. Preservation of the epineurium

    Correct Answer: B

    Explanation:

    Proximal nerve injuries (e.g., at the thigh) are associated with longer reinnervation times and poorer outcomes due to the greater distance that regenerating axons must travel. This increases the risk of permanent motor endplate atrophy before reinnervation occurs.

    [84]

43. Regarding treatment of painful neuroma following digital amputation:

    43a. What is the most common treatment?
    A. Corticosteroid injection
    B. Neuroma resection and burying the nerve end in bone
    C. Neuroma resection and capping with a silicone cap
    D. Nerve reconstruction with conduit

    43b. All of the following is acceptable surgical methods to treat neuroma post amputation where distal stump is not found, EXCEPT:
    A. Centro-central connector-assisted neurorrhaphy
    B. Nerve cap
    C. Relocation nerve grafting
    D. Allograft reconstruction

    Correct Answers: 43a:B, 43b: D

    Explanation:

    Neuroma post amputation can cause intractable pain. Often the nonsurgical treatment is unsatisfactory. Surgical treatment of neuromas after amputation depends on the availability of the distal nerve end. If the distal end is present, nerve reconstruction is preferred, with success influenced by the gap size after neuroma excision. When the distal end is absent, as in most amputations, reconstruction is not possible, and management focuses on burying the proximal nerve stump into nearby tissue—such as muscle, bone, or vein to protect the nerve and reduce symptoms. This can lead to good to excellent results in 82% of the patients.

    [81]

44. A 40-year-old patient undergoes nerve repair for a traumatic ulnar nerve injury at the elbow level. Despite early intervention, recovery is incomplete, with clawing of the hand. What is the most likely cause of this poor outcome?
   A. Extensive scarring around the nerve
   B. Injury location proximal to the cubital tunnel
   C. Incomplete motor reinnervation of intrinsic hand muscles
   D. Delayed tendon transfer

   Correct Answer: C

   Explanation:

   Repair of ulnar nerve often results in incomplete recovery with functional results that are inferior to outcome of radial nerve and median nerve repair. Incomplete motor recovery, particularly of the intrinsic hand muscles, is common in ulnar nerve injuries at the elbow level. Even with early intervention, the long reinnervation distance and the small size of intrinsic hand muscles lead to suboptimal functional recovery.

   [82]

45. One of the following is an advantage of nerve transfer over nerve grafting for brachial plexus injury:
   A. Nerve transfer is more physiologic and make re-learning when muscle power returns easier.
   B. Nerve transfer can provide more motor axons.
   C. Nerve transfer can decrease the time of reinnervation to the targeted muscles.
   D. All of the above

   Correct Answer: C

   Explanation:

   Nerve transfers and nerve grafts each have specific advantages. Nerve transfers are performed distally, near the target muscle's motor point, allowing faster reinnervation with a single, focused repair in healthy tissue, making them ideal for selective muscle recovery, particularly after nerve root avulsion. In contrast, nerve grafts are done proximally at the injury site, following natural anatomy, which aids functional relearning and provides more donor axons, supporting recovery of entire motor groups and sensory function. While nerve transfers are highly targeted, grafts offer broader reinnervation potential and can be performed with basic surgical tools.

   (SSW, p. 2152)

46. The most common nerve injured during volar plating of a distal radius fracture is:
   A. Median nerve
   B. Ulnar nerve
   C. Anterior interosseous nerve
   D. Posterior interosseous nerve

   Correct Answer: A

   Explanation:

   Median nerve injury is a well-documented complication of distal radius fractures and has been reported as the most common complication in some studies, affecting up to 30% of patients. The injury is typically caused by direct compression from fracture fragments and surrounding edema, while less frequently, it may result from laceration by bone fragments or thrombosis of the median artery.

(PNO, p. 145)

47. In a high median nerve injury near the elbow, which of the following muscles remains innervated and can be used as a donor muscle for tendon transfer?
    A. Flexor carpi radialis
    B. Pronator teres
    C. Flexor pollicis longus
    D. Flexor carpi ulnaris

    Correct Answer: D

    Explanation:

    All the mentioned muscles are innervated by the median nerve except the flexor carpi ulnaris which is innervated by the ulnar nerve and is often spared in median nerve injuries. It can be used as a donor muscle for tendon transfers to restore functions such as wrist flexion or thumb opposition in cases of median nerve palsy.

    [83]
48. Patient presented with sharp laceration at the supra-clavicular area. He has flail arm. During exploration of the wound by the general surgeon, the trunks of the brachial plexus were found sharply divided. The next best step in the management is:
    A. Close and plan nerve conduction study (NCS) within 3 weeks
    B. Plan primary or early repair within 72 h
    C. Tack to adjacent planes and plan secondary repair at 2–3 weeks
    D. Prognosis is poor and plan nerve transfer in the future

    Correct Answer: B

    Explanation:

    In open brachial plexus injuries with sharp nerve division, primary or early repair should be performed within 72 h to optimize alignment and functional recovery. This aligns with the need for immediate surgical intervention to prevent retraction and fibrosis.

    (SSW, p. 2149)
49. A 30-year-old female has a forearm injury from a motorcycle accident, resulting in a brachial plexus injury with a blunt, contused nerve and ragged epineurium. The injury is 1 week old.

    What is the recommended treatment for this patient?
    A. Immediate primary repair within 72 h
    B. Begin physical therapy immediately without surgical intervention
    C. Tack to adjacent planes and plan secondary repair at 2–3 weeks
    D. Perform exploration and NAP recordings to assess regeneration

    Correct Answer: C

Explanation:

For open injuries where the nerve is contused and the epineurium is ragged, the nerve should be tacked to adjacent planes and plan a secondary repair after 2–3 weeks. This allows time for inflammation to subside, improving surgical outcomes.

(SSW, p. 2149)

50. A patient with a closed brachial plexus injury has been monitored for 3 months with no signs of recovery. Upon exploration, the nerve was found contused and the nerve action potential (NAP) recordings show no response (-NAP). The lesion is determined to be postganglionic.
What is the next step in treatment?
    A. Perform neurolysis
    B. Perform nerve transfer
    C. Continue with physical therapy
    D. Resect the nerve and perform direct graft repair

Correct Answer: D

Explanation:

For -NAP in a postganglionic lesion, the nerve should be resected and direct graft repair, as there are no functional axons, and grafting can restore continuity for regeneration.

In case of preganglionic injury, nerve transfer is the treatment choice.

(SSW, p. 2149)

51. The main goal in treating adult brachial plexus injury is to:
    A. Restore shoulder flexion, elbow extension and hand function
    B. Restore shoulder abduction, external rotation, elbow flexion, and forearm supination
    C. Restore shoulder abduction, external rotation, elbow extension and forearm pronation
    D. Relieve neuropathic pain only

Correct Answer: B

Explanation:

The primary goals in treating severe adult brachial plexus injuries focus on restoring shoulder abduction, external rotation, elbow flexion, and forearm supination. These movements together enable the patient to perform essential daily activities like holding a food tray, lifting their hand to their mouth, and push open doors while carrying items with their unaffected arm.

(SSW, p. 2146)

52. A 28-year-old man undergoes repair of a radial nerve transection at the mid-humerus level following a laceration. At 12 months post-repair, he has incomplete recovery of wrist extension but good recovery of finger extension. What is the most likely explanation for this outcome?
    A. Poor surgical technique
    B. Proximal axonopathy
    C. Mismatch in fascicular alignment
    D. Delayed surgery beyond 3 months

Correct Answer: C

Explanation:

In peripheral nerve injury repairs, incomplete recovery of specific muscle functions (e.g., wrist extension) with better recovery of others (e.g., finger extension) often results from imperfect fascicular alignment during the repair. Fascicles innervating different muscles may not be perfectly aligned, affecting functional outcomes.

(MPN, p. 164)

53. Injuries to all of the following nerves can cause winging of the scapula, EXCEPT:
    A. Long thoracic nerve
    B. Spinal Accessory nerve injury.
    C. Dorsal Scapular nerve
    D. Suprascapular nerve

    Correct Answer: D

    (MPN, p. 3 and 136) (PNG, p. 172)

54. A 52-year-old male presents with acute pain and weakness in his right shoulder following a recent neck surgery. On examination, his right scapula is noticeably drooping downward and displaced laterally away from the spine. Active shoulder abduction is limited to approximately 50°, and the scapula exhibits winging during attempted shoulder elevation. The surgeon suspects serratus anterior paralysis as the cause.

    Which nerve is primarily involved?
    A. Spinal accessory nerve
    B. Long thoracic nerve
    C. Dorsal scapular nerve
    D. Axillary nerve

    Correct Answer: A

    Explanation:

    The case involved a spinal accessory nerve (SAN) injury, often from surgery at the posterior triangle's apex. It causes immediate pain and major functional loss, with the scapula winging downward and outward due to trapezius paralysis (SAN-innervated). Active shoulder abduction drops to around 50°, and scapular winging appears, frequently misdiagnosed as serratus anterior paralysis (long thoracic nerve). Here, the surgical history, scapular position, and reduced abduction point to SAN injury.

    (PNG, p. 172)

55. A 50-year-old diabetic patient presents with foot drop after a proximal tibial fracture. Electromyography (EMG) 3 months post-injury shows no motor unit recruitment in the tibialis anterior. Which of the following is the best prognostic indicator for functional recovery?
    A. Early use of ankle-foot orthosis
    B. Nerve conduction studies showing preserved sensory function
    C. Early nerve decompression
    D. Muscle reinnervation within 6 months

    Correct Answer: D

Explanation:

Motor reinnervation within 6 months is critical for good functional outcomes, as muscle atrophy becomes irreversible after prolonged denervation. Early detection of motor unit potentials on EMG or improved clinical motor function grading are positive prognostic signs.

(MPN, p. 92)

56. One of the following is salvage procedure for peripheral nerve injury:
    A. Tendon transfer
    B. Muscle transfer
    C. Joint arthrodesis
    D. All of the above

    Correct Answer: D

    (SSW, p. 2147)

57. Patient with supraclavicular plexus stretch injury with clinical picture of upper and middle trucks injury. During supraclavicular exploration, the upper and middle trunks were found scarred. Intraoperative nerve action protentional for the scarred trunks were positive but small in amplitude and relatively slow in conduction. The next appropriate surgical action is:
    A. Neurolysis of upper and middle trunks
    B. Resection of suspected neuroma and repair both trunks with sural nerve grafts
    C. Extend the exposure to infra-clavicular area and explore all brachial plexus divisions
    D. Close and plan for C5 and C6 nerve transfers

    Correct Answer: A

    Explanation:

    Neurolysis of upper and middle trunks is the most appropriate next step, as it addresses the scarred trunks with a positive NAP, aiming to enhance natural regeneration without resorting to more invasive procedures.

    (SSW, p. 2184)

58. The commonest nerve involved in injection injury is:
    A. Femoral nerve from femoral arterial line
    B. Sciatic nerve from gluteal intramuscular injections
    C. Common peroneal nerve from knee injections
    D. Posterior tibial nerve from ankle joint aspiration procedures

    Correct Answer: B

    Explanation:

    Since the gluteal region is the most frequent site for injections, the sciatic nerve is the nerve most commonly affected by injection-related injuries.

    (MPN, p. 22)

59. In a case of high-velocity gunshot wound causing sciatic nerve injury, the nerve is severely damaged with a large defect. What is the most likely outcome if a nerve graft is performed?
    A. Full recovery of motor and sensory function
    B. Full sensory recovery but limited motor recovery
    C. Complete loss of both motor and sensory function
    D. Partial recovery of sensory function but no motor recovery

    Correct Answer: D

    Explanation:

    There are collective evidence that the repair of sciatic nerve injuries tends to result in suboptimal motor and sensory recovery.

    [10]
60. Which peripheral nerve demonstrated the best recovery rate after surgical repair of gunshot wound injuries?
    A. Peroneal nerve
    B. Ulnar nerve
    C. Tibial nerve
    D. Brachial plexus

    Correct Answer: C

    Explanation:

    In a large series of peripheral nerve injury from gunshot wound, the author found that the tibial, median, and femoral nerves showed the best recovery rates, while the peroneal nerve, ulnar nerve, and brachial plexus had the worst.

    [84]
61. A 30-year-old male sustains a gunshot wound to the forearm, resulting in an ulnar nerve lesion. The injury is at the proximal forearm. How does the injury level impact the expected functional recovery?
    A. High-level injuries have better recovery
    B. Injury level has no impact
    C. High-level injuries have poorer recovery
    D. High-level injuries affect only sensation

    Correct Answer: C

    Explanation:

    Peripheral nerve injury can be classified according to the injury levels, high (proximal), intermediate, or low (distal) based on the proximal stump position, with the borderline between high and intermediate at the middle of the arm/forearm. Proximal injury requires longer axonal regeneration to reach hand muscles, increasing the risk of poor outcomes.

    [84]
62. Which nerve transfer is most commonly used to restore shoulder abduction in patients with upper brachial plexus injuries?
    A. Ulnar to axillary nerve transfer
    B. Thoracodorsal to axillary nerve transfer
    C. Radial to axillary nerve transfer
    D. Spinal accessory to suprascapular nerve transfer

    Correct Answer: D

    (SSW, p. 2148)

63. One of the following is CORRECT about end-to-side nerve repair:
    A. It is connecting the distal stump of a transected nerve to the side of an intact adjacent nerve.
    B. It is ideally done for sensory nerve injury.
    C. It has an advantage of recovery of injured nerve without compromising the function of donor nerve.
    D. All of the above

    Correct Answer: D
    (MPN, p. 76)
64. One of the following is FALSE about tubulization technique for nerve injury repair:
    A. It is a repair involves using a conduit to bridge the gap between the injured ends of a nerve.
    B. It is used when the gap between the injured nerve stumps is 3–5 cm.
    C. The conduit could be biological or synthetic.
    D. All of the above

    Correct Answer: B
    Explanation:
    The tubulization technique for nerve injury repair involves using a conduit (biological or synthetic) to bridge the gap between injured nerve ends, guiding axonal regeneration. It is used when the gap between the injured nerve stumps is 3–5 cm.
    (MPN, p. 77)
65. A 42-year-old male has right inguinal hernia repair. Postoperatively he developed sharp burning pain at the right lower abdominal wall and upper medial thigh.

    65a. Which nerve is likely injured?
    A. Ilioinguinal
    B. Iliohypogastric
    C. Genitofemoral
    D. A and B

    65b. The best method to establish the diagnosis is:
    A. The location of Tinel's sign
    B. Location of the sensory loss
    C. Successful nerve block
    D. All of the above

    65c. Patient underwent nerve decompression; however, he still experiences persistent pain. What is the most appropriate next step in management?
    A. Repeat neurolysis with additional mobilization of the nerve
    B. Neurectomy of the ilioinguinal nerve
    C. Dorsal root ganglionectomy at T11-L1
    D. Implantation of a peripheral nerve stimulator

    Answers: 65a: A, 65b: C, 65c: B

Explanation:

Ilioinguinal nerve sensation covers a region in the lower abdominal wall and medial upper thigh. However, injury to the Ilioinguinal and iliohypogastric nerves can both give similar pain. The best diagnostic tool is successful nerve block. Decompression or neurolysis is the first-line surgical approach for nerve entrapment. However, it has a high failure rate (50%). Neurectomy is the recommended next step for patients who fail decompression, especially when the nerve is embedded in extensive scarring. This has a higher success rate (60%) compared to decompression. Dorsal root ganglionectomy is reserved for patients who fail both decompression and neurectomy and who demonstrate significant pain relief from paravertebral nerve blocks.

Peripheral nerve stimulators are not a standard treatment for ilioinguinal neuralgia.

(SPN, p. 165)

66. In femoral nerve injury, which clinical findings indicates intra-pelvic injury site?
    A. Weakness in quadriceps with preserved hip flexion
    B. Isolated sensory loss over the anterior thigh
    C. Absent knee jerk reflex with normal hip adduction
    D. Hip flexion weakness

    Correct Answer: D

    Explanation:

    Hip flexion weakness which (iliopsoas muscle) indicates proximal (intra-pelvic) femoral nerve injury.

    (SPN, p. 182)

67. A patient presents with numbness on the ulnar side of the small finger after a laceration. What should the examiner do to confirm a digital nerve injury?
    A. Check for Tinel sign at the elbow.
    B. Test pinprick sensation at the distal middle phalanx.
    C. Assess two-point discrimination on the forearm.
    D. Evaluate wrist flexion strength.

    Correct Answer: B

    Explanation:

    The absence of pinprick sensation at the distal middle phalanx on the radial or ulnar aspect of the finger suggests a digital nerve injury, necessitating exploration. This is a key diagnostic step for acute injuries to the digital nerves.

    (SPN, p. 109)

68. During repair of a digital nerve laceration, the surgeon uses 9.0 nylon sutures. What type of repair is most appropriate for the proper digital nerves?
    A. Nerve grafting
    B. Neurolysis
    C. Fascicular repair
    D. Epineurial repair

    Correct Answer: D

Explanation:

Epineurial repair is required for small nerve injury like the digital nerves proper usually using 8–0 or 9–0 nylon, while fascicular repair is suggested for common digital nerves which is bigger.

(SPN, p. 109)

69. A 60-year-old patient undergoes digital nerve repair after a laceration. What factor is most likely to negatively impact the outcome?
    A. Simple long laceration
    B. Older age
    C. Surgical intervention by a resident trainee
    D. Male patient

    Correct Answer: B

    Explanation:

    Older age, complex lacerations, and chronicity negatively influence outcomes, with younger patients with simple lacerations having the best prognosis. About 50% achieve two-point discrimination <10 mm.

    (SPN, p. 109)

70. A surgeon is performing sural nerve harvesting for a nerve graft in a 35-year-old patient with a median nerve injury. The procedure begins with an incision posterior to the lateral malleolus. Which of the following steps is critical to ensure a successful harvest while minimizing complications?
    A. Dissecting deep to the sural nerve to avoid damaging the small saphenous vein
    B. Using a continuous suture technique to secure the nerve ends during harvest
    C. Applying a tourniquet at 150 mmHg to reduce bleeding throughout the procedure
    D. Identifying and transecting the medial sural cutaneous nerve proximally before the anastomosis with the lateral branch

    Correct Answer: D

    Explanation:

    The sural nerve harvesting technique begins with a small incision posterior to the lateral malleolus, where the sural nerve lies superficially alongside the small saphenous vein. A critical step is to trace the nerve proximally, identifying the anastomosis site and transecting the medial sural cutaneous nerve contribution before it joins the lateral branch to ensure the longest possible graft (up to 30–50 cm). This prevents incomplete harvest and preserves the nerve's integrity.

    (MPN, p. 78)

71. A 32-year-old patient presented with leg weakness after a gunshot wound. From the following X-ray (Fig. 17.2), which nerve is likely affected?
    A. Sciatic nerve
    B. Tibial nerve
    C. Common peroneal nerve
    D. Deep peroneal nerve

    Correct Answer: C

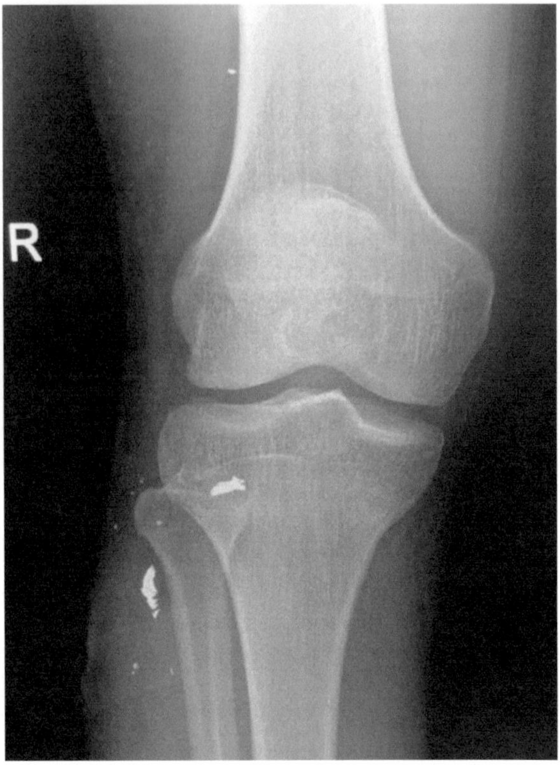

Fig. 17.2 A 32-year-old patient presented with leg weakness after a gunshot wound

Explanation:

The cases showed anterior view of the knee with multiple shrapnels. The biggest one is at the neck of the fibular where common peroneal nerve found (Fig. 17.3).

72. A 41-year-female who was assaulted and hit on the anterior right leg. Three months after the assault, she has severe pain at the distribution of the superficial peroneal nerve. The following picture shows the exposure of the nerve (Fig. 17.4).

The best next step in surgical management is:

A. Dissect the scar seen in the picture
B. Lengthen the fascia around the nerve
C. Decompress the nerve at the transverse crural ligament distally
D. All of the above

Correct Answer: D

Explanation:

The case shows a scar over the superficial peroneal nerve which likely responsible of the patient's symptoms. Dissecting this scar area and compressing the nerve is essential step, however the usual entrapment areas of the nerve need to be addressed to prevent secondary compression due to nerve swelling. The entrapment areas of the superficial nerve is superficial fascial layer that

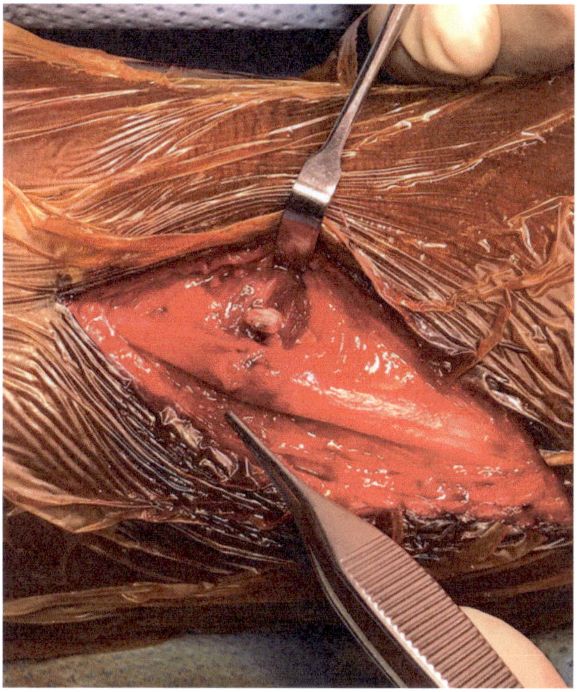

Fig. 17.3 Surgical photography showing the shrapnel and the injured common peroneal nerve

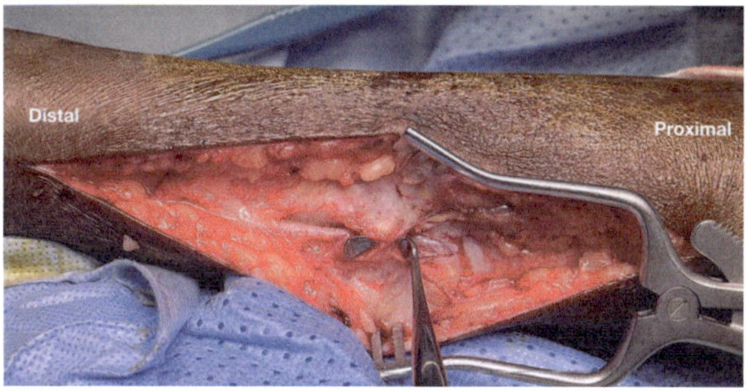

Fig. 17.4 A 41-year-female who was assaulted and hit on the anterior right leg. Three months after the assault she has severe pain at the distribution of the superficial peroneal nerve

encapsulates the nerve distally called the transverse crural ligament. Also, the facial layers around the nerve can serve as entrapments points and need to be lengthened as seen in the following post decompression picture (Fig. 17.5).

73. A 21-year-old male has blast injury to the posterior thigh with massive bleeding. Patient was stabilized with wound packing and suturing and blood transfusion. He reported severe neuropathic pain at the distribution of the sciatic nerve after he was stabilized. Upon exploration of the wound, the sciatic nerve (black arrow) was found strangulated in a stitch (Fig. 17.6) (white arrow).

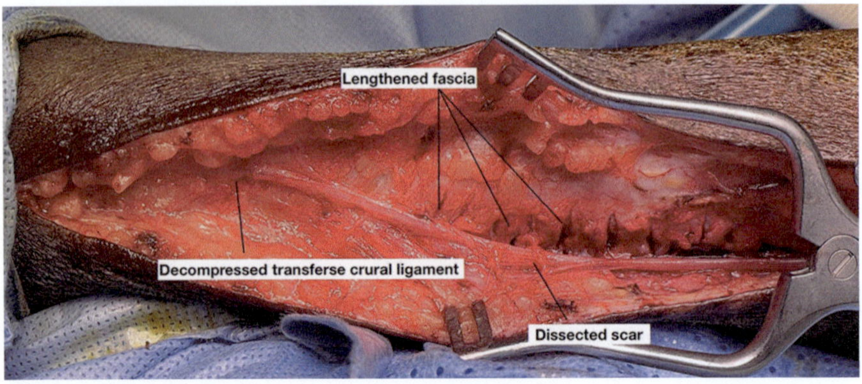

Fig. 17.5 Post decompression of the superficial peroneal nerve

Fig. 17.6 Case 73. Upon exploration of the wound, the sciatic nerve (black arrow) was found strangulated in a stitch

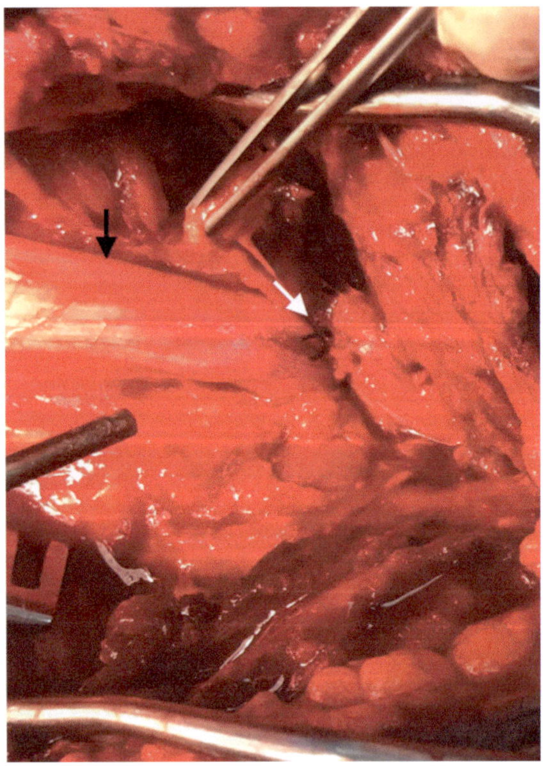

73a. After decompressing the nerve, which factor is most predictive of poor recovery?
A. Type of surgical technique used
B. Timing of surgery beyond 6 months
C. Patient age over 50 years
D. Proximal nerve injury

73b. Which of the following nerves is least commonly affected by iatrogenic injuries?
A. Median nerve
B. Peroneal nerve
C. Femoral nerve
D. Radial nerve

73c. Which iatrogenic peripheral nerve injury has the worst prognosis for functional recovery after surgical treatment?
A. Radial nerve injury
B. Musculocutaneous nerve injury
C. Axillary nerve injury
D. Sciatic nerve injury

Correct Answers: 73a: B, 73b: C, 73c: D

Explanation:

Patients with iatrogenic peripheral nerve injury who underwent surgery after 6 months had a lower rate of satisfactory recovery (67.6%) compared to those who underwent surgery within 6 months (85.4%). Among 122 cases analyzed, the femoral nerve was only injured in 2.5% of cases, making it one of the least commonly affected nerves in iatrogenic injuries. Among these cases, sciatic nerve has the worse outcome.

[85]

74. Which of the following clinical findings indicates median nerve injury above the elbow?
A. Inability to extend the wrist
B. Isolated weakness of thumb opposition with preserved wrist flexion
C. Sensory loss limited to the radial side of the palm
D. Weakness in pronation

Correct Answer: D

Explanation:

Pronator teres and the flexor carpi radialis are the first innervated muscle by the median. Their involvement suggests median nerve injury at or above the elbow.

(SPN, p. 88)

75. A 32-year-old male has an injury to the proximal arm with clinical feature suggests median nerve injury, one of the following is typical in this type of injury?
A. Involvement of ulnar nerve
B. Weakness of wrist extension with preserved finger flexion
C. Isolated weakness of flexor carpi ulnaris with intact finger flexion
D. Weakness of wrist extension due to radial nerve involvement

Correct Answer: A

Explanation:

In the upper arm, the ulnar nerve runs near the median nerve but lies medial to the brachial artery. Consequently, injuries to the brachial artery or surgical procedures involving it may lead to damage to both the median and ulnar nerves. (SPN, p. 86)

76. A 29-year-old has gunshot wound to the ventral forearm. He has radial nerve motor and sensory deficit. Because of persistence deficit, exploration was done after 6 months and the ulnar nerve was in a scar and repair was done with a conduit as in the following picture (Fig. 17.7).

76a: What is the primary mechanism by which a conduit facilitates axonal regeneration?

A. Direct electrical stimulation of regenerating axons
B. Encasing nerve ends to guide axonal sprouting
C. Replacement of Schwann cells with synthetic growth factors
D. Immediate restoration of endoneurial blood supply

76b. What complication is most likely if the conduit resorbs too slowly?

A. Excessive axonal sprouting leading to neuroma formation
B. Rapid clearance of neurotrophic factors from the repair site
C. Compression of the nerve from chronic immune rejection
D. Failure to initiate Schwann cell proliferation

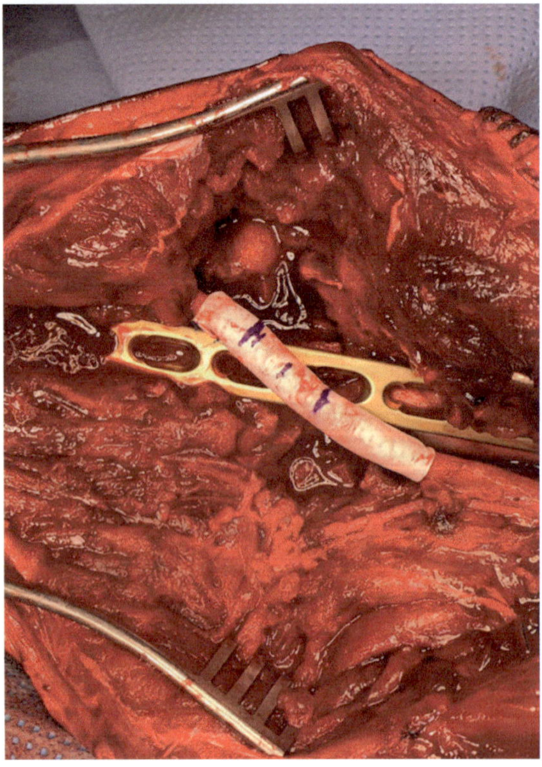

Fig. 17.7 A 29-year-old has gunshot wound to the ventral forearm

76c. After conduit repair and suturing to the inured nerve what is the next critical step to optimize the repair before applying fibrin glue?
  A. Flushing the lumen with saline to remove air bubbles
  B. Measuring the exact nerve diameter to adjust tube size
  C. Applying a tourniquet to reduce bleeding
  D. Suturing the distal stump without tension assessment

76d. What is the most significant limitation of using a conduit for this repair?
  A. Insufficient neurotrophic factors
  B. Length of the nerve defect
  C. Donor-site morbidity
  D. Difficult microsuturing

Correct Answers: 76a: B, 76b: C, 76c: A, 76d: B

Explanation:

Nerve conduit's primary mechanism is **encasing nerve ends to guide axonal sprouting**, protecting and directing regeneration. If resorption is too slow, **compression of the nerve from chronic immune rejection** is the likely complication due to pressure and immune response. The next critical step after suturing the conduit is **flushing the lumen with saline to remove air bubbles**, preventing air entrapment. The main limitation of nerve conduit is the **length of the nerve defect**, as conduits are limited to gaps <3 cm.

(MPN, pp. 79–81)

77. A 25-year-old motorcyclist sustains a high-speed crash, presenting with complete right arm paralysis, drooping eyelid, and a constricted pupil on the right. Exam shows no shoulder shrug on that side.

77a. What is the pattern of his injury?
  A. Postganglionic brachial plexus injury
  B. Preganglionic brachial plexus injury
  C. Spinal cord injury
  D. Mixed injury

77b. EMG is performed 3 weeks post-injury. What the typical findings in this type of injury?
  A. Fibrillations in deltoid with absent sensory nerve action potentials (SNAPs)
  B. Reduced CMAPs in biceps with normal SNAPs
  C. Denervation in trapezius with absent SNAPs
  D. Loss of paraspinal muscle activities

77c. What other diagnostic test help in the diagnosis?
  A. Nerve conduction study
  B. MRI of brachial plexus
  C. CT myelography
  D. Repeat EMG after 6 weeks

Correct Answers: 77a: B, 77b: D, 77c: C

Explanation:

The case is typical preganglionic injury (root avulsion) involves C8–T1 roots proximal to the dorsal root ganglion, causing total arm paralysis, Horner syndrome (ptosis, miosis from T1 sympathetic disruption), and trapezius weakness (spinal accessory nerve involvement). Typical EMG finding is loss of paraspinal muscle activities. Because dorsal root ganglion is intact, sensory nerve action potential (SNAP) will be normal. CT myelography or MRI cervical spine show pseudomeningoceles (dural tears at avulsed roots), a hallmark of preganglionic injury.

(SSW, p. 2129)

78. A 25-year-old cyclist sustains a forearm injury in a crash. On the day of injury, percussion over the radial nerve at the mid-forearm elicits a surge of pins and needles radiating to the dorsum of his hand. Two months later, the Tinel's sign has advanced distally by 5 cm. What does this suggest about the nerve injury?
    A. Neurotmesis with no recovery potential
    B. Conduction block without axonal damage
    C. Entrapment neuropathy with focal demyelination
    D. Axonotmesis with likely spontaneous recovery

    Correct Answer: D

    Explanation:

    A strong Tinel's sign on the day of injury indicates axonal rupture, not just conduction block. Distal advancement of the sign by 2 months suggests regenerating axons, favoring axonotmesis over neurotmesis or static entrapment. Conduction block would not produce a Tinel's sign.

    (PNG, pp. 157–163)

79. A clinician percusses from proximal to distal over the ulnar nerve in a patient with elbow trauma and no initial Tinel's sign. The patient later reports tingling in the pinky when percussion reaches the wrist. What does this suggest about the percussion technique (Tinel's sign)?
    A. Correct method confirming a distal lesion
    B. Incorrect direction of percussion; should be distal to proximal
    C. Accurate approach for deep-seated nerves
    D. Invalid due to patient misreporting

    Correct Answer: B

    Explanation:

    Tinel's sign should be elicited by percussing from distal to proximal starting below the lesion. Proximal-to-distal percussion is incorrect.

    (PNG, pp. 157–163)

80. A 32-year-old male who sustained median nerve injury at the forearm. He presented to the clinic 3 month after nerve graft surgery. He was found to have strong Tinel's sign elicited distal to the suture line of the graft surgery. What is the best interpretation of this finding?
    A. Suggest strong likelihood of successful repair
    B. Sign of neuroma formation at the suture site

C. Indicative of chronic nerve degeneration
D. Suggestive of muscle fibrosis and motor end-plate failure

Correct Answer: A

Explanation:

Distal movement (indicated in this case by suture line) of Tinel's sign on follow up after nerve repair indicates strong likelihood of successful repair. In contrary, a suture line that elicits a stronger Tinel's sign than the area distal to it suggests a high likelihood of repair failure.

(PNG, pp. 157–163)

81. A patient presents with weakness in plantarflexion, inversion of the foot, and toe flexion after a deep laceration to the posterior leg. Which of the following muscles is most likely affected?

A. Extensor digitorum longus
B. Tibialis anterior
C. Flexor digitorum longus
D. Peroneus longus

Correct Answer: C

Explanation:

Flexor digitorum longus is innervated by tibial nerve and responsible for plantar flexion and foot eversion.

(EPN, p. 143)

Peripheral Nerves - Upper Limb 18

1. A 25-year-old male presents with wrist drop and numbness on the dorsum of his right hand after sleeping with his arm over a chair following heavy drinking. Examination reveals weakness in wrist and finger extension (MRC 2/5), preserved elbow extension, and normal median/ulnar sensation. A nerve conduction study shows prolonged latency with normal amplitude, indicating a conduction block.

1a. What is this condition called?
   A. Saturday night palsy
   B. Sunday noon syndrome
   C. Post-drinking palsy
   D. All are used terms.

1b. What is the underlying pathophysiological mechanism of this nerve injury?
   A. Demyelination
   B. Ischemic neuropathy
   C. Axonal degeneration
   D. Neurotmesis

1c. The nerve conduction study finding of prolonged latency with normal amplitude suggests which type of injury?
   A. Axonotmesis
   B. Neuropraxia
   C. Neurotmesis
   D. Wallerian degeneration

Correct Answers: 1a: A, 1b: B, 1c: B

Explanation:

"Saturday night palsy" describes radial nerve compression, often from prolonged pressure on the arm, leading to wrist drop and dorsal hand numbness. The mechanism is ischemia of the nerve leading to demyelination and neuropraxia with evidence of prolonged latency with normal amplitude in a nerve conduction study. Treatment is conservative with observation with wrist splinting.

(MPN, p. 86)

K. F. AlAli, H. T. Hashim, *Spine Surgery and Peripheral Nerve Surgery*,
https://doi.org/10.1007/978-3-031-98543-0_18

2. A 45-year-old female undergoes a cervical lymph node biopsy in the posterior triangle of her left neck for suspected lymphoma. Post-operatively, she reports numbness and tingling over the side of her neck, extending toward her ear and shoulder. On examination, she has sensory loss over the skin posterior to her left ear, along the anterior neck, and over the upper shoulder, with no motor deficits. The surgeon suspects iatrogenic injury to the nerves emerging from Erb's point during the procedure.
   2a. Which nerves emerging from Erb's point are most likely affected, given the patient's sensory loss after the cervical lymph node biopsy?
   A. Lesser occipital, great auricular, and transverse cervical nerves
   B. Phrenic, dorsal scapular, greater occipital nerve
   C. Suprascapular, supraclavicular, and scapular nerves
   D. Accessory and suprascapular nerves
   2b. Which of the following nerves does NOT emerge from Erb's point in this patient's injury region?
   A. Lesser occipital nerve
   B. Great auricular nerve
   C. Supraclavicular nerve
   D. Phrenic nerve
   Correct Answers: 2a: A, 2b: D
   Explanation:
   Erb's point is located 2–3 cm above the clavicle at the sternocleidomastoid's posterior border in the neck's posterior triangle. It is where the cervical plexus (C2–C4) sensory nerves—lesser occipital, great auricular, transverse cervical, and supraclavicular—emerge, but not the phrenic nerve (C3–C5). These nerves are prone to iatrogenic injury during neck procedures, causing sensory deficits.
   (EPN, p. 86 and pp. 112–113)
3. The phenomenon of "double crush syndrome" in peripheral neuropathies refers to:
   A. Two simultaneous fractures compressing a nerve
   B. A proximal compression makes distal nerves more susceptible to injury
   C. Compression of two different nerves causing similar symptoms
   D. Nerve compressed between two bony structures
   Correct Answer: B
   Explanation:
   Double crush syndrome describes a scenario where a proximal nerve compression (e.g., cervical radiculopathy at C6) impairs axonal transport, making the distal nerve (e.g., median nerve at the carpal tunnel) more vulnerable to injury, as seen in this patient's combined neck and wrist symptoms.
   (MPN, p. 131)
4. The most common nerve involved in upper limb peripheral neuropathy secondary to systemic amyloidosis is:
   A. Median nerve
   B. Ulnar nerve

C. Radial nerve
D. Musculocutaneous nerve
Correct Answer: A
Explanation:
Median neuropathy is the most common peripheral nerve manifestation of systemic amyloidosis. It occurs due to amyloid **deposition** within the **flexor retinaculum**, leading to nerve compression.
(NB, p. 822)

5. A 32-year-old male presents with wrist drop, finger extension weakness (MRC 1/5), and numbness on the posterior forearm and lower lateral arm after a fall on his right side. Examination shows intact triceps strength (MRC 5/5), normal deltoid and latissimus dorsi function, and weak supination. A radial nerve palsy was expected.
5a. Where is the most likely site of this patient's radial nerve compression?
A. Axilla
B. Distal humerus
C. Spiral groove
D. Posterior cord
5b. Which finding rules out a posterior cord injury in this patient?
A. Normal posterior forearm sensation
B. Weak brachioradialis muscle
C. Numbness on both volar and dorsal third digits
D. Preserved deltoid and latissimus dorsi strength
Correct Answers: 5a: C, 5b: D
Explanation: The patient's presentation, wrist drop, finger extension weakness, numbness over the posterior forearm and lateral arm, preserved triceps, deltoid, and latissimus dorsi function strongly localizes the lesion to the radial nerve at the spiral groove. This site is distal to the nerve's branches to the triceps (hence triceps strength is preserved) but proximal to branches innervating wrist/finger extensors and sensory fibers to the posterior arm. The preserved function of the deltoid (axillary nerve) and latissimus dorsi (thoracodorsal nerve) rules out a more proximal lesion at the posterior cord, confirming that the injury is localized to the spiral groove of the humerus.
(MPN, p. 40)

6. Which sensory deficit supports a spiral groove radial nerve injury?
A. Numbness on the volar third digit
B. Sensory loss in the posterior forearm
C. Loss of sensation in the deltoid
D. Tingling on the anterior forearm
Correct Answer: B
Explanation:
Spiral groove injuries affect the posterior and lower lateral cutaneous nerves, causing sensory loss in the posterior forearm and lower lateral arm, matching the patient's symptoms.
(MPN, p. 40)

7. What is the most indicative of radial nerve palsy distal to the elbow (forearm)?
   A. Normal extensor carpi radialis longus muscle
   B. Normal extensor carpi radialis brevis muscle
   C. Normal brachioradialis muscle
   D. Normal supinator muscle
   Correct Answer: C
   Explanation:
   Normal strength of the brachioradialis muscle is indicative that radial nerve palsy or injury is beyond the elbow.
   (MPN, p. 41)
8. A 25-year-old man is involved in a high-velocity motorcycle accident and presents with weakness in shoulder abduction, elbow flexion, and loss of sensation over the lateral aspect of the arm and forearm. He also has Horner's syndrome. Cervical MRI is shown (Fig. 18.1). What is the best description of the MRI findings?
   A. Traumatic dural injury with hemorrhage
   B. Ruptured cervical arachnoid cyst
   C. Traumatic spinal epidural hematoma
   D. Cervical nerve root avulsion with pseudomeningocele
   Correct Answer: D
   Explanation:
   The MRI shows extradural CSF signal intensity collection with blood signals indicating CSF leakage following avulsion of multiple nerve roots, shifting the spinal cord to the right. This is typical of findings in pseudomeningocele post-cervical nerve root avulsion.
   (DI, p. 1020)

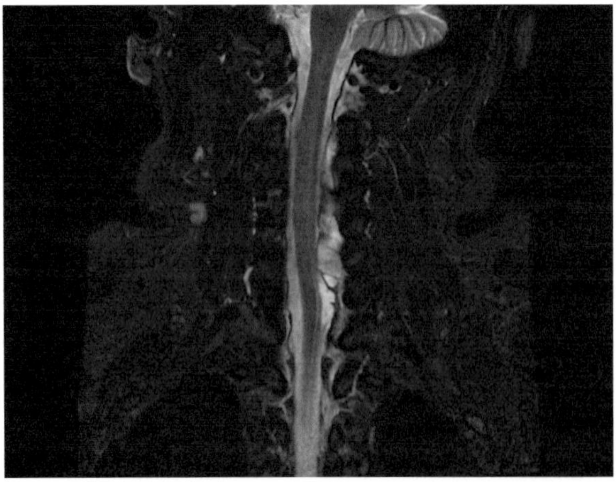

Fig. 18.1 Case 9 cervical MRI

9. The preferred surgical treatment for cubital tunnel syndrome refractory to conservative management is:
   A. Ulnar nerve simple decompression
   B. Medial epicondylectomy
   C. Flexor carpi ulnaris tendon release
   D. Ulnar nerve simple transposition

   Correct Answer: A

   Explanation:

   Simple decompression is as effective as anterior subcutaneous transposition for cubital tunnel syndrome. It is the preferred surgical method, as it is a less invasive procedure.

   [86]
10. The most common tumor of the peripheral nerve?
    A. Neurofibroma
    B. Malignant peripheral nerve sheath tumor
    C. Lipoma
    D. Schwannoma

    Correct Answer: D

    Explanation:

    Schwannomas are the most common peripheral nerve tumors in patients without Neurofibromatosis Type 1 (NF1).

    (MPN, p. 184)
11. Sublimis arch syndrome is different from pronator teres syndrome in:
    A. The pronator teres muscle is not affected in sublimis arch syndrome.
    B. The median nerve is compressed where it passes between the two heads of the pronator teres in sublimis arch syndrome.
    C. The median nerve is compressed between the two heads of the flexor digitorum superficialis in pronator teres syndrome.
    D. Flexion of the median proximal interphalangeal joints precipitates symptoms in sublimis arch syndrome.

    Correct Answer: D

    Explanation:

    Pronator teres syndrome occurs when the median nerve is compressed between the two heads of the pronator teres, but the muscle itself remains unaffected since its nerve supply originates proximal to the compression site. Sensory deficits are often absent, while motor weakness, particularly in flexion of the second and third digits, may be masked by pain. Additionally, the sublimis arch, a fibrotic band between the two heads of the flexor digitorum superficialis, can also compress the median nerve, mimicking pronator teres syndrome. However, symptoms may worsen with forceful flexion of the proximal interphalangeal joints of digits 2–5, distinguishing it from pronator teres syndrome.

    (MPN, p. 31)

12. The most common site of compression for the anterior interosseous nerve is:
    A. Between the two heads of the pronator teres
    B. At the ligament of Struthers
    C. Under the fibrous arch of the flexor digitorum superficialis
    D. At the arcade of Frohse

    Correct Answer: A

    Explanation:

    The primary site of compression is often the tendinous origin of the deep head of the pronator teres. The median nerve then travels beneath the arch of the flexor digitorum superficialis, which can serve as another potential compression site.

    (SPN, p. 92)
13. An 18-year-old female presents with a 5-year history of progressive weakness and atrophy in her right hand, worse with overhead arm use, and dropping objects. Examination reveals atrophy of the thenar eminence and diminished ulnar sensation. What is the most likely diagnosis?
    A. Carpal tunnel syndrome
    B. True neurogenic thoracic outlet syndrome
    C. Ulnar neuropathy
    D. Cervical radiculopathy

    Correct Answer: B

    Explanation:

    The patient's progressive hand atrophy (Gilliatt–Sumner hand), ulnar sensory loss, and provocation with overhead use, without trauma or other limb involvement, align with true neurogenic thoracic outlet syndrome.

    (SPN, p. 51)
14. Regarding neurogenic thoracic outlet syndrome:

    14a. What is the most common cause?
    A. Pancoast tumor
    B. Scalene muscle hypertrophy
    C. Subclavian artery aneurysm
    D. Cervical rib

    14b. In which anatomical passageway does the majority of neurogenic thoracic outlet syndrome compression occur?
    A. Costoclavicular triangle
    B. Subcoracoid space
    C. Interscalene triangle
    D. Supraclavicular fossa

    14c. A 40-year-old male with chronic neck and arm pain after trauma exhibits guarding, give-way weakness, and positive 90-degree abduction/external rotation (AER) test. What distinguishes his presentation from true neurogenic TOS?
    A. Presence of muscle atrophy
    B. Chronic pain syndrome with unreliable neurological findings
    C. Ulnar sensory loss with thenar atrophy
    D. Normal reflexes and pulse changes

14d. What condition should be excluded to confirm true neurogenic TOS in the 18-year-old female patient?

A. Spinal cord neoplasm
B. Brachial plexus tumor
C. Carpal tunnel syndrome
D. All of the above

14e. During surgical decompression for the 18-year-old patient with a cervical rib, which approach allows visualization of the C8–T1 spinal nerves?

A. Transaxillary approach
B. Posterior subscapular approach
C. Anterior supraclavicular approach
D. Subcoracoid approach

Correct Answers: 14a: D, 14b: C, 14c: B, 14d: D, 14e: C

Explanation:

Thoracic outlet syndrome (TOS) is a controversial condition involving compression of the neurovascular bundle in the thoracic inlet, primarily within the interscalene triangle, costoclavicular triangle, or subcoracoid space. The interscalene triangle is the most common site. It manifests in two main neurogenic forms: true neurogenic TOS, a rare, painless condition often seen in young, thin females with atrophy (e.g., Gilliatt–Sumner hand) and sensory loss due to anatomical anomalies like cervical ribs, and disputed neurogenic TOS, a more common, pain-dominant syndrome linked to trauma, featuring diffuse discomfort but minimal objective findings. Vascular TOS, involving arterial or venous compression, is less frequent, though sympathetic symptoms may overlap.

TOS is often a diagnosis of exclusion. The combination of thenar muscle atrophy (median nerve involvement) and ulnar sensory loss is a distinguishing feature of true TOS. The ninety-degree abduction and external rotation (AER) test is used to provoke symptoms and cannot be used alone in the diagnosis of TOS. EMG/NCS shows low-amplitude responses. Imaging (cervical x-ray and MRI/A) is done to detect anomalies or rule out mimics (like carpal tunnel, brachial plexus pathologies, and spinal cord tumors). Management starts conservatively with activity modification and physical therapy, progressing to surgical decompression (e.g., supraclavicular approach) if needed. The outcomes of surgical treatment are variable between a 40% and 90% success rate.

(SPN, pp. 50–54)

15. Regarding Parsonage–Turner Syndrome (PTS)

15a. What is the most common initial symptom?

A. Gradual onset of weakness
B. Abrupt onset of severe pain
C. Muscle atrophy
D. Bilateral arm numbness

15b. Which demographic group is mostly affected by Parsonage–Turner Syndrome?
A. Females
B. Males
C. Children
D. Elderly adults

15c. A patient with PTS has weakness that persists after 3 years. What is the most likely explanation based on typical prognosis?
A. Full recovery is expected in 89% of cases, so this is unusual.
B. Weakness always resolves within weeks, so this is not PTS.
C. Pain, not weakness, resolves in 3 years, making this typical.
D. Upper trunk lesions never recover, explaining the persistence.

15d. Which proceeding condition is LEAST likely to be associated with Parsonage–Turner Syndrome?
A. Recent hepatitis B vaccination
B. Postoperative recovery from spine surgery
C. Chronic lower back pain
D. Systemic lupus erythematosus

15e. What finding on electrodiagnostic studies is characteristic of Parsonage–Turner Syndrome?
A. Demyelination of sensory nerves
B. Normal EMG and NCS results
C. Conduction block in motor nerves
D. Multifocal with axonal loss

15f. A pediatric patient with PTS is less likely to experience which symptom compared to adults?
A. Pain
B. Weakness
C. Atrophy
D. Phrenic nerve involvement

Correct Answers: 15a: B, 15b: B, 15c: A, 15d: C, 15e: D, 15f: A

Explanation:

Parsonage–Turner Syndrome (brachial plexitis) is a sporadic and immune-mediated brachial plexus neuropathy. It commonly affects males and typically monophasic and unilateral. It usually starts with abrupt, severe pain, often nocturnal, followed by weakness and later atrophy, with a patchy distribution favoring motor nerves (e.g., long thoracic, phrenic). It is usually preceded by viral infections, vaccines, or surgery. EMG shows axonal loss. Pain resolves in weeks, while recovery (89% in 3 years) varies by lesion site. Treatment is conservative with corticosteroids offering pain relief but uncertain benefits for strength.

(NB, p. 796)

16. A 30-year-old man presents after sustaining a gunshot wound to the right shoulder, resulting in a brachial plexus injury. A CT angiogram is shown (Fig. 18.2). What is the positive finding in the angiogram that can affect the management?

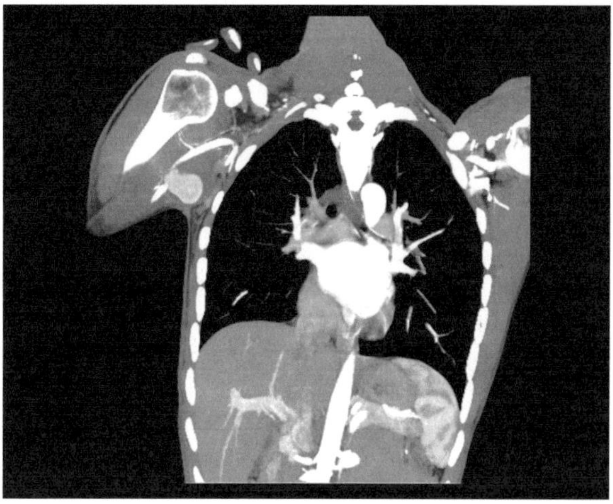

Fig. 18.2 Case 17 CT angiogram

A. Head of humerus necrosis
B. Axillary artery pseudoaneurysms
C. Clavicle fracture
D. All of the above
Correct Answer: B

17. Injury to all of the following nerves can cause winged scapula, EXCEPT?
A. Long thoracic nerve
B. Spinal accessory nerves
C. Dorsal scapular nerve
D. Thoracodorsal nerve
Correct Answer: D
Explanation:
The most common cause of a winged scapula is dysfunction of the serratus anterior muscle, which is supplied by the long thoracic nerve. In rare cases, lateral scapular winging can occur due to injury to the trapezius or rhomboid muscles, innervated by the spinal accessory nerve and dorsal scapular nerve, respectively.
(EPN, p. 89)

18. A 45-year-old typist presents with hand pain and tingling for 6 months. Physical exam shows positive Tinel's sign, but wrist MRI reveals mild synovial thickening unrelated to symptoms. Nerve conduction study (NCS) shows normal median sensory nerve conduction velocity (50 m/s) and motor distal latency (3.8 ms). The provisional diagnosis is carpal tunnel syndrome (CTS); what should the clinician do next?
A. Order a cervical MRI to exclude radiculopathy.
B. Conclude CTS is unlikely due to normal NCS.
C. Perform a comparison of median and ulnar sensory latencies.
D. Recommend immediate carpal tunnel release surgery.
Correct Answer: C

Explanation:

Normal NCS velocities do not rule out CTS, specifically when the patient has a typical clinical picture. Comparing median and ulnar nerve sensory latencies enhances the test sensitivity from 75% to 95%. A latency difference of 0.4 to 0.5 milliseconds is considered abnormal and strongly indicative of carpal tunnel syndrome.

[87]

19. A 35-year-old carpenter with hand pain after repetitive work has a positive Phalen's test. NCS shows median motor distal latency of 4.5 ms (normal <4.2 ms), but sensory velocity is 48 m/s (normal >45 m/s). His physician notes untreated CTS can lead to atrophy. What NCS finding most urgently warrants intervention?
    A. Borderline sensory velocity reduction
    B. Prolonged median motor distal latency
    C. Positive Phalen's test alone
    D. Absence of atrophy on exam

    Correct Answer: B

    Explanation:

    Untreated CTS can progress to weakness and atrophy. Motor latency of 4.5 ms indicates moderate CTS affecting motor fibers, a more advanced stage than sensory-only changes. Sensory velocity is borderline, and Phalen's is nonspecific without NCS. Lack of atrophy does not negate urgency.

    [87]

20. A 50-year-old diabetic patient complains of bilateral hand tingling. NCS shows median sensory latency of 4.0 ms (normal <3.6 ms) and ulnar latency of 3.9 ms (normal <3.4 ms). Median motor latency is 4.3 ms (normal <4.2 ms). What complicates the CTS diagnosis here?
    A. Bilateral symptoms rule out CTS
    B. Motor latency is too mild for CTS
    C. Diabetes invalidates NCS results
    D. Ulnar latency prolongation suggests polyneuropathy

    Correct Answer: D

    Explanation:

    CTS affects only the median nerve, but ulnar latency prolongation (3.9 ms) alongside median changes hints at a generalized process like diabetic polyneuropathy.

    [87]

21. All of the following are predisposing conditions for carpal tunnel syndrome (CTS), EXCEPT:
    A. Renal failure
    B. Pregnancy
    C. Marfan syndrome
    D. Hypothyroidism

    Correct Answer: C

    All are predisposing factors for CTS except Marfan syndrome. Other factors are diabetic neuropathy, polyneuropathies, pregnancy, acromegaly, and amyloidosis.

    (NB, p. 779)

22. Which statement about ulnar nerve compression in Guyon's tunnel is correct?
    A. Zone 1 compression impacts only sensory fibers.
    B. Zone 2 affects sensation alone.
    C. Zone 3 causes motor weakness in hand muscles.
    D. Zone 1 impairs both motor and sensory function.

    Correct Answer: D

    Explanation:

    Ulnar nerve compression at the wrist is uncommon. It occurs in three zones within Guyon's tunnel (Fig. 18.3):

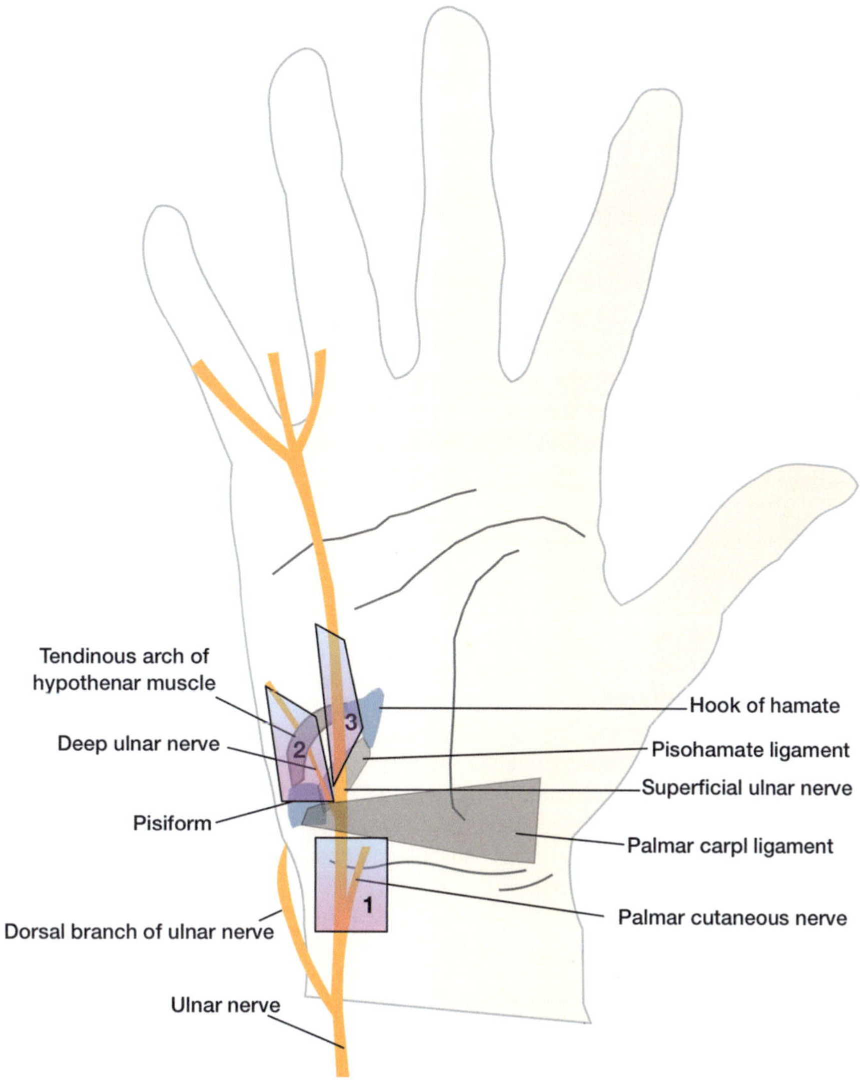

Fig. 18.3 Guyon's canal compression zones

- Zone 1: Affects the nerve before it splits, impacting both motor and sensory functions.
- Zone 2: Involves only the deep motor branch, leading to muscle weakness.
- Zone 3: Affects the superficial sensory branch, causing sensory loss only. (EPN, p. 57)

23. A 42-year-old avid cyclist presents with weakness in his right hand after months of long rides. He reports difficulty gripping his handlebars and numbness in his ring and pinky fingers, but his thumb strength is intact. On exam, he has weakness in finger abduction and adduction, with no clawing of the digits. Sensory loss is confined to the ulnar side of the palm and the ring and pinky fingers, sparing the dorsal hand. Electrodiagnostic studies confirm ulnar nerve dysfunction. Given the anatomy of Guyon's canal, which zone is most likely compressed?
    A. Zone 1
    B. Zone 2
    C. Zone 3
    D. All zones

    Correct Answer: B

    Explanation:

    Finger abduction/adduction means the interossei are weak, and grip trouble suggests motor involvement. The deep motor branch (Zone 2) supplies these. Ring and pinky plus ulnar palm numbness suggest ulnar sensory branch, but the dorsal hand being spared rules out a proximal lesion (like at the elbow). The dorsal cutaneous branch splits off before Guyon's canal. In cyclists, Zone 2 compression often occurs near the hook of the hamate and can indirectly affect sensation if pressure spreads slightly or if there's overlap with Zone 3.

    (EPN, p. 57)
24. One of the following is a differential diagnosis of musculocutaneous nerve palsy:
    A. Biceps tendon rupture
    B. C7 radiculopathy
    C. Herpes zoster
    D. All of the above

    Correct Answer: A

    Explanation:

    Isolated musculocutaneous nerve palsy is uncommon and needs to be differentiated from biceps tendon rupture and C6 radiculopathy. In the biceps tendon, the ruptured tendon can be felt, and the muscle usually retracts proximally. C6 radiculopathy can affect non-musculocutaneous nerve muscles like brachioradialis and latissimus dorsi. It also has different sensory patterns that affect the thumb and index finger, while the sensory pattern of the lateral antebrachial cutaneous nerve extends to the wrist.

    (MPN, p. 25)

25. The most common site of entrapment of the ulnar nerve at the elbow is:
    A. Arcade of Struthers
    B. Cubital tunnel
    C. Between the heads of the flexor carpi ulnaris
    D. Guyon's canal E
    Correct Answer: B
26. The most common cause of median nerve injury at the wrist is:
    A. Laceration
    B. Carpal tunnel syndrome
    C. Pronator syndrome
    D. Anterior interosseous syndrome
    Correct Answer: B
    (MPN, p. 20)
27. A 38-year-old electrician presents with paresthesias in the right fifth and medial fourth digits, reduced grip strength, and clawing of digits IV-V after prolonged elbow flexion during work. Nerve conduction studies reveal a motor conduction velocity of 45 m/s from above elbow to below elbow compared to 58 m/s from below elbow to wrist (W), with a 25% reduction in compound muscle action potential (CMAP) amplitude across the elbow when recording at abductor digiti minimi, but no amplitude change at first dorsal interosseous. Dorsal ulnar cutaneous sensory response is normal. What is the most likely site and pathology?
    A. Cubital tunnel compression with focal demyelination
    B. Wrist level with involvement of the main ulnar nerve trunk
    C. Wrist level entrapment sparing dorsal sensory
    D. Cubital tunnel with Martin–Gruber anomaly
    Correct Answer: A
    Explanation:
    The patient's ulnar neuropathy: paresthesias in digits V and medial IV, weak grip, and clawing from lumbrical weakness worsens with elbow flexion. NCS shows elbow localization: 45 m/s above elbow-to-below elbow vs. 58 m/s BE-to-W (focal slowing, >10 m/s) Normal dorsal ulnar sensory fits elbow, not wrist, with sparing possible. All leads to ulnar nerve compression at the elbow (cubital tunnel syndrome).
    (NB, p. 781)
28. A patient with suspected ulnar nerve palsy is asked to hold a piece of paper between their thumb and index finger. The examiner tries to pull the paper away, and the patient compensates by flexing the thumb at the interphalangeal joint.
    28a. This indicates weakness of which muscle?
    A. Flexor pollicis longus
    B. Adductor pollicis
    C. Abductor pollicis longus
    D. Opponens pollicis

28b. What muscle is compensating for the weakness in this patient?
A. Flexor pollicis longus
B. Adductor pollicis
C. Abductor pollicis brevis
D. Extensor pollicis longus

28c. What is the name of this sign?
A. Jeanne's sign
B. Wartenberg's sign
C. Froment's sign
D. Phalen's sign

Answers: 28a: A, 28b: A, 28c: C

Explanation:

In ulnar nerve injury, the adductor pollicis muscle is weakened or paralyzed, making it difficult for the patient to maintain a pinch grip. To compensate, the flexor pollicis longus, which is innervated by the median nerve, takes over, causing excessive thumb flexion at the interphalangeal joint when attempting to pinch an object. This compensatory mechanism is known as Froment's sign and is a key clinical test for ulnar nerve dysfunction.

(NB, p. 781)

29. The most performed surgical treatment for a patient with a confirmed diagnosis of neurogenic thoracic outlet syndrome and failure of conservative therapy is:
A. First rib resection
B. Scalenectomy
C. Subclavian artery revascularization
D. Cervical rib resection

Correct Answer: D

(SPN, p. 53)

30. A 35-year-old with neurogenic thoracic outlet syndrome undergoes supraclavicular decompression. Post-incision and sternocleidomastoid retraction, how is the phrenic nerve best identified before scalene division?
A. Visual check on middle scalene
B. Stimulation on anterior scalene
C. Palpation near the clavicle
D. Tracing from cervical rib

Correct Answer: B

Explanation:

The phrenic nerve is located through visual inspection and electrical stimulation. It is the only nerve in the neck that runs from lateral to medial, which is an important anatomical feature to help localization. After localization, It is then carefully mobilized medially by incising the fascia over the anterior scalene muscle.

(SPN, p. 53)

31. The most common peripheral nerve sheath tumor in patients with Neurofibromatosis Type 1 (NF 1) is:
    A. Schwannoma
    B. Neurofibroma
    C. Malignant peripheral nerve sheath tumor (MPNST)
    D. Ganglioneuroma

    Correct Answer: B

    Explanation:

    Neurofibromas are a hallmark feature and the most common type of tumor in NF1.

    (NB, p. 421)
32. What is the other name for NF1?
    A. Pseudoxanthoma elasticum
    B. Fabry's disease
    C. Charcot–Marie–Tooth disease
    D. Von Recklinghausen's disease

    Correct Answer: D

    Explanation:

    NF1 is an autosomal dominant condition, also known as von Recklinghausen's disease.

    (NB, p. 421)
33. Where do the neurofibromas typically occur?
    A. Near spinal roots
    B. Distal nerves
    C. Near nerve plexuses
    D. All of the above

    Correct Answer: A

    (NB, p. 421)
34. A 45-year-old woman notices a painless, palpable lump on her forearm. Exam reveals Tinel's sign but no sensory loss. MRI shows a well-encapsulated mass on the ulnar nerve. What's the most likely diagnosis?
    A. Neurofibroma
    B. Schwannoma
    C. Malignant peripheral nerve sheath tumor
    D. Plexiform neurofibroma

    Correct Answer: B

    Explanation:

    Schwannomas, the most common nerve sheath tumors, peak in the 40 s–50 s. They often present as asymptomatic, palpable masses with Tinel's sign and are encapsulated on MRI.

    (NB., p. 663)

35. A 42-year-old man has an asymptomatic median nerve schwannoma in the forearm, stable on serial MRI for 2 years. He is worried about cancer risk. What's the best management and risk profile?
    A. Resect now; high malignant potential
    B. Resect now; common progression to NF2
    C. Monitor; rare malignant transformation
    D. Monitor; frequent recurrence post-resection

    Correct Answer: C

    Explanation:

    Asymptomatic schwannomas can be followed with imaging. Surgical resection is left for cases with growth and/or symptoms. Malignant transformation is rare. NF2 links to bilateral acoustic schwannomas, not peripheral, and recurrence is rare.

    (NB, p. 663)
36. One of the following is CORRECT about malignant transformation of nerve sheath tumors:
    A. Both schwannomas and neurofibromas have a similar rate of malignant transformation.
    B. Neurofibromas have less potential for malignant transformation.
    C. Schwannomas have less potential for malignant transformation.
    D. 40–60% of neurofibromas transform to malignant in 10 years.

    Correct Answer: C

    Malignant transformation of schwannomas is rare, unlike neurofibromas, which have 5–10% of transformation.

    (NB, p. 663)
37. A 55-year-old woman's ulnar nerve mass biopsy shows spindle cells in a myxomatous stroma, no encapsulation, and nerve infiltration. Her sister has NF1. What shifts this from schwannoma to another diagnosis?
    A. Myxomatous stroma with Antoni B pattern
    B. Family history of NF1
    C. Ulnar nerve location
    D. Lack of encapsulation and nerve infiltration

    Correct Answer: D

    Explanation:

    Schwannomas are encapsulated, displacing fascicles, with Antoni A/B patterns. This mass infiltrates, lacks encapsulation, and fits neurofibroma. This is supported by NF1 history, but the pathology pattern is the key in diagnosis.

    (NB, p. 663)

38. One of the following is CORRECT about the epidemiology of peripheral nerve schwannomas:
    A. It is less common than neurofibromas.
    B. It is more common in females.
    C. It peaks at the second and third decades of life.
    D. None of the above

    Correct Answer: B

    Explanation:

    Schwannomas are the most common nerve sheath tumors. They occur more in women and peak at the fourth and fifth decades of life.

    (NB, p. 663)
39. The superficial radial nerve can be compressed at:
    A. The fascial edge of the brachioradialis muscle
    B. Proximal to the radial styloid process approximately 8 cm
    C. Directly at the styloid process
    D. All of the above

    Correct Answer: D

    Explanation:

    The superficial radial nerve is susceptible to compression at two primary sites. The first is at the **fascial edge of the brachioradialis**. The second is **approximately 8 cm proximal to the radial styloid or directly at the styloid**, where the nerve lies superficially and is highly vulnerable to external pressure, like in tight gloves, watches, or tight bracelets or bands.

    (SSW, p. 2192)
40. Paralabral cysts can cause compression to the following nerve:
    A. Suprascapular nerve
    B. Medial cord of the brachial plexus
    C. Musculocutaneous nerve
    D. All of the above

    Correct Answer: A

    Explanation:

    Paralabral cysts are cysts containing fluid located within the glenoid labrum of the shoulder. It can compress the suprascapular nerve and rarely the axillary nerve.

    [88]
41. The most common site for suprascapular nerve entrapment is:
    A. Suprascapular notch
    B. Cervical origin
    C. Spinoglenoid notch
    D. Glenoid notch

    Correct Answer: A

    Explanation:

    The suprascapular nerve is vulnerable to entrapment at three key locations along its course: the cervical origin, suprascapular notch, and spinoglenoid notch. Among these, the suprascapular notch is the most common site of compression.

(PNN, p. 823)

42. The most distinct clinical feature of Guyon's tunnel syndrome is:
    A. Spare flexor carpi ulnaris muscle
    B. Spare sensation over the palm and dorsum of the hand
    C. Spare sensation over volar fifth finger
    D. A and B

    Correct Answer: D

    Explanation:

    Guyon's tunnel syndrome typically presented with preserved function of the flexor carpi ulnaris and flexor digitorum profundus, as well as preservation of the sensation over the palm and dorsum of the hand, since the sensory branches arise proximal to the wrist.

    (MPN, p. 35)

43. In the Riche–Cannieu anastomosis, the median nerve:
    A. Anastomoses with the deep ulnar branch in the palm
    B. Anastomoses with the ulnar nerve in the proximal forearm
    C. Anastomoses with the ulnar nerve in the distal forearm
    D. The anterior interosseous branch anastomoses with the ulnar nerve

    Correct Answer: A

    Explanation:

    The Riche–Cannieu anastomosis is a neuronal connection between the deep branch of the ulnar and median nerves in the thenar muscles of the hand. It allows ulnar nerve fibers to innervate muscles typically supplied by the median nerve, potentially preserving thumb function in median nerve palsy.

    (MPN, p. 30)

44. A 40-year-old man has weak thumb opposition after a forearm injury. Electrodiagnostic studies show normal median nerve conduction to the forearm but reduced thenar CMAP amplitude when stimulating the median nerve at the wrist. Ulnar nerve stimulation at the wrist activates the abductor pollicis brevis. What explains this presentation?
    A. Carpal tunnel syndrome with median nerve compression
    B. Ulnar neuropathy at Guyon's canal
    C. Radial nerve injury affecting thumb extension
    D. Martin–Gruber anastomosis involving thenar muscles

    Correct Answer: D

    Explanation:

    In a Martin–Gruber anastomosis, nerve fibers meant for the median nerve-innervated thenar muscles (opponens pollicis, abductor pollicis brevis, and flexor pollicis brevis) travel via the anterior interosseous branch, cross to the ulnar nerve, and then return to the thenar motor branch in the palm to supply these muscles.

    (MPN, p. 30)

45. What is the other name for the anterior interosseous nerve entrapment?
    A. Kiloh–Nevin syndrome
    B. Wartenberg syndrome
    C. Parsonage–Turner syndrome
    D. Pronator teres syndrome
    Correct Answer: A
    (SSW, p. 185)
46. In the literature, the differences between endoscopic versus open carpal tunnel release is:
    A. Endoscopic procedures have more recurrence.
    B. Open procedure has more incisional pain.
    C. There is no difference in the outcome between the two procedures.
    D. The learning curve of the endoscopic procedure is steeper.
    Correct Answer: C
    Explanation:
    In a randomized clinical trial for open decompression vs. endoscopic decompression for carpal tunnel syndrome, there were no differences in the outcome between the two procedures.
    [9]
47. The most common cause of isolated teres minor muscle atrophy is:
    A. Quadrilateral space syndrome
    B. Axillary nerve compression
    C. Rotator cuff tear
    D. Cervical radiculopathy
    Correct Answer: A
    Explanation:
    Quadrilateral space syndrome is an uncommon cause of posterolateral shoulder pain, resulting from compression of the axillary nerve and the posterior circumflex humeral artery within the quadrilateral space. It can affect teres minor muscles.
    (DI, p. 1025)
48. In scalene muscle syndrome, the part of the brachial plexus at higher risk is:
    A. Upper brachial plexus roots (C5-C7)
    B. Lower brachial plexus roots (C8-T1)
    C. All of brachial plexus roots (C5-T1)
    D. Brachial plexus roots and cords
    Correct Answer: B
    Explanation:
    Scalene muscle syndrome is a form of neurogenic thoracic outlet syndrome caused by compression of the brachial plexus (and sometimes the subclavian artery) between the anterior and middle scalene muscles in the neck. The lower brachial plexus roots are commonly involved.
    (TS, p. 41)

49. A 32-year-old typist reports numbness and tingling on the back of her right thumb for 3 months, worse after long shifts. Exam shows no weakness or thenar atrophy, and sensation is intact in the palm. Nerve conduction studies are normal for median and ulnar nerves.

49a. What is the involved peripheral nerve?

A. Ulnar nerve
B. Median nerve
C. Radial sensory nerve
D. Lateral antebrachial cutaneous nerve

49b. What is the name of this syndrome?

A. Wartenberg's syndrome
B. Carpal tunnel syndrome
C. De Quervain's syndrome
D. Distal radial syndrome

Answers: 49a:C, 49b: A

Explanation:

Wartenberg's syndrome is a rare condition of entrapment of the radial sensory nerve due to repetitive trauma or local compression (e.g., typist, tight watches, or bracelets). Because it is similar to meralgia paresthetica, it is called cheiralgia paresthetica.

(PNN, p. 1097)

50. The most common cause of ulnar nerve entrapment at the wrist (Guyon's canal syndrome) is:

A. Repetitive trauma
B. Ulnar artery thrombosis
C. Ganglion cyst
D. A and C

Correct Answer: D

Explanation:

A frequent cause of ulnar neuropathy at the wrist is chronic repetitive trauma. This can result from external pressure, such as prolonged cycling or repeated use of tools like screwdrivers. Additional causes include fractures of the hook of the hamate, metacarpals, or pisiform, as well as ulnar artery thrombosis. Ganglion cysts are another common source of ulnar nerve compression within Guyon's canal.

(MPN, p. 111)

51. Regarding the "OK" sign

51a. Which nerve is being tested?

A. Median nerve
B. Ulnar nerve
C. Anterior interosseous nerve
D. Posterior interosseous nerve

51b. Which muscles are usually weak when OK sign is positive?

A. Flexor pollicis longus and flexor digitorum profundus
B. Extensor pollicis brevis and extensor indicis

C. Abductor pollicis brevis and opponens pollicis
D. Flexor carpi radialis and pronator teres

Correct answers: 51a: C, 51b: A

Explanation:

During the clinical examination, the patient is asked to form an "OK" sign by touching the tips of the thumb and index finger. In anterior interosseous nerve dysfunction, due to weakness of the flexor pollicis longus and flexor digitorum profundus, the patient uses the pads instead of the tips, resulting in a flattened "O."

(MPN, p. 31)

52. A 45-year-old farmer reports forearm pain and thumb weakness for 4 months, worse after milking cows. Exam shows weak thumb flexion and numbness in the palm and radial fingers, with pain on resisted forearm pronation.

52a. What is the most likely diagnosis?
A. Carpal tunnel syndrome
B. Pronator teres syndrome
C. Anterior interosseous syndrome
D. Radial tunnel syndrome

52b. Where does the median nerve most commonly get compressed in this condition?
A. Under the carpal tunnel
B. Between flexor carpi radialis and palmaris longus
C. Between the pronator teres heads
D. Proximal to the cubital fossa

52c. What is the most likely cause of this condition?
A. Static fibrous band
B. Trauma-induced Volkmann's contracture
C. Dynamic compression from repetitive pronation
D. Hypertrophy of flexor digitorum superficialis

52d. What sensory finding distinguishes this condition from other conditions affecting the same nerve?
A. Sensory loss in the palm
B. Numbness in the thenar eminence only
C. Tingling in the dorsal hand only
D. No sensory disturbance

52e. What is the most appropriate surgical treatment for this patient?
A. Sublimis arch release
B. Pronator teres release
C. Median nerve transposition
D. A and B

Correct Answers: 52a: B, 52b: C, 52c: C, 52d: A, 52e: D

Explanation:

Pronator teres syndrome (PTS) occurs when the median nerve is compressed between the two heads of the pronator teres, but the muscle itself remains unaffected since its nerve supply originates proximal to the compression site. The typical etiology is repetitive compression during supination or elbow extension, like in cow milkers in this case. PTS causes sensory loss in the palm, unlike in carpal tunnel syndrome, where palm sensation is spared due to proximal branching of the palmar cutaneous branch of the median nerve. Treatment is usually conservative; however, if it fails in 3–6 months, surgery is indicated. Surgical decompression involves wide forearm exposure of the median nerve with sectioning the tendinous arch of the flexor digitorium superficialis (sublimis arch) and pronator teres release (Fig. 18.4).

(TS, pp. 101–104)

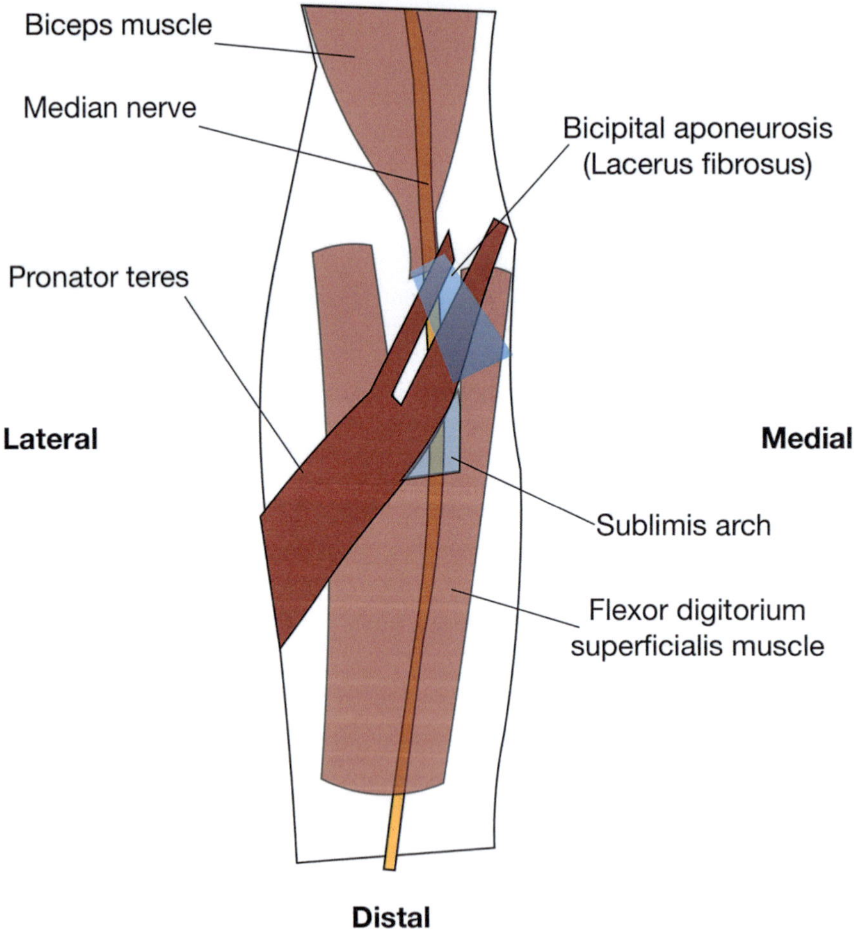

Fig. 18.4 illustration of the median nerve in the proximal forearm. For the purpose of simplification, the superficial flexor muscles of the forearm are not included. The illustration shows the main compressive sites for pronator teres syndrome (pronator teres two heads, lacerus fibrosus, sublimis arch)

53. One of the following is a provocative test for pronator teres syndrome:
    A. Resisted elbow flexion with forearm
    B. Resisted forearm pronation with elbow extended.
    C. resisted contraction of flexor digitorium superficialis to middle finger
    D. All of the above

    Correct Answer: D

    Explanation:

    Provocative tests for pronator teres syndrome include Tinel's sign at ventral proximal forearm, resisted elbow flexion with forearm for compression at bicipital aponeurosis, resisted forearm pronation with elbow extended for compression at two heads of pronator teres, and resisted contraction of flexor digitorium superficialis (FDS) to the middle finger for compression at FDS fibrous arch.

    (TS, pp. 101–104)
54. Scapular winging due to long thoracic nerve injury is caused by:
    A. Loss of serratus anterior muscle action
    B. Loss of latissimus dorsi muscle action
    C. Both A and B
    D. None of the above

    Correct Answer: A

    Explanation:

    The most common cause of a winged scapula is dysfunction of the serratus anterior muscle, which is supplied by the long thoracic nerve.

    (EPN, p. 89)
55. The following indicates a proximal median nerve injury:
    A. Flexion of median proximal interphalangeal joints weakness
    B. Flexion of the thumb at the interphalangeal joint weakness
    C. Abduction of the thumb weakness
    D. Forearm pronation weakness

    Correct Answer: D

    Explanation:

    The first muscle innervated by the median nerve is the pronator teres, which often arises above the elbow. Involvement of the flexor carpi radialis also suggests median nerve injury at or above the elbow. The pronator teres action is forearm pronation.

    (MPN, p. 31)
56. A 40-year-old violinist reports forearm pain and weak finger extension for 3 months, worse after playing. Examination shows no sensory loss, normal wrist extension, and pain distal to the lateral epicondyle.

    56a. What is the most likely diagnosis?
    A. Lateral epicondylitis
    B. Posterior cord compression
    C. Supinator syndrome
    D. Radial nerve palsy proximal to the elbow

56b. Where is the most common compressive site in this condition?
A. Proximal to the lateral intermuscular septum
B. Under the arcade of Frohse
C. Between brachialis and brachioradialis
D. Distal to the extensor carpi radialis brevis origin

56c. What is the most frequent etiology of this condition in this patient?
A. Traumatic radial artery aneurysm
B. Lipoma in the supinator canal
C. Thickened fascia above the elbow.
D. Dynamic compression from repetitive movement

56d. What EMG finding would confirm the diagnosis in this case?
A. Fibrillations in brachioradialis with normal SNAPs
B. Denervation in extensor indicis with intact radial SNAPs
C. Reduced CMAPs in extensor carpi radialis longus with sensory loss
D. Normal EMG in hand extensors

56e. After 2 months of persistent symptoms despite rest, what is the next step?
A. Surgical decompression of the affected nerve
B. Corticosteroid injection into the nerve
C. Continue physical therapy
D. Anesthetic block for long-term relief

Correct Answers: 56a: C, 56b: B, 56c: D, 56d: B, 56e: A

Explanation:

This case shows typical supinator syndrome, also known as radial tunnel syndrome. It involves posterior interosseous nerve (PIN) compression under the supinator's tendinous arch (arcade of Frohse), causing forearm pain and finger extension weakness without sensory loss. Wrist extension is spared. It is typically caused by dynamic compression from repetitive supination. The NCS usually shows reduced compound muscle action potentials (CMAPs) in radial-innervated muscles distal to especially in extensor digitorum, extensor indicis, and extensor pollicis longus. EMG shows denervation in extensor digitorum communis (EDC), extensor indicis, and extensor pollicis longus. It shows intact radial SNAPs.

Initial treatment is by avoiding repetitive movement, plus physical therapy. Corticosteroid injection might relieve the symptoms. Surgical decompression of the PIN is indicated if symptoms persist despite conservative treatment.

(TS, pp. 107–110)

57. The most common cause of spontaneous radial nerve compression at the arm is:
A. Strenuous muscular exercise
B. Mass lesions
C. External compression (Saturday night palsy)
D. Old trauma

Correct Answer: A

Explanation:

Spontaneous compression of the radial nerve at the arm is commonly caused by strenuous exercise. Other causes include previous trauma, mass lesions, and external compression like in Saturday night pals.

(SSW, p. 2191)

58. The usual cause of ape hand deformity is
    A. Proximal median nerve injury
    B. Proximal ulnar nerve injury
    C. Distal median nerve injury
    D. Anterior interosseous nerve injury

    Correct Answer: C

    Explanation:

    Ape deformity involves weak thumb opposition, which occurs in distal median nerve injury.
59. The nerve involved in a patient with a "guitar player's palsy" is:
    A. Ulnar nerve
    B. Median nerve
    C. Anterior interosseous nerve
    D. Posterior interosseous nerve

    Correct Answer: D

    Explanation:

    Inability to use fingers in guitar playing or any activities involving the repetitive extension of the fingers is typical for posterior interosseous nerve palsy.

(TS, pp. 107–110)

60. The hyperabduction syndrome is the compression of:
    A. Roots of the brachial plexus
    B. Trunks of the brachial plexus
    C. Cords of the brachial plexus
    D. All of the above

    Correct Answer: C

    Explanation:

    The hyperabduction syndrome caused by repeated or prolonged hyperabduction of the arm can cause stretching of the neurovascular bundle (commonly brachial plexus cords) beneath the pectoralis minor tendon and the coracoid process.

    (TS, p. 44)

Peripheral Nerves - Lower Limb

19

1. A patient presents with deep peroneal nerve palsy. Despite typical weakness in dorsiflexion, you notice no sensory loss over the web space between the first and second toes. What is the most likely explanation for the absence of sensory loss?
   A. Anomalous innervation by the superficial peroneal nerve
   B. Complete axonotmesis of the deep peroneal nerve
   C. Incomplete lesion sparing sensory fibers
   D. Presence of Martin–Gruber anastomosis

   Correct Answer: A

   Explanation:

   There is high variability in innervating the sensory of first web space of the foot. It is usually innervated by the deep peroneal nerve; however, it can be supplied by an anomalous superficial peroneal nerve.

   [89]
2. A 35-year-old hiker presents with painless foot drop and numbness on the dorsum of his right foot after a long trek. Exam reveals weak ankle dorsiflexion and toe extension, with an abnormal gait.

   2a. What is the most likely diagnosis?
   A. L5 radiculopathy
   B. Sciatic nerve injury
   C. Common peroneal nerve entrapment
   D. Deep peroneal nerve neuropathy

   2b. What are the other risk factors for this condition?
   A. Repetitive squatting
   B. High-heeled shoe use
   C. Regular stretching of the knee
   D. All of the above

K. F. AlAli, H. T. Hashim, *Spine Surgery and Peripheral Nerve Surgery*,
https://doi.org/10.1007/978-3-031-98543-0_19

2c. What surgical position is considered a common risk factor for this condition?

A. Supine position
B. Prone position
C. Lithotomy
D. All are correct.

2d. What is the typical gait abnormality for this condition?

A. Steppage gait
B. Antalgic gait
C. Trendelenburg gait
D. Spastic gait

Correct Answers: 2a: C, 2b: A, 2c: C, 2d: A

Explanation:

The most common cause of painless foot drop is common peroneal nerve entrapment/neuritis at the fibular head. Risk factors are most often related to trauma, followed by behavioral factors. Traumatic injuries such as knee dislocations or fibular fractures. Behavioral causes like prolonged leg-crossing or repetitive squatting. The most common surgical position that is considered a risk factor is the lithotomy position. The foot drop causes steppage of slapping gait with toe dragging that causes difficulties in walking and climbing stairs with frequent falling.

[90] (PNN, pp. 2229–2230)

3. One of the following signs can help differentiate L5 radiculopathy from common peroneal nerve entrapment:

A. Weakness of foot dorsiflexion
B. Loss of sensation over the dorsum of the foot
C. Negative Tinel's sign at the fibular neck
D. Normal inversion

Correct Answer: D

Explanation:

Inversion of the foot is primarily mediated by the tibialis posterior, which is innervated by the tibial nerve (L5). This muscle is affected in L5 radiculopathy but spared in peroneal neuropathy, making preserved inversion a helpful distinguishing sign in favor of common peroneal nerve entrapment.

[90]

4. Which structures commonly contribute to common peroneal nerve entrapment?

A. Flexor retinaculum and tibialis posterior
B. Aponeuroses of tibialis posterior
C. Aponeuroses of the soleus and peroneus longus muscles
D. All of the above

Correct Answer: C

Explanation:

The common peroneal nerve (CPN) is most frequently compressed at the peroneal tunnel, where it curves around the neck of the fibula. The arch is formed by the aponeurotic fibers of the soleus and peroneus longus muscles.

(PNN, p. 2242)

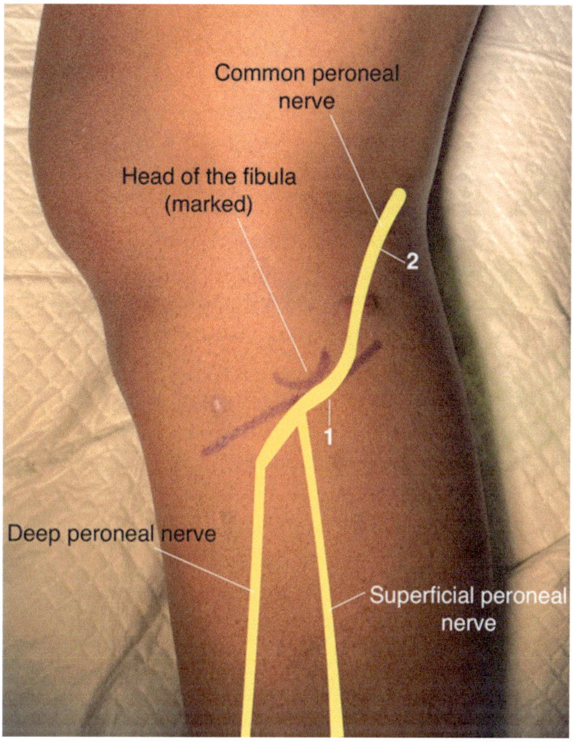

Fig. 19.1 Surgical picture of a posterio-lateral knee illustrating the course of the common peroneal nerve around the fibular head. The 2 entrapment points are [1] the aponeuroses of the soleus and peroneus longus muscles and (2) the muscular septum between the gastrocnemius and biceps femoris muscles

5. What other entrapment points are there for the common peroneal nerve?
   A. Between the gastrocnemius and biceps femoris muscles
   B. Within the adductor canal
   C. Under the pes anserinus tendon
   D. Between the popliteus and semimembranosus muscles

   Correct Answer: A

   Explanation:

   The common peroneal nerve can be entrapped at a muscular septum (posterior-lateral) between the gastrocnemius and biceps femoris muscles (number 2 in the picture below)

   (PNN, p. 2242) (Fig. 19.1).

6. A patient is diagnosed with L5 radiculopathy based on clinical and imaging findings. However, he has full strength in foot dorsiflexion but weakness in hip abduction. Which of the following muscles is primarily responsible for this pattern of weakness?
   A. Tensor fasciae latae
   B. Gluteus maximus
   C. Gluteus medius
   D. Quadratus femoris

   Correct Answer: C

Explanation:

L5 radiculopathy is caused by L5 nerve root compression, which contributes to the lumbosacral plexus. L5 innervates muscles via the sciatic and superior gluteal nerves. L5 radiculopathy usually causes ankle dorsiflexion weakness (tibialis anterior, deep peroneal nerve) and foot eversion weakness (peroneus longus/brevis, superficial peroneal nerve). This patient has intact dorsiflexion strength with isolated weakness in hip abduction. The gluteus medius, innervated by the superior gluteal nerve (L4–L5, mostly L5), serves as the principal hip abductor. Selective compression of the L5 root, potentially preserving sciatic nerve fibers reaching the peroneal part while affecting the superior gluteal nerve, accounts for the picture of this case.

(EPN, p. 199)

7. A 32-year-old female patient with a history of breast cancer and DVT and on anticoagulation. She developed sudden difficulty adducting the thigh and pain in the symphysis pubis radiating to the medial knee.

7a. Which nerve has been most likely affected?

A. Pudendal nerve
B. Femoral nerve
C. Superior gluteal nerve
D. Obturator nerve

7b. What is the likely etiology of this presentation?

A. Possible pregnancy
B. Pelvic hematoma
C. Retroperitoneal or intrapelvic tumors
D. Pelvic fracture

7c. What is the name of the sign of the pain in the symphysis pubis radiating to the medial knee?

A. Howship–Romberg sign
B. Finkelstein's sign
C. Romberg–Tinel sign
D. Howship–Klass sign

7e. What is the typical gait disturbance usually found in this condition?

A. Waddling gait
B. Ataxic gait
C. Steppage gait
D. Circumduction gait

Correct Answers: 7a: D, 7b: B, 7c: A, 7e: D

Explanation:

The case is obturator tunnel syndrome. The obturator nerve is vulnerable to injury from various pelvic disorders and compression within the obturator tunnel. It may be affected by pelvic fractures, hematomas (especially with anticoagulation), retroperitoneal or intrapelvic tumors, and even pregnancy. Obturator tunnel syndrome presents with deep, non-localized pain radiating from the pubic region to the medial knee, often worse at rest. A key feature is medial knee pain (Howship–Romberg sign), due to compression of the posterior branch of the obturator nerve. Prolonged compression may lead to adductor weakness and a circumduction gait, though some adductors are partially spared by femoral and sciatic innervation.

(TS, pp. 209–212)

8. After prolonged surgery in the lithotomy position, a patient develops persistent numbness and foot drop. Electrodynamic studies have shown a lesion in the deep peroneal nerve, with normal superficial peroneal function. Which muscle is most likely to be spared?
   A. Tibialis anterior
   B. Extensor digitorum longus
   C. Peroneus longus
   D. Extensor hallucis longus

   Correct Answer: C

   Explanation:

   The deep peroneal nerve innervates tibialis anterior (ankle dorsiflexion), extensor digitorum longus (toe extension), and extensor hallucis longus (toe extension). The superficial peroneal nerve supplies the peroneus longus and brevis (foot eversion), making (C) the right answer.
9. A 42-year-old runner presents with left leg weakness and numbness after a disc herniation at L4–L5. Exam shows weak foot dorsiflexion and hip abduction, with sensory loss over the lateral calf. The medial hamstring reflex is absent on the left, but the Achilles reflex is intact. What does the absent medial hamstring reflex most likely indicate in this L5 radiculopathy case?
   A. Isolated L5 root compression sparing S1
   B. Concurrent S1 radiculopathy
   C. Sciatic nerve involvement distal to the plexus
   D. Normal variant unrelated to the pathology

   Correct Answer: A

   Explanation:

   The medial hamstring reflex, mediated by the L5 nerve root via the sciatic nerve's tibial division to the semitendinosus and semimembranosus, is absent, consistent with L5 root pathology, as corroborated by observed weakness in dorsiflexion (tibialis anterior) and hip abduction (gluteus medius). Preservation of the Achilles reflex, innervated by S1 through the tibial nerve, excludes S1 involvement, localizing the lesion to L5. This aligns with L4–L5 disc herniation selectively compressing the L5 root. Although reflex reliability may vary, the findings unequivocally indicate isolated L5 radiculopathy.

   (SS, p. 174) [92]
10. When performing medial hamstring reflex, the patient should be positioned:
    A. Supine
    B. Lateral
    C. Prone
    D. All of the above are correct.

    Correct Answer: C

Explanation:

To test the medial hamstring reflex with the patient in the prone position, place your index finger over the medial hamstring tendon, just above the knee. Then tap your finger with a tendon hammer and observe for contraction of the semitendinosus and semimembranosus muscles.

[92]

The two cases above (9 and 10) highlight the importance of differentiating between lumbar radiculopathy and peripheral neuropathy. It is crucial to master lower limb examinations for radiculopathy and peripheral nerves.

11. What needle EMG finding can help differentiate common peroneal nerve neuropathy from high sciatic neuropathy?
    A. Normal findings at the short head of biceps femoris
    B. Normal findings at tibialis anterior only
    C. Fibrillations in all hamstring muscles
    D. Normal findings at extensor digitorum brevis only

    Correct Answer: A

    Explanation:

    A normal short head EMG favors distal common peroneal neuropathy; however, a comprehensive EMG approach is needed.

    EMG of the biceps femoris, short head, alone cannot definitively differentiate high sciatic neuropathy from common peroneal neuropathy without comparing findings with tibial-innervated muscles. An abnormal short head EMG with normal tibial muscles suggests proximal common peroneal neuropathy, while abnormalities in both indicate high sciatic neuropathy.

    [91]

12. In the popliteal entrapment syndrome, the following nerve is entrapped:
    A. Common peroneal nerve
    B. Tibial nerve
    C. Saphenous nerve
    D. None of the above

    Correct Answer: D

    Explanation:

    The popliteal artery, vein, and tibial nerve pass through the popliteal fossa; however, unlike other entrapment syndromes, the popliteal entrapment syndrome affects mainly the tibial artery and spares the tibial nerve.

    (TS, p. 233)

13. A 52-year-old with L2-L3 discitis and psoas abscess. He has severe burning pain at the lateral thigh. The likely explanation of this presentation is?
    A. Meralgia paresthetica
    B. Psoas muscle stretch
    C. Obturator nerve irritation
    D. L2 radicolopathy

    Correct Answer: A

Explanation:

The lateral femoral cutaneous nerve originates from L2 and L3 nerve roots. After that, it travels beneath the psoas muscle and emerges laterally, crossing the iliac bone within a fibrous tunnel formed by a fold in the iliacus fascia. It then courses toward the medial side of the anterior superior iliac spine (ASIS) and passes beneath the inguinal ligament. Any compression at its course is called meralgia paresthetica, causing numbness and pain at the anterior-lateral thigh. One of the etiologies of meralgia paresthetica is psoas abscess.

(TS, p. 225–227)

14. The most common cause of meralgia paresthetica is:
    A. Psoas abscess
    B. Obesity
    C. Pregnancy
    D. Idiopathic

    Correct Answer: D

    Explanation:

    All the listed options are possible causes of meralgia paresthetica. Obesity is a common cause; however, in most cases the cause is idiopathic.

    (PNN, p. 1988)

15. What is the crucial step in the surgical treatment of meralgia paresthetica?
    A. Splitting the inferior edge of the inguinal ligament
    B. Releasing the pes anserinus tendon
    C. Complete split of the inguinal ligament
    D. Splitting the sartorius muscle with fascia lata overlying the nerve

    Correct Answer: A

    Explanation:

    The lateral femoral cutaneous nerve passes underneath the inguinal ligament and then pierces the fascia lata overlying the sartorius muscle. During surgical decompression, the nerve is identified where it pierces the fascia lata. Then the fascia lata is split (not the sartorius muscle) and extended proximally till reaching the inferior edge of the inguinal ligament, where it is also split (where the nerve exists).

    (SPN, p. 169)

16. A 28-year-old avid runner presents with burning pain and tingling in the medial ankle and sole of her left foot, worsening with runs. Exam reveals a positive Tinel's sign at the medial ankle and mild sensory loss on the heel. Symptoms persist after 6 weeks of rest and NSAIDs.

    16a. What's the most likely diagnosis?
    A. Plantar fasciitis
    B. Tarsal tunnel syndrome
    C. S1 radiculopathy
    D. Morton's neuroma

16b. Which nerve is affected?

A. Medical calcaneal nerve
B. Medial plantar nerve
C. Anterior tibial nerve
D. Posterior tibial nerve

16c. Which physical finding is most consistently reported in this condition?

A. Motor weakness of intrinsic foot muscles
B. Positive Tinel's sign
C. Painless atrophy of plantar muscles
D. Negative dorsiflexion-eversion test

16d. Which statement is CORRECT regarding the role of EMG/NCS in this condition?

A. NCS/EMG is highly sensitive.
B. NCS/EMG has low specificity and misses structural causes.
C. NCS/EMG is unreliable due to frequent false negatives.
D. NCS/EMG only confirms idiopathic cases.

16e. Another patient has a similar clinical picture and was found to have calcaneal osteochondroma. What is the best treatment for this patient?

A. Sectioning the deep fascia of the abductor hallucis muscle
B. Release of the flexor retinaculum of the ankle only
C. Release of the sustentaculum tali
D. All of the above

16 f. What factor most likely predicts the outcome in this condition?

A. Absence of a mass effect in the medial ankle
B. Long history of symptoms pre-surgery
C. Younger age at intervention
D. Unilateral presentation

Correct Answers: 16a: B, 16b: D, 16c: B, 16d: C, 16e: D, 16f: B

Explanation:

This case shows a typical clinical picture of tarsal tunnel syndrome, with burning pain and tingling in the medial ankle and foot sole and positive Tinel's sign at the medial ankle with sensory loss on the heel. The tarsal tunnel syndrome is a compression of the posterior tibial nerve and its branches. It is usually underdiagnosed and with unknown etiology. The diagnosis is mainly clinical, and electrodiagnostic studies are unreliable due to frequent false negatives. Tinel's sign at the tarsal tunnel is the most consistent clinical finding. Treatment is usually conservative with good results. If it fails, surgery is indicated by decompression of the flexor retinaculum near the medial malleolus down to the sustentaculum tali and sectioning the deep fascia of the abductor hallucis muscle. Prognosis is not favorable when etiology is unknown and there is a long duration of the symptoms.

[93]

17. What can predict failure of conservative management in tarsal tunnel syndrome?
    A. Slow nerve conduction of the posterior tibial nerve
    B. Presence of isolated heel pain without nerve conduction abnormalities
    C. Normal EMG and nerve conduction studies despite ongoing symptoms
    D. Preservation of intrinsic foot muscle strength with no sensory loss

    Correct Answer: A

    Explanation:

    The electrodiagnostics are unreliable in the diagnosis if tarsal tunnel syndrome; however, the positive finding of slow nerve conduction of the posterior tibial nerve can predict failure of conservative management.

    [93]

18. A 26-year-old woman with a history of hemophilia presents with progressive thigh weakness and pain. She has difficulty standing from a seated position and weakness in hip flexion.

    18a. What nerve is most likely involved?
    A. Obturator nerve
    B. Sciatic nerve
    C. Superior gluteal nerve
    D. Femoral nerve

    18b. What is the most likely etiology?
    A. Inguinal hernia
    B. Aortic aneurysm
    C. Pelvic mass
    D. Pelvic hematoma

    18c. What are the possible entrapment sites for this nerve?
    A. Iliacus compartment
    B. Inguinal ligament
    C. Lateral epicondyle of the femur
    D. A and B

    18e. The affected nerve also can be entrapped in the muscular lacuna. What are the boundaries of this structure?
    A. The liopectineal arch and the inguinal ligament ventrally and the iliac bone and iliopsoas muscle dorsally
    B. The sacrotuberous ligament and piriformis muscle ventrally, and the ischial spine and gluteus maximus dorsally
    C. The femoral sheath and adductor longus ventrally, and the vastus medialis and femur dorsally
    D. The transverse intermuscular septum and sartorius ventrally, and the femoral artery and nerve dorsally

    Correct Answers: 18a: D, 18b: D, 18c: D, 18e: A

    Explanation:

    The case is typical for femoral nerve involvement with hip flexion weakness. Because of the history of hemophilia, pelvic hematoma is the likely etiology of the femoral nerve entrapment. The femoral nerve can be entrapped in the iliacus compartment and inguinal ligament and when passing through the muscular lacuna canal. The muscular lacuna canal is the lateral compartment of the thigh beneath the inguinal ligament. It is bounded by the liopectineal arch and the inguinal ligament ventrally and the iliac bone and iliopsoas muscle dorsally.

(PNN, pp. 1840–1851)

19. In exposing the femoral nerve in the thigh, the following fascia must be opened first:
    A. Cribriform fascia
    B. Sartorius fascia
    C. Popliteal fascia
    D. Iliacus fascia

    Correct Answer: D

    Explanation:

    During femoral nerve exposure in the thigh, the iliacus fascia must be incised to access the nerve. Failure to do so may lead to searching in the wrong compartment, delaying identification and dissection.

    (SPN, p. 82)

20. A 35-year-old male presents to the emergency department with a 3-day history of progressive weakness and numbness starting in his feet and today involving his thighs. He reports difficulty walking and climbing stairs. Two weeks prior, he had a mild respiratory infection that resolved. On exam, he exhibits symmetric distal lower limb muscle weakness, absent deep tendon reflexes, and reduced sensation to pinprick in a stocking-glove pattern.

    20a. What is the likely diagnosis?
    A. Guillain–Barré Syndrome
    B. Chronic inflammatory demyelinating polyneuropathy
    C. Diabetic polyneuropathy presenting with gradual progression and preserved reflexes
    D. Spinal cord compression

    20b. What is the pathological hallmark of this condition?
    A. Neuronal degeneration due to viral infection
    B. Progressive degeneration of the cerebral cortex
    C. Autoimmune loss of myelin sheath
    D. Accumulation of Lewy bodies in motor neurons

    Correct Answers: 20a: A, 20b: C

    Explanation:

    This case illustrates the importance of differential diagnosis in lower extremity weakness beyond peripheral nerve entrapment or injury. Guillain–Barré syndrome has a typical presentation of distal lower extremity weakness and then ascending weakness (like in the case) that might reach upper extremities. It is caused by autoimmune demyelination due to recent viral infection.

    (DI, p. 656)

21. A 35-year-old runner presents with numbness over the dorsum of the foot and weakness in foot eversion. Symptoms are worsened by prolonged walking and

relieved with rest. On examination, Tinel's sign is positive over the anterolateral aspect of the lower leg. What is the most likely diagnosis?

A. Entrapment of the superficial peroneal nerve
B. Entrapment of the deep peroneal nerve
C. Chronic exertional compartment syndrome
D. L5 radiculopathy

Correct Answer: A

Explanation:

The case shows typical superficial peroneal nerve entrapment with numbness over the dorsum of the foot and weakness in foot eversion. Also, the positive Tinel's sign over the anterolateral aspect of the lower leg is a typical finding.

(TS, p. 246)

22. What is the most common etiology of entrapment of the superficial peroneal nerve?

A. Iatrogenic
B. Muscle hernia
C. Lipoma
D. Trauma

Correct Answer: D

Explanation:

All mentioned answers are possible causes of entrapment of the superficial peroneal nerve; however, trauma is the most common. Trauma to the anterior leg can lead to inflammation and swelling, which both lead to compression and entrapment of the nerve.

(TS, p. 245)

23. Being superficial contributes to the incidence of entrapment of the superficial peroneal nerve. One of the following also contributes to this:

A. Fixed course at distal leg
B. Its passage near the tarsal tunnel
C. Its close association with the fibula
D. Its penetration of the intermuscular septum of the posterior compartment

Correct Answer: A

Explanation:

Dynamic compression, influenced by the functional anatomy of the leg, increases the risk of superficial peroneal nerve entrapment. Because the nerve has a fixed course, forced foot inversion and extension can stretch it over the fascial border, exacerbating compression. Also, the nerve is more fixed when piercing the crural fascia and continues subcutaneously.

(TS, p. 245)

24. All of the following can cause deep peroneal nerve entrapment EXCEPT:

A. Osteophytes from osteoarthritis
B. Playing soccer
C. High-heeled shoes
D. Severe flat feet

Correct Answer: D

Explanation:

Deep peroneal nerve entrapment is commonly caused by repetitive foot activity in runners, dancers, and kicking sports like soccer, especially with tight lacing or extreme plantarflexion. Mechanical factors include high-heeled shoes, tight footwear or casts, and pes cavus, which increases tension under the inferior extensor retinaculum. Though less common, osteophytes from osteoarthritis may also contribute. Trauma, such as direct blows, ankle sprains, or ankle surgeries, can also precipitate entrapment.

(PNN, p. 2303)

25. Which of the following statements best reflects current evidence regarding the surgical treatment of painful lower limb diabetic peripheral neuropathy through nerve decompression?
    A. Nerve decompression has shown no long-term benefit over sham surgery in randomized controlled trials.
    B. Surgical decompression is only effective when both lower limbs are operated on simultaneously.
    C. Nerve decompression has demonstrated sustained pain reduction in multiple RCTs, with superior long-term outcomes compared to control or sham procedures.
    D. Surgical decompression is contraindicated in all patients with symmetrical diabetic neuropathy due to lack of anatomical targets.

    Correct Answer: C

    Explanation:

    Over the past decade, multiple randomized controlled trials have supported the effectiveness of nerve decompression surgery in treating painful diabetic peripheral neuropathy (DPN). Across these studies, patients who underwent nerve decompression reported significant and sustained reductions in pain compared to control groups. While early outcomes sometimes showed similar improvements in both treated and sham-operated limbs, long-term follow-up consistently favored decompressed nerves, indicating a true therapeutic benefit.

    [94–96]

26. What is a common site of entrapment for the medial branch of the deep peroneal nerve?
    A. Beneath the inferior extensor retinaculum
    B. At the anterior intermuscular septum
    C. Beneath the extensor hallucis brevis tendon
    D. Over the lateral part of the talonavicular joint

    Correct Answer: C

    Explanation:

    The medial branch of the deep peroneal nerve is commonly entrapped beneath the extensor hallucis brevis tendon at the first and second tarsometatarsal joints.

    (PNN, p. 2316)

27. Which of the following positions maximally stretches the deep peroneal nerve over the talonavicular joint?
    A. Dorsiflexion of the foot with plantar flexion of the toes
    B. Plantar flexion of the foot with dorsiflexion of the toes
    C. Inversion of the foot with dorsiflexion of the toes
    D. Eversion of the foot with plantar flexion of the toes

    Correct Answer: B

    Explanation:

    According to a cadaver study, plantar flexion of the foot with dorsiflexion of the toes.

    Stretch the deep peroneal nerve over the talonavicular joint.

    (PNN, p. 2316)
28. Which of the following is a common symptom of medial branch deep peroneal nerve entrapment?
    A. Weakness of the ankle
    B. Dull pain in the first toe
    C. Deep ache radiating to the ankle and leg
    D. Foot drop

    Correct Answer: B

    Explanation:

    The medial terminal branch of the deep peroneal nerve provides sensory innervation to the adjacent sides of the first two toes and the web space between them. Entrapment of this nerve causes first toe dull pain, often worse after activity.

    (PNN, p. 2316)
29. What is the term used for deep peroneal nerve entrapment at the ankle beneath the inferior extensor retinaculum?
    A. Anterior tarsal tunnel syndrome
    B. Posterior tarsal tunnel syndrome
    C. Lateral compartment syndrome
    D. Talonavicular dysfunction

    Correct Answer: A

    Explanation:

    Entrapment of the deep peroneal nerve in the ankle underneath the inferior extensor retinaculum is called anterior tarsal syndrome, a term that is uncommonly used. Commonly the condition is called deep peroneal nerve entrapment (Fig. 19.2).

    (PNN, p. 2316)
30. One of the following is a special provocative clinical test for deep peroneal nerve entrapment:
    A. Tinel's sign
    B. Ankle flexion sign
    C. Ankle eversion sign
    D. Squeeze test

    Correct Answer: D

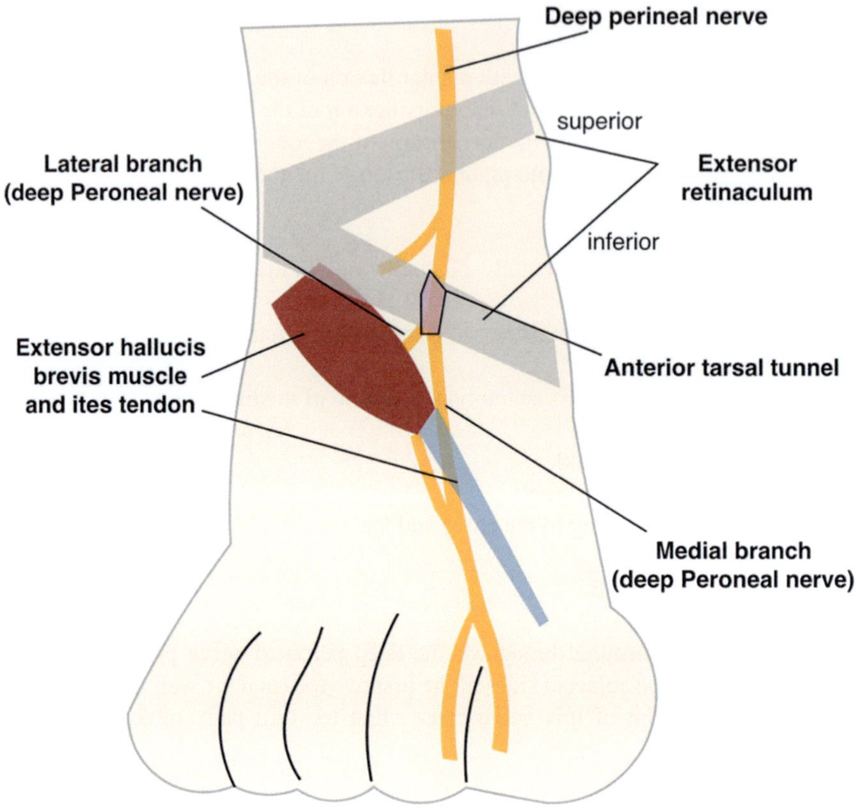

Fig. 19.2 Illustration of distal deep peroneal nerve course and entrapment points. It shows anterior tarsal tunnel formed by the inferior extensor retinaculum, where the nerve can be entrapped. Also, it shows medial branch of the deep peroneal nerve entrapment beneath the extensor hallucis brevis tendon

Explanation:

The squeeze test can replicate and diagnose deep peroneal nerve entrapment by compressing the metatarsal heads together while simultaneously squeezing the nerve from both above and below. Tinel's sign is helpful but not specific for this nerve.

(PNN, P. 2319)

31. A patient presents with loss of plantar sensation and an inability to curl the toes following ankle trauma. X-ray reveals a fracture of the medial malleolus. Which of the following is NOT an entrapment point for this nerve?
   A. Popliteal fossa
   B. Tarsal tunnel
   C. Lower edge of the gastrocnemius muscle
   D. Lateral edge of medial malleolus

   Correct Answer: D

Explanation:

This case shows injury of the tibial nerve (loss of plantar sensation and an inability to curl the toes) at the medial ankle from fracture of the medial malleolus. The question is about the entrapment points of the tibial nerve, which includes the popliteal fossa, the tarsal tunnel, and the lower edge of the gastrocnemius muscle.

(PNN, p. 2458)

32. Entrapment of tibial nerve at the popliteal fossa can result from:
    A. Baker's cyst
    B. Compression by the iliotibial band
    C. Tarsal tunnel inflammation
    D. Lateral meniscus tear

    Correct Answer: A

    Explanation:

    The tibial nerve can be entrapped, usually due to a mass like a Baker's cyst or popliteal artery aneurysm.

    (PNN, p. 2458)

33. A 52-year-old female with a history of thrombophlebitis presents with burning pain at the posterior and lateral ankle and foot.

    33a. Which nerve is affected?
    A. Lateral plantar nerve
    B. Posterior tibial nerve
    C. Sural nerve
    D. Anterior tibial nerve

    33b. What is the likely etiology of the nerve entrapment in this case?
    A. Previous trauma
    B. Thrombophlebitis
    C. Unknown etiology
    D. All are possible causes.

    33c. What is the typical entrapment point for this nerve?
    A. When piercing crural fascia
    B. Posterior to the lateral malleolus
    C. Distal one-third of the leg
    D. None of the above

    Correct Answers: 33a: C, 33b: B, 33c: A

    Explanation:

    The sural nerve supplies the cutaneous innervation of the posterior and lateral aspects of the ankle and foot. Possible causes of entrapment of this nerve are trauma, leg swelling like in thrombophlebitis or pitting edema, and external pressure (boots); sometimes the etiology is unknown. In this case, there is a clear explanation of the entrapment, thrombophlebitis. Typically, the sural nerve is entrapped where it pierces the crural fascia and becomes superficial.

    (PNN, p. 2378) (TS, p. 251)

34. A 45-year-old female office worker presents with chronic pain in her right buttock that radiates down the back of her leg, describing it as a burning sensation. She reports difficulty sitting for long periods and discomfort when getting out of bed. On examination, flexion of the hip test reproduces her symptoms.

34a. What is the most likely diagnosis?
- A. Lumbar spinal stenosis
- B. Piriformis syndrome
- C. Hamstring injury
- D. Sacroiliac joint dysfunction

34b. What is the primary anatomical cause of such condition?
- A. Compression of the femoral nerve by the piriformis muscle
- B. Entrapment of the sciatic nerve at the level of the ischial tuberosity
- C. Inflammation of the sacroiliac joint
- D. Hypertrophy of the gluteus maximus muscle

34c. Which of the following is a common risk factor for developing this condition?
- A. Prolonged standing
- B. Sitting for extended periods
- C. Excessive knee flexion
- D. Frequent ankle dorsiflexion

34d. What is a typical symptom of this condition that distinguishes it from other differential diagnoses?
- A. Pain worsened by coughing or sneezing
- B. Bilateral leg weakness
- C. Loss of bladder control
- D. Sciatic numbness and tingling with gluteal pain

34e. Which of the following is a recommended initial treatment?
- A. Immediate surgical decompression
- B. Long-term bed rest for 2 weeks
- C. Short-term rest and physical therapy
- D. High-dose steroid therapy

34 f. Which anatomical variation can predispose an individual to this condition?
- A. A bipartite piriformis muscle
- B. A shortened sciatic nerve
- C. Absence of the sacrotuberous ligament
- D. Hypertrophy of the femoral nerve

34 g. What is the most common complication associated with surgical intervention for this condition?
- A. Infection
- B. Chronic hip dislocation
- C. Sciatic nerve injury
- D. Pulmonary embolism

Correct Answers: 34a: B, 34b: A, 34c: B, 34d: D, 34e: C, 34f: A, 34 g: C

Explanation:

The clinical case describes a middle-aged woman with gluteal pain radiating down the leg, worsened by sitting and reproduced by the hip flexion, which aligns with piriformis syndrome. It is a condition of sciatic nerve entrapment by the piriformis muscle at the ischial tuberosity. Risk factors include prolonged sitting, common among office workers. The FAIR test (flexion, adduction, and internal rotation of the hip) is a key diagnostic tool, stretching the piriformis to reproduce symptoms. Symptoms like gluteal pain with numbness and tingling along the sciatic nerve differentiate it from lumbar stenosis, which may involve more spinal-related signs. Initial treatment focuses on rest and physical therapy. Anatomical variations like a bipartite piriformis muscle can predispose individuals to this condition by altering nerve compression dynamics. Surgery, reserved for refractory cases, carries a risk of sciatic nerve injury, the most common complication due to the nerve's proximity to the surgical site.

[97]

35. A patient is diagnosed with L4 radiculopathy. Which of the following clinical findings would help distinguish L4 radiculopathy from a femoral nerve injury?
    A. Weakness in knee extension
    B. Absent patellar reflex
    C. Weakness in hip flexion
    D. Weakness on hip adduction

    Correct Answer: D

    Explanation:

    Both femoral neuropathy and L4 radiculopathy may cause quadriceps weakness, loss of the patellar reflex, and medial leg numbness, but L4 radiculopathy additionally affects the thigh adductors (obturator nerve), anterior tibialis (deep peroneal nerve), and posterior tibialis muscles (tibial nerve).

    [98]

36. A soccer player presents with pain and weakness in dorsiflexion after an ankle injury. MRI shows edema of the extensor retinaculum and compression of a nerve. Which nerve is most likely involved?
    A. Tibial nerve
    B. Deep peroneal nerve
    C. Superficial peroneal nerve
    D. Sural nerve

    Correct Answer: B

    (See question 29 answer.)

37. A patient complains of weakness in hip abduction and foot dorsiflexion. Which of the following tests would best distinguish between a high sciatic nerve lesion and L5 radiculopathy?
    A. MRI of the lumbar spine
    B. Nerve conduction study of the peroneal nerve
    C. Electromyography of the gluteus medius
    D. Lumbar CT myelogram

    Correct Answer: C

Explanation:

The gluteus medius is innervated by the superior gluteal nerve, a branch of L5 that comes off the lumbosacral plexus before the sciatic nerve forms. Therefore, if EMG shows denervation in the gluteus medius, the lesion is at the L5 root or plexus level, not the sciatic nerve.

[99]

38. A patient undergoes a knee arthroscopy and develops foot drop. Postoperative EMG shows isolated damage to the deep peroneal nerve. Which muscle would still function normally?
    A. Tibialis anterior
    B. Extensor hallucis longus
    C. Peroneus longus
    D. Extensor digitorum longus

    Correct Answer: C

    Explanation:

    All of the muscles are innervated by the deep peroneal nerve except peroneus longus, which is innervated by the superficial peroneal nerve.

    (EPN, p. 154)

39. A 42-year-old man presents with burning pain and numbness over the lateral aspect of his right calf. Symptoms worsen with walking. On exam, Tinel's sign is positive lateral to the biceps femoris tendon. Motor strength and reflexes are normal. A local anesthetic injection provides temporary relief.

39a. The affected nerve is a branch of which peripheral nerve?
   A. Tibial nerve
   B. Common peroneal nerve
   C. Sural nerve
   D. Femoral nerve

39b. All of the following have been reported as causes of entrapment of the affected nerve EXCEPT:
   A. Piercing through the biceps femoris tendon
   B. Compression by peri-popliteal cystic bursitis
   C. Fibrous band of tissue
   D. Compression beneath the flexor retinaculum

39c. Which clinical feature best supports a diagnosis of entrapment?
   A. Weakness of plantar flexion
   B. Absent ankle reflex
   C. Numbness and burning pain over the lateral calf
   D. Numbness between the first and second toes

39d. What is the most likely diagnosis?
   A. L5 radiculopathy
   B. Common peroneal nerve entrapment
   C. Lateral sural cutaneous nerve entrapment
   D. Sural nerve entrapment

Correct Answers: 39a: B, 39b: D, 39c: C, 39d: C

Explanation:

The case is typical entrapment of the lateral sural cutaneous nerve (LSCN), which is a sensory branch of the common peroneal nerve, providing cutaneous innervation to the lateral calf (typical clinical feature for the diagnosis). The LSCN can be entrapped due to the biceps femoris tendon, peri-popliteal cystic bursitis, or a fibrous band of tissue over its course. The flexor retinaculum is relevant for tarsal tunnel syndrome involving the tibial nerve.

(PNN, p. 2429)

40. Which of the following clinical signs would help differentiate between a high sciatic nerve pathology and common peroneal nerve injury in a patient with foot drop?
    A. Weakness in plantarflexion
    B. Weakness in dorsiflexion
    C. Loss of sensation over the dorsum of the foot
    D. Loss of Achilles reflex

    Correct Answer: A

    Explanation:

    Weakness in plantarflexion helps differentiate a high sciatic nerve injury from a common peroneal nerve injury. The sciatic nerve innervates both the tibial and common peroneal divisions, so an injury high in the sciatic nerve would affect plantarflexion (tibial nerve) and dorsiflexion (peroneal nerve). In contrast, an isolated common peroneal nerve injury affects only dorsiflexion and eversion, sparing plantarflexion.

    [100]
41. What else can differentiate between a high sciatic nerve injury and common peroneal nerve injury in a patient with foot drop? (No choices)

    Answer: Tinel's sign at the buttock

    Explanation:

    Provocative tests like Tinel's sign can help identify location of the entrapment or nerve pathology in most cases. In deep nerve like sciatic nerve, percussion needs to be stronger than in superficial nerves.

    [100]
42. A 60-year-old patient develops a painless foot drop. All of the following can cause painless foot drop EXCEPT:
    A. ALS (amyotrophic lateral sclerosis)
    B. Acute inflammatory demyelinating polyneuropathy (AIDP)
    C. Charcot–Marie Tooth (CMT)
    D. Myasthenia gravis

    Correct Answer: D

    Explanation:

    This question illustrates the importance of extensive differential diagnosis of painless foot drop beyond mononeuropathy. ALS (amyotrophic lateral sclerosis), acute inflammatory demyelinating polyneuropathy (AIDP), and Charcot–Marie Tooth (CMT) can all present as painless foot drop. Myasthenia gravis refers to a chronic autoimmune neuromuscular disorder characterized by fluctuating muscle weakness and fatigability, especially with activity, and does not present as foot drop.

[100]

43. A 49-year-old obese female patient presents with pain and numbness over the lateral thigh, which worsens with prolonged standing. Physical examination reveals no motor deficits. Which of the following tests would confirm the diagnosis?
   A. Tinel's sign at the medial malleolus
   B. More history and clinical examination
   C. Nerve conduction study
   D. MRI of the lumbar spine

   Correct Answer: B

   Explanation:

   The patient has a typical presentation of meralgia paresthetica, which is a compression of the lateral femoral cutaneous nerve. This condition is usually diagnosed based on history and clinical examination. Typically, the patient is middle-aged and overweight with numbness and pain at the anterolateral thigh that worsens with standing, hip extension, or tight clothing. The clinical examination reveals no motor deficit. Electrodiagnostic study results are variable and difficult to perform in obese patients.

   (PNN, pp. 1988–1990)

44. One of the following is CORRECT regarding the use of Tinel's sign in meralgia paresthetica:
   A. Sensitivity and specificity are both around 85%.
   B. A negative Tinel's sign reliably excludes lateral femoral cutaneous nerve entrapment.
   C. Tinel's sign has high sensitivity but low specificity.
   D. Tinel's sign has a low yield in meralgia paresthetica.

   Correct Answer: A

   Explanation:

   Tinel's sign can be valuable in the diagnosis of meralgia paresthetica (MP). According to a case series of 30 electrophysiologically proven patients with MP, the sensitivity and specificity are both around 85%. The tine's sign was elicited by tapping just below the anterior superior iliac spine.

   [101]

45. A 25-year-old man presents with foot drop and sensory loss over the dorsum of the foot. He has a positive Tinel's sign at the fibular head. Which structure is most likely compressing the nerve?
   A. Extensor digitorum longus
   B. Tibialis anterior
   C. Peroneus longus
   D. Gastrocnemius

   Correct Answer: C

Explanation:

This is a typical presentation of common peroneal nerve compression at the fibular head. The nerve is commonly trapped at the fibular tunnel, formed by fibers from aponeuroses of the soleus and peroneus longus muscles.

(PNN, p. 2242)

46. A 65-year-old man presents with progressive difficulty walking, frequent tripping, weakness in ankle dorsiflexion, and sensory loss over the lateral lower leg and dorsum of the foot. His medical history includes chronic alcohol use. Which of the following is the most likely cause of his neuropathy?
    A. Alcoholic Polyneuropathy
    B. Amyotrophic Lateral Sclerosis (ALS)
    C. B12 Deficiency
    D. Guillain–Barré Syndrome

    Correct Answer: A

    Explanation:

    Chronic alcohol use can lead to alcoholic polyneuropathy, which typically affects the distal nerves in a symmetric pattern. Symptoms include weakness, sensory loss, and motor deficits, with the lower limbs commonly involved first. This condition is a direct result of the neurotoxic effects of alcohol and associated nutritional deficiencies, particularly thiamine (vitamin B1).

    (NB, p. 323)

47. A patient presents with numbness over the medial thigh and weakness in thigh adduction. During the pelvic exam, the obturator nerve is found to be entrapped. Which structure is likely compressing the nerve?
    A. Femoral artery
    B. Pubic bone
    C. Adductor longus muscle
    D. Psoas major muscle

    Correct Answer: B

    Explanation:

    The obturator nerve passes through the obturator foramen in the pelvic bone and can be entrapped from inflammatory changes or osteophytes of the pubic bone.

    (TS, pp. 209–212)

    (See question 7 answer)

48. Which of the following is most likely to result in isolated paralysis of the quadriceps muscle without affecting sensation in the leg?
    A. L3 radiculopathy
    B. Femoral nerve compression
    C. Sciatic nerve injury
    D. Obturator nerve injury

    Correct Answer: A

    Explanation:

    An L3 radiculopathy can result in isolated weakness of the quadriceps muscle (primarily L2–L4 nerve roots, especially L3) without necessarily affecting cutaneous sensation in the leg, particularly in early or mild cases. In contrast, femoral nerve compression would typically affect both quadriceps strength and anterior thigh sensation, since it carries both motor and sensory fibers. Sciatic nerve injury does not affect the quadriceps.

(SS, p. 33)

This question emphasizes the importance of mastering all levels of lumbar radiculopathy disorders, which are important differential diagnoses in lower extremity peripheral nerve conditions.

49. A patient who underwent knee arthroscopy developed pain and paresthesia over the lower medial knee. Which of the following is the most likely cause?
    A. Main trunk saphenous nerve
    B. Anterior femoral cutaneous branch
    C. Superficial peroneal nerve
    D. Infrapatellar branch of the saphenous nerve

    Correct Answer: D

    Explanation:

    Entrapment or injury of the infrapatellar branch of the saphenous nerve causes typical lower medial knee pain. It commonly occurs after knee surgery.

    (MPN, p. 46)

50. The following condition can also cause entrapment of the infrapatellar branch of the saphenous nerve:
    A. Pes anserinus bursa
    B. Popliteal artery entrapment
    C. Lateral meniscus tear
    D. Common peroneal nerve compression at the fibular neck

    Correct Answer: A

    Explanation:

    Pes anserinus bursa is inflammation of the bursa located between the tibia and tendons of the hamstring muscle in the medial knee, near the course of the infrapatellar branch of the saphenous nerve.

    (PNN, p. 1888)

51. All of the following can cause injury or entrapment of the proximal saphenous nerve EXCEPT:
    A. Femoral artery aneurysms
    B. Direct trauma to the medial thigh
    C. Femoral catheterization
    D. Trochanteric bursitis

    Correct Answer: D

    Explanation:

    The saphenous nerve route is from the inguinal ligament when it comes from the femoral nerve and then courses in the medial thigh. Any pathology in its course can cause entrapment, like femoral artery aneurysms, direct trauma to the medial thigh, or femoral vessel artery catheterization. Trochanteric bursitis affects the lateral thigh, away from the saphenous nerve course.

    (PNN, p. 1888)

52. In a patient with a history of diabetes, weakness in dorsiflexion of the foot and loss of sensation over the dorsum of the foot and lateral shin are present. Which of the following would most likely differentiate diabetic neuropathy from common peroneal nerve entrapment?
   A. Positive Tinel's sign at the fibular head
   B. Sensory loss over the sole of the foot
   C. Nerve conduction study
   D. Weakness in plantarflexion

   Correct Answer: C

   Explanation:

   Entrapment neuropathy is common in diabetic patients. Lower limb diabetic neuropathies can present, especially in early stages, as common peroneal nerve entrapment with typical clinical pictures like foot drop, positive Tinel's sign, and the same sensory abnormalities. Nerve conduction study is the primary diagnostic tool to differentiate both.

   [102]
53. A 62-year-old male with a 15-year history of poorly controlled type 2 diabetes presents with a 6 month history of numbness and burning pain in his feet. He reports difficulty healing a small cut on his toe. On examination, he has reduced sensation to pinprick in a stocking distribution and absent ankle reflexes.

   53a. Which of the following is a major predisposing factor for the development of this disease?
   A. History of coronary heart disease
   B. Poor hyperglycemic control
   C. Female sex
   D. Young age

   53b. What is the primary pathological mechanism of nerve damage in this disease?
   A. Direct toxicity of elevated plasma glucose to nerves
   B. Autoimmune destruction of myelin sheaths
   C. Compression of nerves by surrounding tissues
   D. Deficiency of essential nerve nutrients

   53c. Which of the following best describes the typical pattern of nerve damage in this disease?
   A. Multifocal demyelination
   B. Length-dependent axonal degeneration
   C. Proximal motor neuropathy
   D. Selective large-fiber demyelination

   53d. A typical patient with this disease is most likely to present initially with which of the following symptoms?
   A. Proximal muscle weakness
   B. Loss of joint position sense
   C. Neuropathic pain and paresthesias in the feet
   D. Asymptomatic gait ataxia

53e. Which finding on electromyography (EMG) would be atypical for this disease?
A. Fibrillation potentials in distal muscles
B. Neurogenic motor unit potentials
C. Evidence of length-dependent axonal loss
D. Multifocal conduction block and reduced nerve conduction velocities

53 f. Which of the following is a recommended treatment for neuropathic pain in this disease?
A. Gabapentin
B. High-dose corticosteroids
C. Beta-blockers
D. Surgical nerve decompression

53 g. In a less common large-fiber variant of this disease, a patient might present with:
A. Severe neuropathic pain in the feet
B. Early muscle atrophy with ataxia
C. Prominent small-fiber sensory loss
D. Painless paresthesias and gait sensory ataxia

53 h. What is the most likely diagnosis?
A. Peripheral artery disease
B. Diabetic polyneuropathy
C. Lumbar radiculopathy
D. Vitamin B12 deficiency

Correct Answers: 53a: B, 53b: A, 53c: B, 53d: C, 53e: D, 53f: A, 53 g: D. 53 h: B

Explanation:

The case describes a patient with long-standing, poorly controlled diabetes who presents with distal sensory loss, neuropathic pain, poor healing of wounds, and mild autonomic symptoms (dizziness), consistent with diabetic polyneuropathy. Predisposing factors include poor hyperglycemic control. The pathogenesis involves direct glucose toxicity to nerves, leading to length-dependent axonal degeneration. High glucose can also lead to microvascular disease of the nerves. Initial symptoms typically involve small-fiber damage, causing neuropathic pain and paresthesias in the feet. Atypical EMG findings like multifocal conduction block suggest alternative diagnoses, as diabetic polyneuropathy is predominantly axonal. Treatment of neuropathic pain often involves tricyclic antidepressants (like amitriptyline) or anticonvulsants (like gabapentin). The less common large-fiber variant of diabetic polyneuropathy presents with painless paresthesias and sensory ataxia, reflecting selective large-fiber involvement.

(NB, pp. 823–834)

54. A 42-year-old woman presents with weakness in hip abduction and internal rotation after a pelvic mass excision. MRI of the lumbar spine is normal. Which nerve has most likely been injured?
    A. Femoral nerve
    B. Sciatic nerve
    C. Superior gluteal nerve
    D. Inferior gluteal nerve

    Correct Answer: C

    Explanation:

    The superior gluteal nerve innervates the gluteus medius, gluteus minimus, and tensor fasciae latae, which are responsible for hip abduction and internal rotation. Injury to this nerve, often during pelvic or gluteal surgeries, can cause weakness in these movements. The normal lumbar MRI rules out radiculopathy.

    (PNN, p. 1719)
55. One of the following is a typical location for superior gluteal nerve entrapment?
    A. Between the gluteus medius and gluteus minimus muscles
    B. Between the piriformis and quadratus femoris muscles
    C. Within the sacroiliac joint capsule near the posterior sacrum
    D. In the greater sciatic foramen inferior to the piriformis muscle

    Correct Answer: A

    Explanation:

    The superior gluteal nerve can be entrapped within the fascial plane between the gluteus medius and minimus muscles due to shearing forces generated by forced external rotation of the leg. Entrapment can also occur at the superior edge of the piriformis muscle.

    (PNN, p. 1727)
56. One of the following is CORRECT regarding inferior gluteal nerve entrapment:
    A. It causes weakness to all gluteal muscles.
    B. It usually occurs in conjunction with superior gluteal nerve entrapment.
    C. Piriformis muscle hypertrophy is not a cause of entrapment.
    D. All of the above are correct.

    Correct Answer: B

    Explanation:

    Inferior gluteal nerve entrapment leads to buttock pain and gluteal muscle weakness, and it often occurs alongside entrapments of the superior gluteal nerve, posterior femoral cutaneous nerve, or sciatic nerve. Although rare or possibly under-recognized, it is most commonly seen following buttock trauma or surgical procedures such as hip operations.

    (PNN, p. 1743)

References

Spine Studies References[1]

1. *Mazur MD, Mumert ML, Bisson EF, Schmidt MH. Avoiding pitfalls in anterior screw fixation for type II odontoid fractures. Neurosurg Focus 2011;31(4):E7. https://doi.org/10.3171/2011.7.FOCUS11135.
2. Masevnin S, Ptashnikov D, Michaylov D, Meng H, Smekalenkov O, Zaborovskii N. Risk factors for adjacent segment disease development after lumbar fusion. Asian Spine J. 2015;9(2):239–44. https://doi.org/10.4184/asj.2015.9.2.239.
3. Khelifa A, Berchiche L, Aichaoui F, Lagha N, Asfirane N, Morsli A. Traumatic cervical spine spondyloptosis: a systematic review. J Craniovertebr Junction Spine. 2022;13(1):9–16. https://doi.org/10.4103/jcvjs.jcvjs_132_21.
4. *Weinstein JN, Tosteson TD, Lurie JD, et al. Surgical versus nonoperative treatment for lumbar spinal stenosis four-year results of the spine patient outcomes research trial. Spine (Phila Pa 1976). 2010;35(14):1329–1338. https://doi.org/10.1097/BRS.0b013e3181e0f04d.
5. Pairojboriboon S, Niruthisard S, Chandhanayingyong C, Monsereenusorn C, Poopan S, Lo SL. A comparison of transforaminal lumbar interbody fusion (TLIF) cage material on fusion rates: a systematic review and network meta-analysis. World Neurosurg X. 2024;23:100392. Published 2024 May 25. https://doi.org/10.1016/j.wnsx.2024.100392.
6. *Fehlings MG, Tetreault LA, Wilson JR, Kwon BK, Burns AS, Martin AR, et al. A clinical practice guideline for the Management of Patients with Acute Spinal Cord Injury: recommendations on the timing (≤24 hours versus >24 hours) of Decompressive surgery. Global Spine Journal. 2017;7(3_suppl):195S–202S. https://doi.org/10.1177/2192568217706367.
7. Goyal K, Sunny JT, Gillespie CS, et al. A systematic review and meta-analysis of vertebral artery injury after cervical spine trauma. Global Spine Journal. 2024;14(4):1356–68. https://doi.org/10.1177/21925682231209631.
8. AlAli KF. Minimally invasive tubular microdiscectomy for recurrent lumbar disc herniation: step by-step technical description with safe scar dissection. J Orthop Surg Res. 2023;18:755. https://doi.org/10.1186/s13018-023-04226-1.
9. MacDermid JC, Richards RS, James H, er al. Endoscopic versus open carpal tunnel release: a randomized trial. J Hand Surg Am. 2003;28(3):475–80. https://doi.org/10.1053/jhsu.2003.50080.
10. Turkman A, Thanaraaj V, Soleimani-Nouri P, Harb E, Thakkar M. Outcomes of sciatic nerve injury repairs: a systematic review. Eplasty. 2023;23:e42. Published 2023 Jul 14

[1] References studies (must know studies marked with*)

K. F. AlAli, H. T. Hashim, *Spine Surgery and Peripheral Nerve Surgery*,
https://doi.org/10.1007/978-3-031-98543-0

11. Radcliff K, Hilibrand A, Lurie JD, et al. The impact of epidural steroid injections on the outcomes of patients treated for lumbar disc herniation: a subgroup analysis of the SPORT trial. J Bone Joint Surg Am. 2012;94(15):1353–8. https://doi.org/10.2106/JBJS.K.00341.
12. Betsch MW, Blizzard SR, Shinseki MS, Yoo JU. Prevalence of degenerative changes of the atlanto-axial joints. Spine J. 2015;15(2):275–80. https://doi.org/10.1016/j.spinee.2014.09.011.
13. Lei T, Shen Y, Wang LF, Cao JM, Ding WY, Ma QH. Cerebrospinal fluid leakage during anterior approach cervical spine surgery for severe ossification of the posterior longitudinal ligament: prevention and treatment. Orthop Surg. 2012;4(4):247–52. https://doi.org/10.1111/os.12007.
14. Guerin P, El Fegoun AB, Obeid I, et al. Incidental durotomy during spine surgery: incidence, management and complications. A retrospective review. Injury. 2012;43(4):397–401. https://doi.org/10.1016/j.injury.2010.12.014.
15. Vaccaro AR, Karamian BA, Levy HA, et al. Update on upper cervical injury classifications: the new AO upper cervical spine classification system. Clin Spine Surg. 2022;35(6):249–55. https://doi.org/10.1097/BSD.0000000000001215.
16. Cirillo JI, Ricciardi GA, Alvarez Lemos FL, Guiroy A, Yurac R, Schnake K. Treatment of unilateral cervical facet fractures without evidence of dislocation or subluxation: a narrative review and proposed treatment algorithm. EFORT Open Rev. 2024;9(3):202–9. Published 2024 Mar 5. https://doi.org/10.1530/EOR-23-0161.
17. Avila MJ, Farber SH, Rabah NM, et al. Nonoperative versus operative management of type II odontoid fracture in older adults: a systematic review and meta-analysis. J Neurosurg Spine. 2023;40(1):45–53. Published 2023 Sep 29. https://doi.org/10.3171/2023.6.SPINE22920.
18. Murphy RF, Mooney JF 3rd. Complications following spine fusion for adolescent idiopathic scoliosis. Curr Rev Musculoskelet Med. 2016;9(4):462–9. https://doi.org/10.1007/s12178-016-9372-5.
19. Lee MJ, Hacquebord J, Varshney A, et al. Risk factors for medical complication after lumbar spine surgery: a multivariate analysis of 767 patients. Spine (Phila Pa 1976). 2011;36(21):1801–6. https://doi.org/10.1097/brs.0b013e318219d28d.
20. Sarwahi V, Payares M, Wendolowski S, et al. Pedicle screw safety: how much anterior breach is safe?: a cadaveric and CT-based study. Spine (Phila Pa 1976). 2017;42(22):E1305–10. https://doi.org/10.1097/BRS.0000000000002153.
21. Mobbs RJ, Phan K, Malham G, Seex K, Rao PJ. Lumbar interbody fusion: techniques, indications and comparison of interbody fusion options including PLIF, TLIF, MI-TLIF, OLIF/ATP. LLIF and ALIF J Spine Surg. 2015;1(1):2–18. https://doi.org/10.3978/j.issn.2414-469X.2015.10.05.
22. Zdeblick TA, Zou D, Warden KE, McCabe R, Kunz D, Vanderby R. Cervical stability after foraminotomy. A biomechanical in vitro analysis. J Bone Joint Surg Am. 1992;74(1):22–7.
23. Chen F, Liu X, Wang G, Sun J, Cui X. Anatomic relationship of bony structures in pedicle-rib unit and its significance. World Neurosurg. 2020;139:e691–9. https://doi.org/10.1016/j.wneu.2020.04.108.
24. Nunley PD, Cavanaugh DA, Kerr EJ 3rd, et al. Heterotopic ossification after cervical Total disc replacement at 7 years-prevalence, progression, clinical implications, and risk factors. Int J Spine Surg. 2018;12(3):352–61. Published 2018 Aug 15. https://doi.org/10.14444/5041.
25. McNamara AL, Dickerson EC, Gomez-Hassan DM, Cinti SK, Srinivasan A. Yield of image-guided needle biopsy for infectious discitis: a systematic review and meta-analysis. AJNR Am J Neuroradiol. 2017;38(10):2021–7. https://doi.org/10.3174/ajnr.A5337.
26. Siddiqui Abdul H. StatPearls. https://www.ncbi.nlm.nih.gov/books/NBK482221/
27. Hsu CY, Yu CW, Wu MZ, Chen BB, Huang KM, Shih TT. Unusual manifestations of vertebral osteomyelitis: intraosseous lesions mimicking metastases. AJNR Am J Neuroradiol. 2008;29(6):1104–10. https://doi.org/10.3174/ajnr.A1003.
28. Gabay C, Kushner I. Acute-phase proteins and other systemic responses to inflammation [published correction appears in N Engl J med 1999 Apr 29;340(17):1376]. N Engl J Med. 1999;340(6):448–54. https://doi.org/10.1056/NEJM199902113400607.

29. Hadgaonkar S, Rathi P, Vincent V, Shyam A, Sancheti P. Actinomycotic infection of spine - a rare disease with diagnostic challenge, an update on spinal infection. J Orthop Case Rep. 2021;11(1):72–8. https://doi.org/10.13107/jocr.2021.v11.i01.1970.
30. Tyagi R. Spinal infections in children: a review. J Orthop. 2016;13(4):254–8. Published 2016 Jun 24. https://doi.org/10.1016/j.jor.2016.06.005.
31. *Patchell RA, Tibbs PA, Regine WF, et al. Direct decompressive surgical resection in the treatment of spinal cord compression caused by metastatic cancer: a randomised trial. Lancet 2005;366(9486):643–648. https://doi.org/10.1016/S0140-6736(05)66954-1.
32. Baker S, Fairchild A. Radiation-induced esophagitis in lung cancer. Lung Cancer (Auckl). 2016;7:119–27. Published 2016 Oct 13. https://doi.org/10.2147/LCTT.S96443.
33. Bydon M, Mathios D, Macki M, et al. Long-term patient outcomes after posterior cervical foraminotomy: an analysis of 151 cases. J Neurosurg Spine. 2014;21(5):727–31. https://doi.org/10.3171/2014.7.SPINE131110.
34. Sofianos DA, Briseño MR, Abrams J, Patel AA. Complications of the lateral transpsoas approach for lumbar interbody arthrodesis: a case series and literature review. Clin Orthop Relat Res. 2012;470(6):1621–32. https://doi.org/10.1007/s11999-011-2088-3.
35. Lewandrowski KU, Dowling Á, Calderaro AL, et al. Dysethesia due to irritation of the dorsal root ganglion following lumbar transforaminal endoscopy: analysis of frequency and contributing factors. Clin Neurol Neurosurg. 2020;197:106073. https://doi.org/10.1016/j.clineuro.2020.106073.
36. *Fisher CG, DiPaola CP, Ryken TC, et al. A novel classification system for spinal instability in neoplastic disease: an evidence-based approach and expert consensus from the spine oncology study group. Spine (Phila Pa 1976). 2010;35(22):E1221–E1229. https://doi.org/10.1097/BRS.0b013e3181e16ae2.
37. *Weill A, Chiras J, Simon JM, Rose M, Sola-Martinez T, Enkaoua E. Spinal metastases: indications for and results of percutaneous injection of acrylic surgical cement. Radiology 1996;199(1):241–247. https://doi.org/10.1148/radiology.199.1.8633152.
38. Boriani S, Weinstein JN, Biagini R. Primary bone tumors of the spine. Terminology and surgical staging. Spine (Phila Pa 1976). 1997;22(9):1036–44. https://doi.org/10.1097/00007632-199705010-00020.
39. Teomita K, Kawahara N, Kobayashi T, Yoshida A, Murakami H, Akamaru T. Surgical strategy for spinal metastases. Spine (Phila Pa 1976). 2001;26(3):298–306. https://doi.org/10.1097/00007632-200102010-00016.
40. Gerszten PC, Mendel E, Yamada Y. Radiotherapy and radiosurgery for metastatic spine disease: what are the options, indications, and outcomes? Spine (Phila Pa 1976). 2009;34(22 Suppl):S78–92. https://doi.org/10.1097/BRS.0b013e3181b8b6f5.
41. Yamazaki T, McLoughlin GS, Patel S, Rhines LD, Fourney DR. Feasibility and safety of en bloc resection for primary spine tumors: a systematic review by the spine oncology study group. Spine (Phila Pa 1976). 2009;34(22 Suppl):S31–8. https://doi.org/10.1097/BRS.0b013e3181b8b796.
42. Marchi PB, Pinheiro RP, Peria FM, Toledo VN, Costa HRT, Defino HLA. Unknown primary tumor sites in spinal metastases: prevalence, clinical features, treatment outcomes, and survival. Coluna/Columna. 2021;20(1):64–7. https://doi.org/10.1590/S1808-185120212001243891.
43. Wang Y, Liao SC, Dai GG, Jiang L. Resorption of upwardly displaced lumbar disk herniation after nonsurgical treatment: a case report. World J Clin Cases. 2020;8(19):4609–14. https://doi.org/10.12998/wjcc.v8.i19.4609.
44. *Vaccaro AR, Lehman RA Jr, Hurlbert RJ, et al. A new classification of thoracolumbar injuries: the importance of injury morphology, the integrity of the posterior ligamentous complex, and neurologic status. Spine (Phila Pa 1976). 2005;30(20):2325–2333. https://doi.org/10.1097/01.brs.0000182986.43345.cb.
45. *Recommendations of WFNS Spine Committee 2019: Recommendations for Clinical Assessment and Classification of Spinal Cord Injury (SCI). https://wfns-spine.org/spinal-cord-injury-recommendations

46. Spine section of The American Association of Neurological Surgeons (AANS)/Congress of Neurological Surgeons (CNS). Guidelines for the management of acute cervical spine and spinal cord injuries. 2017. https://www.cns.org/guidelines/browse-guidelines-detail/introduction
47. Fehlings MG, Wilson JR, Tetreault LA, et al. A clinical practice guideline for the Management of Patients with Acute Spinal Cord Injury: recommendations on the use of methylprednisolone sodium succinate. Global Spine Journal. 2017;7(3_suppl):203S–11S. https://doi.org/10.1177/2192568217703085.
48. McCormack T, Karaikovic E, Gaines RW. The load sharing classification of spine fractures. Spine (Phila Pa 1976). 1994;19(15):1741–4. https://doi.org/10.1097/00007632-199408000-00014.
49. Gopinath P. Lumbar segmental instability: points to ponder. J Orthop. 2015;12(4):165–7. Published 2015 Oct 8. https://doi.org/10.1016/j.jor.2015.09.005.
50. Denis F. The three column spine and its significance in the classification of acute thoracolumbar spinal injuries. Spine. 1983;8:817–31.
51. Si Y, Zhang H, Han S, et al. Clinical features and pathogenesis of scoliosis due to spinal astrocytoma. Oncol Lett. 2023;25(4):140. Published 2023 Feb 21. https://doi.org/10.3892/ol.2023.13726.
52. Cunha SC, Eid F, et al. Human tail with occult spinal dysraphism and dermal sinus in children, Journal of Pediatric Surgery Case Reports. 2023;90:102554.
53. Kwon JH, Chinthala AS, Arnold JC, Witten AJ, Bohnstedt BN. Management of Type III occipital condyle fractures. J Clin Med. 2024;13(24):7639. https://doi.org/10.3390/jcm13247639.
54. Vaccaro AR, Hulbert RJ, Patel AA, et al. The subaxial cervical spine injury classification system: a novel approach to recognize the importance of morphology, neurology, and integrity of the disco-ligamentous complex. Spine (Phila Pa 1976). 2007;32(21):2365–74. https://doi.org/10.1097/BRS.0b013e3181557b92.
55. Fehlings MG, Vaccaro A, Wilson JR, et al. Early versus delayed decompression for traumatic cervical spinal cord injury: results of the surgical timing in acute spinal cord injury study (STASCIS). PLoS One. 2012;7(2):e32037. https://doi.org/10.1371/journal.pone.0032037.
56. Stiell IG, Clement CM, McKnight RD, et al. The Canadian C-spine rule versus the NEXUS low-risk criteria in patients with trauma. N Engl J Med. 2003;349(26):2510–8. https://doi.org/10.1056/NEJMoa031375.
57. Pan Q, Yu H, He X, et al. Lumbar sympathetic trunk injury: an underestimated complication of oblique lateral Interbody fusion. Orthop Surg. 2023;15(4):1053–9. https://doi.org/10.1111/os.13692.
58. Joseph SC, Elias R, Shane Tubbs R. Chapter 25—variations of the intracranial Dural venous sinuses. In: Tubbs RS, editor. Anatomy, imaging and surgery of the intracranial Dural venous sinuses. Elsevier; 2020. p. 205–20. ISBN 9780323653770.
59. Wu CC, Jin HM, Yan YZ, et al. Biomechanical role of the thoracolumbar ligaments of the posterior ligamentous complex: a finite element study. World Neurosurg. 2018;112:e125–33. https://doi.org/10.1016/j.wneu.2017.12.171.
60. Aly MM, Al-Shoaibi AM, Aljuzair AH, Issa TZ, Vaccaro AR. A proposal for a standardized imaging algorithm to improve the accuracy and reliability for the diagnosis of thoracolumbar posterior ligamentous complex injury in computed tomography and magnetic resonance imaging. Global Spine J. 2023;13(3):873–96. https://doi.org/10.1177/21925682221129220.
61. *Fehlings MG, Tetreault LA, Riew KD, Middleton JW, Wang JC. A clinical practice guideline for the Management of Degenerative Cervical Myelopathy: introduction, rationale, and scope. Global Spine J. 2017;7(3_suppl):21S–7S. https://doi.org/10.1177/2192568217703088.
62. Bydon M, Alvi MA, Goyal A. Degenerative lumbar spondylolisthesis: definition, natural history, conservative management, and surgical treatment. Neurosurg Clin N Am. 2019;30(3):299–304. https://doi.org/10.1016/j.nec.2019.02.003.
63. Nguyen HS, Sharma A, Doan N, Gelsomino M, Shabani S, Maiman D. Central cord syndrome in a patient with systemic sclerosis and cervical calcinosis: case report and review of literature [published correction appears in spinal cord Ser cases. 2016 Jul 21;2:16019. https://

doi.org/10.1038/scsandc.2016.19]. Spinal Cord Ser Cases. 2016;2:15029. Published 2016 Jan 7. https://doi.org/10.1038/scsandc.2015.29.

64. Mitchell BA, Chi JA, Driskill EK, et al. A matched-cohort analysis of outcomes in patients with hereditary hemochromatosis after anterior cervical discectomy and fusion. World Neurosurg. 2024;184:e25–31. https://doi.org/10.1016/j.wneu.2023.11.050.
65. Lubicky JP. The spine in Osteogenesis Imperfecta. Spine Deformity. 2012;1(1, Supplement):124–32., ISSN 2212-134X. https://doi.org/10.1016/j.jspd.2012.04.006.
66. Schmidt RF, Goldstein IM, Liu JK. Ossified ligamentum flavum causing spinal cord compression in a patient with acromegaly. J Clin Neurosci. 2013;20(11):1599–603. https://doi.org/10.1016/j.jocn.2012.10.033.
67. Pollock L, Ridout A, Teh J, et al. The musculoskeletal manifestations of Marfan syndrome: diagnosis, impact, and management. Curr Rheumatol Rep. 2021;23(11):81. Published 2021 Nov 26. https://doi.org/10.1007/s11926-021-01045-3.
68. Hu RMD, FRCSC. Severe spinal degeneration in Wilson's disease. Spine. 1994;19(3):372–5.
69. Nirupam N, Pemde H, Chandra J. Spinal epidural hematoma in a patient with hemophilia B presenting as acute abdomen. Indian J Hematol Blood Transfus. 2014;30(Suppl 1):54–6. https://doi.org/10.1007/s12288-013-0245-4.
70. Chen W, et al. Progress and perspective of TBX6 gene in congenital vertebral malformations. Oncotarget. 2016;7(35):57430–41.
71. Charalampidis A, Jiang F, Wilson JRF, Badhiwala JH, Brodke DS, Fehlings MG. The use of intraoperative neurophysiological monitoring in spine surgery. Global Spine J. 2020;10(1 Suppl):104S–14S. https://doi.org/10.1177/2192568219859314.
72. Strommen JA, Crum BA. Intraoperative monitoring with free-running EMG. In: Handbook of clinical neurophysiology, vol. 8. Elsevier; 2008. p. 396–403., ISSN 1567-4231, ISBN 9780444518248. https://doi.org/10.1016/S1567-4231(07)08027-6.
73. Chang MC, Park D. Findings of Electrodiagnostic studies in moderate to severe lumbar central spinal stenosis-Electrodiagnostic studies in lumbar central spinal stenosis. Healthcare (Basel). 2021;9(2):164. Published 2021 Feb 3. https://doi.org/10.3390/healthcare9020164.
74. Ghatol D, Widrich J. Intraoperative Neurophysiological Monitoring. [Updated 2023 Jul 24]. In: StatPearls [Internet]. Treasure Island (FL): StatPearls Publishing; 2025 Jan. Available from: https://www.ncbi.nlm.nih.gov/books/NBK563203/. Jason M. Allen, Barry J. Greer, David G. Sorge, Scot E. Campbell. MR imaging of neuropathies of the leg, ankle, and foot. Magn Reson Imaging Clin N Am, volume 16, Issue 1, 2008, Pages 117–131., ISSN 1064-9689, https://doi.org/10.1016/j.mric.2008.02.006.
75. Kerver AL, Leliveld MS, den Hartog D, Verhofstad MH, Kleinrensink GJ. The surgical anatomy of the infrapatellar branch of the saphenous nerve in relation to incisions for antero medial knee surgery. J Bone Joint Surg Am. 2013;95(23):2119–25. https://doi.org/10.2106/JBJS.L.01297.
76. Lung K, Lui F. Anatomy, Abdomen and Pelvis: Superior Gluteal Nerve. [Updated 2023 Aug 14]. In: StatPearls [Internet]. Treasure Island (FL): StatPearls Publishing; 2025 Jan. Available from: https://www.ncbi.nlm.nih.gov/books/NBK535408/#
77. Felici N, Alban A. Timing of surgery in peripheral nerve injury of the upper extremity. J Hand Surg (European Volume). 2024;49(6):712–20. https://doi.org/10.1177/17531934241240867.
78. Kiernan MC, et al. Chapter 15—nerve excitability: a clinical translation. In: Aminoff MJ, editor. Aminoff's Electrodiagnosis in clinical neurology. 6th ed. W.B. Saunders; 2012. p. 345–65. ISBN 9781455703081.
79. Martins RS, Bastos D, Siqueira MG, Heise CO, Teixeira MJ. Traumatic injuries of peripheral nerves: a review with emphasis on surgical indication. Arq Neuropsiquiatr. 2013;71(10):811–4. https://doi.org/10.1590/0004-282X20130127.
80. Kim T-H, Jo G-Y, Kim W, Do H-K. Complex regional pain syndrome type II caused by iatrogenic lateral dorsal cutaneous nerve injury: a case report. Medicine. 2021;100(49):e28108. https://doi.org/10.1097/MD.0000000000028108.

81. Eberlin KR, Ducic I. Surgical algorithm for neuroma management: a changing treatment paradigm. Plast Reconstr Surg Glob Open. 2018;6(10):e1952. Published 2018 Oct 16. https://doi.org/10.1097/GOX.0000000000001952.
82. Woo A, Bakri K, Moran SL. Management of ulnar nerve injuries. J Hand Surg Am. 2015;40(1):173–81. https://doi.org/10.1016/j.jhsa.2014.04.038.
83. Sridhar K. Tendon transfer for median nerve palsy. Indian J Plast Surg. 2011;44(2):357–61. https://doi.org/10.4103/0970-0358.85357.
84. Secer HI, Daneyemez M, Tehli O, Gonul E, Izci Y. The clinical, electrophysiologic, and surgical characteristics of peripheral nerve injuries caused by gunshot wounds in adults: a 40-year experience. Surg Neurol. 2008;69(2):143–52. https://doi.org/10.1016/j.surneu.2007.01.032.
85. Rasulić L, Savić A, Vitošević F, et al. Iatrogenic peripheral nerve injuries-surgical treatment and outcome: 10 years' experience. World Neurosurg. 2017;103:841–851.e6. https://doi.org/10.1016/j.wneu.2017.04.099.
86. Zlowodzki M, Chan S, Bhandari M, Kalliainen L, Schubert W. Anterior transposition compared with simple decompression for treatment of cubital tunnel syndrome. A meta-analysis of randomized, controlled trials. J Bone Joint Surg Am. 2007;89(12):2591–8. https://doi.org/10.2106/JBJS.G.00183.
87. Rosario NB, De Jesus O. Electrodiagnostic Evaluation of Carpal Tunnel Syndrome. [Updated 2023 Aug 23]. In: StatPearls [Internet]. Treasure Island (FL): StatPearls Publishing; 2025 Jan. Available from: https://www.ncbi.nlm.nih.gov/books/NBK562235/
88. Gupta R, Kapoor L, Shagotar S. Arthroscopic decompression of paralabral cyst around suprascapular notch causing suprascapular neuropathy. J Clin Orthop Trauma. 2015;6(3):184–6. https://doi.org/10.1016/j.jcot.2015.03.007.
89. Cook S, Manning C, et al. Deep and superficial sensory nerve conduction to the first dorsal web space of the foot. Translational Research in Anatomy. 2022;29:100226., ISSN 2214-854X. https://doi.org/10.1016/j.tria.2022.100226.
90. Fortier LM, Markel M, Thomas BG, Sherman WF, Thomas BH, Kaye AD. An update on peroneal nerve entrapment and neuropathy. Orthop Rev (Pavia). 2021;13(2):24937. Published 2021 Jun 19. https://doi.org/10.52965/001c.24937.
91. Reife MD, Coulis CM. Peroneal neuropathy misdiagnosed as L5 radiculopathy: a case report. Chiropr Man Therap. 2013;21(1):12. Published 2013 Apr 22. https://doi.org/10.1186/2045-709X-21-12.
92. Esene IN, Meher A, Elzoghby MA, El-Bahy K, Kotb A, El-Hakim A. Diagnostic performance of the medial hamstring reflex in L5 radiculopathy. Surg Neurol Int. 2012;3:104. https://doi.org/10.4103/2152-7806.100862.
93. Rodríguez-Merchán EC, Moracia-Ochagavía I. Tarsal tunnel syndrome: current rationale, indications and results. EFORT Open Rev. 2021;6(12):1140–7. Published 2021 Dec 10. https://doi.org/10.1302/2058-5241.6.210031.
94. Rozen SM, Wolfe GI, Vernino S, et al. Effect of lower extremity nerve decompression in patients with painful diabetic peripheral neuropathy: the diabetic neuropathy nerve decompression randomized, observation group and placebo surgery-controlled clinical trial. Ann Surg. 2024;280(1):35–45. https://doi.org/10.1097/SLA.0000000000006228.
95. van Maurik JFMM, van Hal M, van Eijk RPA, Kon M, Peters EJG. Value of surgical decompression of compressed nerves in the lower extremity in patients with painful diabetic neuropathy: a randomized controlled trial. Plast Reconstr Surg. 2014;134(2):325–32. https://doi.org/10.1097/PRS.0000000000000369.
96. Best TJ, Best CA, Best AA, Fera LA. Surgical peripheral nerve decompression for the treatment of painful diabetic neuropathy of the foot—a level 1 pragmatic randomized controlled trial. Diabetes Res Clin Pract. 2019;147:149–56. https://doi.org/10.1016/j.diabres.2018.08.002.
97. Hicks BL, Lam JC, Varacallo MA. Piriformis Syndrome. [Updated 2023 Aug 4]. In: StatPearls [Internet]. Treasure Island (FL): StatPearls Publishing; 2025 Jan-. Available from: https://www.ncbi.nlm.nih.gov/books/NBK448172/

98. Amir Ahmadian, Naomi Abel, Elias Dakwar. Chapter 35—injuries to the nerves of the abdominopelvic region. Editor(s): R. Shane Tubbs, Elias Rizk, Mohammadali M. Shoja, Marios Loukas, Nicholas Barbaro, Robert J. Spinner. Nerves and nerve injuries. Academic Press, 2015, Pages 545–555., ISBN 9780128026533, https://doi.org/10.1016/B978-0-12-802653-3.00084-1.
99. Burakgazi AZ, Kelly JJ, Richardson P. The electrodiagnostic sensitivity of proximal lower extremity muscles in the diagnosis of L5 radiculopathy. Muscle Nerve. 2012;45(6):891–3. https://doi.org/10.1002/mus.23361.
100. Nori SL, Stretanski MF. Foot Drop. [Updated 2024 Feb 12]. In: StatPearls [Internet]. Treasure Island (FL): StatPearls Publishing; 2025 Jan-. Available from: https://www.ncbi.nlm.nih.gov/books/NBK554393/
101. Paneyala S, Chandrashekhar NS, Sundaramurthy H, Prashant A, Krishna L. Efficacy of clinical tests in the diagnosis of Meralgia Paresthetica: a case control study. Case Rep Med. 2024;2024:5191280. Published 2024 Dec 9. https://doi.org/10.1155/carm/5191280.
102. Rota E, Morelli N. Entrapment neuropathies in diabetes mellitus. World J Diabetes. 2016;7(17):342–53. https://doi.org/10.4239/wjd.v7.i17.342.

Spine Books References

103. **GB**: Greenberg Handbook of neurosurgery e 10th.
104. **SS**: Devlin. Spine secrets e 3rd.
105. **BSA**: Osborn et al. Imaging anatomy: Brain and spine. e 1st.
106. **DI**: Ross and Moore. Diagnostic imaging: spine. e 4th.
107. **SSW**: Alfredo Quinones-Hinojosa. Schmidek and Sweet: Operative Neurosurgical Techniques . V2. e 7th.
108. **CAS**: Gregory D. Cramer & Susan A. Darby. Clinical Anatomy of the Spine, Spinal Cord, and ANS. e 3rd.
109. **CN:** Anil Nanada. Complications in neurosurgery 1st edition.
110. **RP**: https://radiopaedia.org
111. **UP**: Uptodate.com.
112. **RSS**: Gregory D. Schroeder. Revision spine surgery. CRC. 2020.
113. **NSE**: Harrop J. Neurosurgery by example: spinal neurosurgery. Oxford University Press. 2019.
114. **TS**: Tunnel syndromes: Peripheral Nerve Compression Syndromes. CRC. 2000.
115. **MPN**: Socolovsky M. Manual of Peripheral Nerve Surgery: From the Basics to Complex Procedures. Thieme. 2018.
116. **BS:** Benzel E. et al. Spine Surgery Techniques, Complication Avoidance, and Management. 5th ed. 2021.
117. **RS:** Garfin S. et al. Rothman-Simeone: The Spine. 7th ed. 2017.
118. **EM**: Rhee J. Emory's Illustrated Tips and Tricks in Spine Surgery. LWW. 1st Edition. 2019.
119. **SB**: Patel V. et al. Spine surgery basics. Springer. 2014.
120. **ES**: Lui, Tun Hing. Endoscopy of the Spine: Principle and Practice. 1st Edition. Springer. 2023.
121. MISS: Perez-Cruet, M. An Anatomic Approach to Minimally Invasive Spine Surgery. Thieme, 2018.
122. **HS:** Baal A. Handbook of Spine Surgery 3rd Edition. Thieme; 3rd edition 2024.
123. **CA:** Cramer G. et al. Clinical Anatomy of the Spine, Spinal Cord, and ANS. 3rd edition, 2014.
124. **NB:** Nima Mowzoon, Kelly D. Flemming. Neurology Board Review: An Illustrated Study Guide, 1st Edition, CRC, 2007.
125. **EPN:** Russell, Stephen. Examination of Peripheral Nerve Injuries: An Anatomical Approach, 2nd Edition. 2015.
126. **ABN:** Alberstone, Cary D., et al., editors. Anatomic Bases of Neurologic Diagnosis. Thieme Medical Publishers. Second edition. 2023.

127. **PNG**: Birch, Rolfe. Peripheral Nerve Injuries: A Clinical Guide. Springer. 2012.
128. **FCN:** Mtui, Estomi. Fitzgerald's Clinical Neuroanatomy and Neuroscience 8th Edition. 2020.
129. **PNO**: Christopher J. Overvi. Peripheral Nerve Issues after Orthopedic Surgery: A Multidisciplinary Approach to Prevention, Evaluation, and Treatment, Springer. 2022.
130. **SPN:** Midha, R., Zager, E. Surgery of Peripheral Nerves. A case-based approach. Thieme. 2008.
131. **OPN**: Maniker, Allen H. Operative Exposures in Peripheral Nerve Surgery. Thieme. 2004.
132. **PNN**: Trescot, Andrea M. Peripheral Nerve Entrapments: Clinical Diagnosis and Management. Kindle Edition. Thieme. 2016.

MIX
Papier aus verantwortungsvollen Quellen
Paper from responsible sources
FSC® C105338

If you have any concerns about our products,
you can contact us on
ProductSafety@springernature.com

In case Publisher is established outside the EU,
the EU authorized representative is:
Springer Nature Customer Service Center GmbH
Europaplatz 3, 69115 Heidelberg, Germany

Printed by Libri Plureos GmbH
in Hamburg, Germany